CHEMOTHERAPY

Volume 2
Laboratory Aspects
of Infections

CHEMOTHERAPY

Volume 1 **Clinical Aspects of Infections**
Prophylaxis; life-threatening infections; infection in leukaemia;
surgical infection; anaerobic infection; respiratory and urinary
tract infections; amikacin.

Volume 2 **Laboratory Aspects of Infections**
Sensitivity testing; assay methods; animal models of infection;
sisomycin; tobramycin.

Volume 3 **Special Problems in Chemotherapy**
Tuberculosis; genital tract infections; antibiotic resistance and
mode of action; topical chemotherapy and antisepsis.

Volume 4 **Pharmacology of Antibiotics**
Tissue concentrations; pharmacokinetics; untoward effects of antibiotics.

Volume 5 **Penicillins and Cephalosporins**
Penicillins and cephalosporins; betalactamases; new agents.

Volume 6 **Parasites, Fungi, and Viruses**
Parasitic infections; fungal infections; chemotherapy of viruses;
co-trimoxazole.

Volume 7 **Cancer Chemotherapy I**
Symposia — new drugs and approaches; cell and pharmacokinetics;
potentiators of radiotherapy; in vitro screening systems;
immunological aspects.

Volume 8 **Cancer Chemotherapy II**
Free papers — new drugs and approaches; cell and pharmacokinetics;
mechanisms of action; new analogues; cancer chemotherapy of specific organs.

CHEMOTHERAPY

Volume 2
Laboratory Aspects
of Infections

Edited by
J.D. Williams
The London Hospital Medical College
London, U.K.

and
A.M. Geddes
East Birmingham Hospital
Birmingham, U.K.

Springer Science+Business Media, LLC

Library of Congress Cataloging in Publication Data

International Congress of Chemotherapy, 9th, London, 1975.
   Laboratory aspects of infections.

   (Chemotherapy; v. 2)
   1. Antibiotics — Testing — Congresses. 2. Microorganisms, Effect of antibiotics on
— Congresses. 3. Antibiotics — Analysis — Congresses. 4. Diseases — Animal models —
Congresses. I. Williams, John David, M.D. II. Geddes, Alexander McIntosh. III. Title.
IV. Series.
RM260.2.C45   vol. 2   [RM265.2]   615'.58s   [616.9]   76-1949
ISBN 978-1-4684-7655-2   ISBN 978-1-4684-7653-8 (eBook)
DOI 10.1007/978-1-4684-7653-8

Proceedings of the Ninth International Congress of Chemotherapy
held in London, July, 1975 will be published in eight volumes,
of which this is volume two.

© 1976 Springer Science+Business Media New York
Originally published by Plenum Press, New York in 1976
Softcover reprint of the hardcover 1st edition 1976

CHEMOTHERAPY

Proceedings of the
9th International Congress of Chemotherapy
held in London, July, 1975

Preface

The International Society of Chemotherapy meets every two years to review progress in chemotherapy of infections and of malignant disease. Each meeting gets larger to encompass the extension of chemotherapy into new areas. In some instances, expansion has been rapid, for example in cephalosporins, penicillins and combination chemotherapy of cancer - in others slow, as in the field of parasitology. New problems of resistance and untoward effects arise; reduction of host toxicity without loss of antitumour activity by new substances occupies wide attention. The improved results with cancer chemotherapy, especially in leukaemias, are leading to a greater prevalence of severe infection in patients so treated, pharmacokinetics of drugs in normal and diseased subjects is receiving increasing attention along with related problems of bioavailability and interactions between drugs. Meanwhile the attack on some of the major bacterial infections, such as gonorrhoea and tuberculosis, which were among the first infections to feel the impact of chemotherapy, still continue to be major world problems and are now under attack with new agents and new methods.

From this wide field and the 1,000 papers read at the Congress we have produced Proceedings which reflect the variety and vigour of research in this important field of medicine. It was not possible to include all of the papers presented at the Congress but we have attempted to include most aspects of current progress in chemotherapy.

We thank the authors of these communications for their cooperation in enabling the Proceedings to be available at the earliest possible date. The method of preparation does not allow for uniformity of typefaces and presentation of the material and we hope that the blemishes of language and typographical errors do not detract from the understanding of the reader and the importance of the Proceedings.

K. HELLMANN, Imperial Cancer Research Fund
A. M. GEDDES, East Birmingham Hospital
J. D. WILLIAMS, The London Hospital Medical College

Contents

Introductory Comments 1
   J. C. Sherris

Control of Antibiotic-Sensitivity Testing in Britain 7
   R. Blowers and D. F. J. Brown

Control of Antibacterial Susceptibility Testing:
      Standardization and Proficiency Testing
      in Canada 13
   I. B. R. Duncan

Antibiotic Sensitivity Testing in Australia and
      New Zealand 19
   S. M. Bell

Problems of Standardization of Media 33
   H. Neussel

Effects of Medium on the Results of Antimicrobial
      Sensitivity Testing 41
   J. Bou Casals

Influence of Four Commercial Sensitivity Media on
      In Vitro Activity of Several Antibiotics 47
   G. Th. J. Fabius and R. P. Mouton

A Spot Plate Method for Antibiotic-Bacterial Killing
      Rates 55
   S. H. Zinner, R. B. Provonchee, and K. S. Elias

Usefulness of Commercially Available Media to
      MIC-Determinations of Trimethoprim 61
   B. van Klingeren and A. Rutgers

Thymidine and the Assessment of Co-Trimoxazole
      Action in Liquid Media 67
   R. Then

Antibacterial Susceptibility Testing on Anaerobes   71
    K. Watanabe, K. Ninomiya, I. Mochizuki, T. Miwa,
    H. Imamura, S. Kobata, K. Ueno, and S. Suzuki

Sensitivity Testing of Mixed Infections   77
    M. Taufer and J. Zangger

A Diffusion Disc Susceptibility Test for 5-Fluorocytosine . .   81
    C. Utz and S. Shadomy

The Susceptibility of Clostridia from the Antarctic Soil
        to Antibiotics   89
    T. Miwa, I. Mochizuki, K. Watanabe, S. Kobata,
    H. Imamura, K. Ninomiya, K. Ueno, and S. Suzuki

Brief Antibiotic Exposure and Effect on Bacterial Growth . .   95
    P. J. McDonald, W. A. Craig, and C. M. Kunin

Trimethoprim and Rifampicin: In Vitro Activities
        Separately and in Combination   103
    D. W. Kerry, J. M. T. Hamilton-Miller, and
    W. Brumfitt

A ^{125}I-based Radioimmunoassay for Serum Gentamicin   107
    R. A. A. Watson, E. J. Shaw, and C. R. W. Edwards

Fluorimetric Assay of Tetracycline Mixtures in Plasma   111
    D. Hall

Assay of Antibiotics with Agar Diffusion Technique   115
    A.-S. Malmborg

A New Assay Technique for Antibiotics   125
    M. J. Harber and A. W. Asscher

The Problem of Antibiotic Mixtures in Serum Samples   133
    D. S. Reeves and H. A. Holt

Some Factors Influencing the Assay of Gentamicin   143
    J. D. Jarvis and T. W. C. Leung

Assay of Gentamicin and Tobramycin by a Reliable
        2-1/2 hour Klebsiella Plate Method   147
    D. C. Shanson, C. Hince, and J. V. Daniels

Punch Hole Method. A Simplified Bio-Assay Technique
        of Antibiotic Concentrations   155
    S. Kondo

The Assay of Serum Aminoglycoside Concentrations by
        the (^{14}C) - Acetyl Transferase Techniques 159
    J. M. Broughall and D. S. Reeves

Immunochemical Study of the Structural Specificity of
        an Antigentamycin Antiserum, Useful Also for
        Radioimmunoassay of Sisomycin 165
    S. Jonsson

Serum Activity Determination as Connecting Link
        Between Experiment and Clinic 169
    E. Freerksen and M. Rosenfeld

Animal Models in the Assessment of Antimicrobial
        Agents: What Should We Expect of Them? 177
    F. O'Grady

Local Lesions 183
    G. N. Rolinson

Intraperitoneal Challenge 191
    K. R. Comber, C. D. Osborne, and R. Sutherland

Endocarditis 197
    L. R. Freedman and G. Demierre

The Usefulness of Experimental Models of Urinary Tract
        Infections in the Assessment of Chemotherapeutic
        Compounds 205
    D. M. Ryan

An Animal Model for Intestinal Infections 219
    E. Boehni

Animal Models in the Assessment of Antimicrobial
        Agents: Salmonellosis 229
    E. W. Hook

Animal Models and Pharmacokinetics 235
    G. E. Mawer

Use of an In Vitro Model of the Urinary Bladder in
        the Investigation of Bacterial Response to
        Antibiotics 241
    D. Greenwood

Experimental Intra-Abdominal Sepsis 249
    J. G. Bartlett, A. B. Onderdonk, T. Louie, and
    S. L. Gorbach

Comparative Effects of Amoxycillin and Ampicillin
    in the Treatment of Experimental Mouse
    Infections 259
    K. R. Comber, C. D. Osborne, and R. Sutherland

Model of Pleuropneumonia in Rats 267
    Ch. Krüger, R. Commichau, and W. Henkel

Murine Meningoencephalitis Caused by Ps. aeruginosa
    or Kl. pneumoniae as an Experimental
    Chemotherapeutic Model 273
    E. N. Padeiskaya, S. N. Kutchak, and G. N. Perchin

Animal Experiments on Current Antibiotics 281
    W. Ritzerfeld, R. Koschmieder, and W. Drees

Effect of Carbenicillin on Pseudomonas Infection 289
    P. A. Hunter, G. N. Rolinson, and D. A. Witting

Comparison of Carfecillin and Carbenicillin on
    Experimental Urinary Tract Infection 295
    M. Hatala, J. Morávek, O. Schück, V. Prát,
    M. Liška, and J. Spousta

Model of Experimental Cystitis in Albino Wistar Rats 303
    Ch. Krüger, H. Freiesleben, K. Sack, and R. Commichau

Pathogenesis of an Experimental Pyelonephritis Model
    in the Mouse and Its Use in the Evaluation
    of Antibiotics 311
    K. R. Comber

Chronic E. coli Nephritis in Rats: Model for Assessment
    of Activity of Antimicrobial Agents 317
    R. Commichau, H. Freiesleben, K. Sach,
    Ch. Krüger, and W. Henkel

Combined Therapy of Anti-Endotoxin (OEP) antibody and
    Gentamicin in the Immunosuppressed Mice with
    Pseudomonas aeruginosa Infection 323
    K. Haranaka, K. Sugane, and K. Mashimo

Investigations on Circulatory Tolerance of
    Doxycycline (Vibravenous®) and Rolitetracycline
    (Reverin®) in Waking Minipigs 331
    G. Tauberger, M. Schoog, W. Mehren, G. Mergler,
    and M. Moussawi

An In Vitro Comparison of Sisomicin with Gentamicin
    and Tobramycin 335
    S. Shadomy and C. Utz

Bacteriological and Clinical Evaluation of Sisomicin,
        A New Aminoglycoside Antibiotic   345
    G. F. Abbate, I. Alagia, V. Leonessa, and P. Altucci

Pharmacokinetics of Sisomicin in Patients with
        Renal Impairment   355
    G. Heinecke, K. Finke, and E. Renner

Serum and Tissue Levels of Sisomicin in Dogs   367
    M. Scheer

Sisomicin Treatment of Urinary Tract Infections   375
    G. A. Dale and C. E. Cox

Parenteral Sisomicin for Surgical Infections   389
    H. H. Stone, L. D. Kolb, and C. E. Geheber

Clinical Trial of Sisomycin: Evaluation of Two
        Different Dosages   395
    M. Jonsson, E. Bengtsson, S. Jonsson, I. Julander,
    and G. Tunevall

In Vivo Activity of Sisomicin in Mice   403
    M. Scheer

New Data on Pharmacology of Gentamicin   409
    D. Zhelyazkov, K. Ivanova, N. Gueorguiev,
    R. Marinova, A. Beltcheva, M. Mangurova, and
    N. Temnyalov

Bacteriological, Clinical, and Pharmacological
        Investigations with Tobramycin   417
    E. Iván, A. E. Nagy, and K. N. Csatáry

The Urinary Excretion of Tobramycin and Gentamicin   421
    M. J. Wood and W. Farrell

Pharmacokinetics and Ototoxicity of Gentamicin,
        Tobramycin and Amikacin   427
    P. Federspil and E. Tiesler

Clinical Experience on Tobramycin   431
    S. Ishiyama, I. Nakayama, H. Iwamoto, S. Iwai,
    I. Murata, and M. Ohashi

Evaluation of Tobramycin in Severe Injury Tract
        Infection   437
    A. H. Bennett

Butirosin - Pharmacodynamics and Clinical Experience 441
    W. E. Kunsman and W. J. Holloway

Action Mechanism of 3,4-dideoxykanamycin B (DKB) on
        Some Gram-Negative Bacteria 453
    S. Oka, K. Oizumi, F. Ariji, K. Konno, and
    K. Fukushi

Use of 3,4-dideoxykanamycin B (DKB) in Various
        Infections 457
    S. Oka

List of Contributors 461

INTRODUCTORY COMMENTS

J. C. Sherris

Department of Microbiology and Immunology
University of Washington
Seattle, Washington 98195 U.S.A.

SUMMARY

Improvements in susceptibility testing require better definition
of reagents, test conditions, control strain maintenance and qualitative interpretative criteria. Quality control and external proficiency testing are keys to better performance at the operating level
and will be discussed in the symposium. Developments in mechanization
and automation are accelerating, and procedures designed to give
results on the same day the test is set up are being developed. The
need for agreed reference standards is again pointed up by these
developments.

There have been increasing efforts in different countries during
the past five or six years to improve regional performance of clinical
susceptibility testing. Approaches have varied from attempts to
improve reproducibility in absolute terms with methodological and
reagent standardization to those which focus more on reproducibility
of "qualitative" or "clinical" categorizations and on comparisons
with control strains, with less emphasis on the procedure employed.
Examples of both will be described in this symposium. Unfortunately,
despite these advances, we are still in a situation in which agreement on reference dilution procedures has not been achieved and in
which MIC results may differ considerably between procedures in
different laboratories.

The fundamental problems with susceptibility testing have been
the method dependency of results, the absence of fixed standards, and
the lack of agreed criteria for interpretation. The results of both
dilution and diffusion procedures are influenced, in varying degrees,
by variations of inoculum, medium constitution, pH, and incubation

temperature and duration. In addition, diffusion test results are influenced by disc content and by any substantial growth rate differences in the organisms tested. Without agreed standards or procedures, it is therefore hardly surprising that interlaboratory reproducibility studies in the past showed some quite striking diversities (Hoffman, et al., 1958; Report, 1965; Survey, 1968; McCracken and Palmer, 1969; Ericsson and Sherris, 1971). That results were tolerable at all was probably due to the fact that many pathogens are often highly susceptible or highly resistant to the earlier introduced antimicrobics, and these properties frequently permitted discrimination with even poorly standardized test systems. Clear cut bimodal distributions of susceptibility are less marked or absent with other antimicrobics such as the cephalosporins and broader spectrum penicillins, and with some species which are now seen more commonly in infections in the compromised host. These considerations increase the importance of higher levels of reproducibility.

Better absolute reproducibility can be obtained. Test conditions can be standardized including such components as medium volume, pH, incubation conditions, etc. Antimicrobic disc contents, which were shown to vary excessively in the past in North America (Branch et al., 1957; Greenberg et al., 1957) can be controlled. They are now subject to batch certification regulations in North America and their perfor- mance can be assured within established limits (which could still be tightened). Endpoint reading is more prone to subjectivity, but difficulties can be reduced by establishing prefixed criteria, some- times by simple manipulations such as reading diffusion plates through the back rather than the front, or by reading broth endpoints with relatively simple photometric devices. Inocula can be standardized with various levels of precision depending on the care which is expended or the equipment that is available. In recent studies in our laboratories by Dr. Marie Coyle, duplicate tests with two readers on two successive days were made of a large number of isolates by means of an agar overlay technique using a photometrically adjusted inoculum. Among 294 sets of 8 observations, only 8 (2.7%) had a range of >3 mm for the 8 readings, a level of precision which is considera- bly greater than we have achieved before.

The largest single problem in achieving reproducibility in absolute terms remains the medium. Individual products of single manufacturers usually show good reproducibility from batch to batch (Brenner and Sherris, 1972; Barry and Effinger, 1974); however, as will be considered elsewhere in this meeting, products of some manu- facturers may yield results considerably different from those of others, particularly with antimicrobics affected by divalent cations or by total salt content. These include the aminoglycosides, the tetracyclines, and the polymyxins. Similarly, differences in thy- midine content of media may substantially influence the endpoint clarity and absolute results with the sulfonamides and trimethoprim (R. Ferone et al., 1975).

Intermanufacturer reproducibility of presently used media could be greatly improved if performance limits were established. This should not be too burdensome because batches can be adjusted to meet particular performance requirements. For example, divalent cation content can be manipulated to adjust the gentamicin vs. Pseudomonas aeruginosa performance of MH media of low magnesium and calcium content to conform to a reference batch or yield results within a predetermined range with control strains (Reller et al., 1974; Sherris and Aitken, 1975, unpublished data). Improvement in performance of complex media with sulfonamides and trimethoprim can be attained by enzymic inactivation of thymidine (R. Ferone et al., 1975). Clearly, however, the problem would be greatly simplified with the use of better defined media at least to the point of full descriptions of manufacturing procedures of complex components such as peptones.

In studies by an international collaborative group, it was shown that even when the same medium, reagents, and strains are tested with a standard protocol, there can be very substantial variation between the results of different laboratories (Ericsson and Sherris, 1971). This illustrated clearly the need for standard or control strains, and Chabbert defined the criteria for their selection (Chabbert, 1971). Specific recommendations for control strains have now been made in different countries, but their value depends on their stability under storage conditions. Coyle has recently compared 15 strains of S. aureus and E. coli, which were sent to her by laboratories in different parts of the United States. Each organism was originally derived from the "Seattle" strain (ATCC 25923 and 25922). The strains were maintained under a variety of conditions, some of which were suboptimal. All were tested in duplicate on two occasions by the diffusion test mentioned above, and compared with a strain derived directly from ATCC. Among the staphylococci, one was a penicillinase producer of different phage type to the ATCC strain. All others were of the same phage type and gave zone diameters within 2 mm of the standard with all antimicrobics except the penicillins and cephalothin. Three strains gave penicillin zones which exceeded the others by 3.5 - 7 mm, although all were within the FDA performance range (Fed. Reg., 1972; Fed. Reg., 1973). One strain of E. coli differed in biotype from the ATCC strain and one gave several divergent results. The remaining 13 yielded only 4 results among 113 which differed from the ATCC strain by more than 1 mm, and none that differed by 2 mm or more. Reller (1974) made deliberate attempts to cause variation in proposed Pseudomonas aeruginosa control strains by repeated subculture under adverse conditions and failed. It thus appears that quite high levels of reproducibility of performance with standard strains can be obtained under operating conditions in different laboratories if storage and use conditions are well defined, and this is obviously critical for methods that depend on results relative to standard strains as well as for quality control of procedures that seek reproducibility in absolute terms.

The ultimate test of success in improving susceptibility test performance is at the operating level in the clinical or public health laboratory and several papers in this symposium bear on quality control and performance evaluation. With procedures in which reproducibility is sought in absolute terms, performance limits for control strains need to be established and met within the laboratory. For all procedures, external proficiency test evaluation is an invaluable adjunct and is now being used increasingly. Not only can it measure acceptable performance in relationship to results of reference or referee laboratories, but a detailed analysis of the results can often indicate the nature of the problem in an individual laboratory with poor performance. Performance evaluation systems in clinical microbiology generally can be a most effective educational tool when there is immediate follow-up explanations of sources of error.

Interpretative categories for susceptibility test results have to be determined from several considerations. Relationship of in vitro inhibitory concentrations to blood or other body fluid levels are useful, but when taken alone can be a considerable oversimplification. Distribution of susceptibilities among strains or variants of known responsiveness must also be considered. The borderlines of categories are ultimately best judgment decisions, taking into account these several components. They should be agreed and clearly defined by workers with special knowledge in the field. There have been few well designed studies to test the validity of particular categorical schemes, although much clinical operating experience has been gained. An essential prerequisite to better controlled studies on new agents is methodological reproducibility to provide a better data base.

While work has been continuing in standardization and performance evaluation of traditional methods, there have been a number of new developments towards automated and mechanized procedures (Automation, 1975) and commercially produced test systems which only require inoculation. Some of these have considerable promise and some would appear to be modifiable so that their benefits could be achieved without the use of expensive hardware. Such procedures should reduce the technical errors associated with "hand" methods. Devices now available or under development include procedures for automatically distributing pre-fixed broth volumes, adding antimicrobics, usually as elution discs, and for reading results photometrically or by changes in electrical impedence (Automation, 1975). Automatic particle counting devices have also been developed for measuring microbial growth or inhibition (Isenberg et al., 1971). It seems probable that many devices can be developed to the point of significant utility and accuracy for susceptibility testing in relationship to established methods if overnight reading is employed. Their greatest potential use, however, is in providing results on the day on which the test is set up. To date, efforts to equate rapid to overnight results have focussed on modifying the concentrations of antimicrobic used in the test. Results in our laboratory indicate that better equivalence will result by using heavier inocula for the early-read test, and we believe this approach merits further exploration (Lampe et al., 1975). The need for reference standards is again clear.

Despite these developments, diffusion testing is likely to remain a mainstay for smaller laboratories for several years to come. Performance can be improved and more selective use could almost certainly offset any added cost of better reagents, quality control and proficiency testing. It is to be hoped that the interchange of information and experience in this symposium will be an added stimulus to the further work that is needed to continue to improve susceptibility testing methodology and utility.

REFERENCES

Automation in microbiology and immunology (1975), Hedén, C.-G., and T. Illéni, eds. John Wiley & Sons, Publishers.

Barry, A. L., and Effinger, L. J. (1974), Am. J. Clin. Pathol., 62, 113.

Branch, A., Starkey, D. H., Power, E. E., and Greenberg, L. (1957), In Antibiotics Annual 1956-57. Antibiotica, Inc., N.Y., p. 898.

Brenner, V. C., and Sherris, J. C. (1972), Antimicrob. Ag. Chemother., 1, 116.

Chabbert, Y. A. (1971), In Ericsson, H. M., and Sherris, J. C. Antibiotic sensitivity testing. Report of an international collaborative study. Acta Pathol. et Microbiol. Scandinav., Section B, Suppl. No. 217.

Ericsson, H. M., and Sherris, J. C. (1971), Antibiotic sensitivity testing. Report of an international collaborative study. Acta Pathol. et Microbiol. Scandinav., Section B, Suppl. No. 217.

Federal Register (1972), Rules and regulations. Antibiotic susceptibility discs. Fed. Regist. 37, 20525-20529.

Federal Register (1973), Rules and regulations. Antibiotic susceptibility discs--correction. Fed. Regist. 38, 2576.

Ferone, R., Bushby, S. R. M., Burchall, J. J., Moore, W. D., and Smith, D. (1975), Antimicrob. Ag. Chemother., 7, 91-98.

Greenberg, L., Fitzpatrick, K. M., and Branch, A. (1957), Canad. M. A. J., 76, 194.

Hoffman, R. V., Jr., Jackson, G. G., and Turner, M. P. (1958),
       J. Lab. Clin. Med., 51, 873.

Isenberg, H. D., Reichler, A., and Wiseman, D. (1971), Appl.
       Microbiol., 22, 980.

Lampe, M. F., Aitken, C. L., Dennis, P. G., Forsythe, P. S.,
       Patrick, K. E., Schoenknecht, F. D., and Sherris, J. C.   (1975),
       Antimicrobial Ag. Chemother., in press.

McCracken, L. M., and Palmer, P. H. (1969), N. Z. med. J., 70, 390.

Reller, L. B., Schoenknecht, F. D., Kenny, M. A., and Sherris, J. C.
       (1974), J. Infect. Dis., 130, 454-463.

Report on antibiotic sensitivity test trial organized by the
       Bacteriology Committee of the Assoc. of Clin. Pathologists
       (1965), J. clin. Path., 18, 1.

Survey of antibiotic sensitivity testing (1968), Med. J. Aust.,
       2, 171.

CONTROL OF ANTIBIOTIC-SENSITIVITY TESTING IN BRITAIN

R. Blowers and D.F.J. Brown

Clinical Research Centre, Harrow HA1 3UJ and
Central Public Health Laboratory, Colindale, NW9 5HT
United Kingdom

More than ten years ago the Bacteriology Committee of the
Association of Clinical Pathologists saw the need for a survey of
antibiotic-sensitivity testing in Britain. The committee therefore organised a trial that was reported in 1965 by the convenor of
this symposium, Dr Joan Stokes. One hundred and fifty four laboratories performed 3386 tests on four organisms; 46% of the laboratories returned results including at least one error, and 3.4%
of all results were wrong. This early trial also provided
indications of the methods that were more likely to yield correct
results, and clearly showed the need for nationwide and continuous
control of sensitivity testing. This has not yet been fully
achieved but is being steadily approached by the National Quality-
control Service for Microbiology. The service was formed by the
amalgamation of two pilot schemes - one run by Dr Stokes and
Dr James Whitby with support from the Department of Health and the
other by the Public Health Laboratory Service. It is concerned
with all aspects of diagnostic microbiology but an important part
of its work is to encourage accuracy and consistency of sensitivity
testing and the sensible reporting of results, and to relate the
accuracy of results to the methods that are used.

ACCURACY OF METHODS IN ROUTINE USE

Participating laboratories have been sent usually three
preserved cultures each month for examination and reporting in
their usual way. For organisms on which sensitivity tests were
relevant, the results were entered on computer cards and were
analysed according to a programme that gave scores for correctness
of result and relevance of the report. The "correct" results were

initially determined by the findings of the issuing laboratory but
confirmed by the majority findings of the participating laboratories.
In the very few instances of difference between the intended and the
majority findings, the results were not included in the scoring and
analysis. For tests on each organism, laboratories were awarded
points as follows:

(a) up to three appropriate drugs of choice for each strain,
    +2 points when right, -2 when wrong;

(b) other appropriate drugs to a maximum of eight,
    +1 when right, -2 when wrong;

(c) duplicate tests with similar drugs,
    0 when right, -2 when wrong;

(d) inappropriate tests,
    -2 regardless of answer.

The appropriateness of drugs for various species and two
broad clinical situations was decided, with fairly generous
latitude, by the organising committee and was made known to all
participating laboratories. The performance of 93 laboratories in
tests on 14 organisms during 1971-73 are shown in table I. Future
surveys may show whether participation in this scheme improves the
performance of laboratories.

There has been general agreement that external quality control
of results is useful. But the validity of awarding scores for the
relevance of reports, which is sometimes a matter of opinion, has
been questioned. The organising committee has tried to meet this
objection by deducting marks only for gross irrelevancies with
which no-one should disagree.

Percent of possible score	40-49	50-59	60-69	70-79	80-89	90-94
Number of laboratories	4	8	18	39	20	4

Table I. Distribution of antibiotic-sensitivity scores by 93

laboratories

RELATION OF METHODS TO RESULTS OF DIFFUSION TESTS

From these studies it is not yet possible to recommend a complete system for sensitivity testing by the diffusion method. There have been, however, clear associations between the results and some points of technique. Some of these are briefly described below.

The Use of Controls

The value of comparing test zones with those of sensitive control organisms has been evident throughout the series but is more significant for some organisms and some drugs than for others. It is well illustrated by the results from a sulphonamide-sensitive strain of Klebsiella sp. from urine, shown in table II.

This analysis does not differentiate between the various methods of using control organisms and relating their zone sizes to those of the organisms being tested. At least twelve different methods have been recorded so far, and continued studies may differentiate between the results from them.

Ampicillin Content of Discs

The amount of ampicillin in paper discs has ranged from $2\,\mu g$ to $25\,\mu g$. High-content discs are often used for tests on urinary pathogens because high concentrations of ampicillin can be attained in urine. But misleading results have been obtained when high-content discs were used for testing pathogens from sites that can be reached by antibiotic only in the blood-stream. Table III shows the results of testing an ampicillin-resistant Bacteroides sp. (MIC = $32\,\mu g$ per ml) with discs of various strengths (Blowers et al., 1973).

Number of tests done	Number of reports: Correct (sensitive)	Incorrect (resistant)
79 with controls	63	16 (20%)
15 without controls	8	7 (47%)

Table II. Frequency of correct and incorrect results from tests done with and without controls

Ampicillin content of disc	Number of	
	Tests	Errors
2 µg	23	1 (4%)
10 µg	14	1 (7%)
25 µg	23	7 (30%)
		(P < 0·05)

Table III. Frequency of incorrect results in relation to

ampicillin-content of discs

There is no significant difference between the results from
2-µg and 10-µg discs, but when 25-µg discs were used diminished
zone size indicating resistance was easily missed even when compared with the zone of a fully sensitive control organism.

Use of Cephaloridine Discs

Many laboratories reported the sensitivity of Staphylococcus
aureus to cephaloridine despite the fact that staphylococci show
virtually complete cross-resistance to methicillin and cephaloridine.
It was clear, however, that tests with cephaloridine discs were
much less reliable than those with methicillin. Table IV shows
that when a methicillin/cephaloridine-resistant strain of Staph.aureus
was   distributed to the participating laboratories, errors from
cephaloridine testing were ten times as frequent as those from
methicillin testing. In another series of tests on a methicillin-
resistant strain of Staph. aureus, 10 laboratories reported it to
be resistant to cephaloridine and 10 reported it to be sensitive.
The committee therefore recommended that staphylococci should not
be tested against cephaloridine (Blowers et al., 1973).

Drug	Number of	
	Tests	Errors
Methicillin	175	3 (1·7%)
Cephaloridine	47	8 (17%)

Table IV. Frequency of incorrect results from tests done with

methicillin and cephaloridine

Blood in Media for Tests on Sulphonamides

It is widely recommended that diffusion tests with sulphonamides should be done on media containing blood, which neutralises
sulphonamide inhibitors in the medium. Nevertheless, many laboratories did these tests on blood-free media. Table V shows that
their results, for a sulphonamide-sensitive <u>Klebsiella</u> sp. from
urine, were more likely to be wrong.

These four examples do not exhaust the possibilities of
evaluating sensitivity-test methods by analysis of quality-control
results. As the amount of material from the Microbiology Quality-
control Laboratory accumulates, it will be possible to determine
the effect of other and perhaps lesser variations of technique.
However, quicker indications can sometimes be obtained from
specially designed trials rather than by observing the results from
laboratories who have chosen their own methods. Such trials have
often been conducted in research laboratories where all the methods
can be performed to near perfection, and where technical staff are
free from the pressures of routine diagnostic work. The Public
Health Laboratory Service and the Clinical Research Centre of the
Medical Research Council therefore made a joint study of the results
from four widely-used sensitivity-test methods, in 36 routine
laboratories of various sizes throughout Britain. The four methods
were: a) comparison of zone-size with control on a separate plate;
b) comparison of zone-size with control on the same plate (Stokes
and Waterworth, 1972); c) the Kirby-Bauer method (Bauer <u>et al.</u>,
1966); and d) the Ericsson method (AB Biodisk, 1971). The findings
of this study are being reported at this Congress by D.F.J. Brown
and D. Kothari so are not described here.

We have presented this paper on behalf of the PHLS Quality-
control Committee and are grateful to the committee for all its
work. The committee particularly thanks Mrs J.E. Blair and

Medium	Number of	
	Tests	Errors
With lysed blood	42	5 (11%)
Without blood	12	8 (40%)

Table V. Frequency of incorrect results from tests done on media

with and without lysed blood

Mr W.B. Fletcher for the data analyses,   its secretary Dr J.D.
Abbott,   the directors and staff of the 93 participating
laboratories, and   Dr P.B. Crone, director of the Microbiology
Quality-control Laboratory, for permission to use the results from
some of the later surveys.

REFERENCES

AB Biodisk. The Paper Disc Method. 1971, Stockholm.

Association of Clinical Pathologists (1965). Report on antibiotic-
sensitivity test trial organized by the Bacteriology Committee of
the Association of Clinical Pathologists. J.clin.Path. 18, 1.

Bauer, A.W., Kirby, W.M.M., Sherris, J.C., and Turck, M. (1966).
Antibiotic susceptibility testing by a standardized single disc
method. Amer.J.clin.Path. 45, 493.

Blowers, R., Stokes, E.J., and Abbott, J.D. (1973). Antibiotic-
sensitivity tests. Brit.med.J. 3, 47.

Stokes, E.J. and Waterworth, P.M. (1972). Antibiotic sensitivity
tests by diffusion methods. Assn.Clin.Path. Broadsheet no.55.

CONTROL OF ANTIBACTERIAL SUSCEPTIBILITY TESTING:

STANDARDIZATION AND PROFICIENCY TESTING IN CANADA

I.B.R. Duncan

University of Toronto, Canada

Sunnybrook Medical Centre, Toronto, Canada.   M4N 3M5

Serious interest in the standardization of susceptibility testing in Canada goes back more than 20 years. From 1952 onwards standardized methods were established in the Veterans' hospitals of Canada (Branch et al. 1964) under the direction of Dr. Arnold Branch, who was one of the participants in the International Collaborative Study. As early as 1957 the Canadian federal government set up measures to control the potency of susceptibility test discs sold in Canada (Greenberg and Fitzpatrick 1958), following Greenberg's demonstration (Greenberg et al. 1957) that most discs then on the Canadian market varied widely from their labelled potencies. These early approaches twoards standardization probably did much to improve the quality of susceptibility testing throughout the country, but because medicine in Canada is under provincial rather than federal jurisdiction, they did not lead to any nationally recommended standard methods. Instead proficiency testing of existing methods has been developed at the provincial level.

At present 4 of the 10 provinces have compulsory proficiency testing programs in which every bacteriology laboratory must participate under provincial law; these are British Columbia, Alberta, Manitoba, and Ontario. All four were set up by laboratory physicians themselves under the aegis of their provincial College of Physicians or Medical Association, and the provincial governments make use of them for the licensing of laboratories. Two other provinces have centrally organized proficiency programs in which only a proportion of the province's laboratories take part, and 4 provinces have no local programs. However, many individual laboratory directors in provinces without compulsory programs participate in those of the American Society of Clinical Pathologists or the College of American Pathologists. Although there is no compulsion

to do so, most Canadian Laboratories would appear to use the disc
diffusion method recommended by the F.D.A. and the National Committee for Clinical Laboratory Standards in the U.S.

ONTARIO PROFICIENCY TESTING PROGRAM

The Ontario program was originally established by the laboratory physicians of the province as part of a voluntary laboratory
accreditation scheme administered by the Ontario Medical Association. In January 1975 participation in the program was made a
compulsory part of the licensing of all laboratories in the
province; inspection and licensing of laboratories had been introduced in 1973 by the provincial government at a time when there
was a great increase in the number of private out-patient laboratories in Ontario. Approximately 300 laboratories take part in
the microbiology proficiency testing program; half are hospital
laboratories and half are private laboratories serving the needs
of family physicians' and specialists' private office practice.
The hospitals range from tertiary referral university hospitals
with over 1,000 beds to simple community hospitals with under 100
beds. The results from the Ontario proficiency testing program
are probably therefore representative of the sort of work being
done in the various kinds of laboratories in the country. I am
very grateful to the Microbiology Committee of the O.M.A. Laboratory Proficiency Testing Program for permission to report the
results of the first 6 months of compulsory testing. Four freeze-
dried bacteria are sent out every 6 weeks for identification and
susceptibility testing. Tests are done by the laboratory's regular
method against the antimicrobial agents considered appropriate in
that laboratory for the particular organism identified, and they
are reported simply as sensitive, intermediate or resistant. The
results from all the laboratories are centrally assessed by a
computer program which takes the results of a number of reference
laboratories of known high quality as being "correct". Each
laboratory receives a copy of its own findings, the correct results,
and the results reported by all participating laboratories. It is
from these print-out sheets that I have compiled the data for this
report.

Defining the testing of one bacterium against one antibiotic
as one test, an analysis was made of the percentages of laboratories obtaining correct results in the first 100 tests done from
Jan. to May 1975. This data, which covers tests with 14 bacteria
and 18 antimicrobials, gives a broad impression of the general
quality of the work being done in the province. In 27 tests 98-
100% of laboratories were correct, in 28 tests 95-97% were correct,
in 14 tests 90-94% were correct, and in 7 tests 80-89% were
correct. Thus 24 tests were poorly done in that less than 80% of
participating laboratories reported correct results. Of the 24, 12

were tests with either sulphonamides or trimethoprim. It is by no means unexpected to find that results for these two agents were much poorer than for other antimicrobials, but is is disappointing that so many laboratories, left to make their own decisions on the agents against which they would choose to test the proficiency testing organisms, would still do perfunctory susceptibility testing with sulphonamide and trimethoprim rather than avoid testing them altogether. When the results for all agents except sulphonamides and trimethoprim are analysed, 80% of the tests were found to have been done correctly by 90% of laboratories or more. Tests with gentamicin were well done, and tetracycline testing was almost as satisfactory. More laboratories were in error with ampicillin and cephalothin testing; the errors with these antibiotics arose almost always with bacteria having M.I.C.s close to the break-point. Variations in bacterial inoculum were presumably responsible. The results of a number of individual tests were interesting. A penicillinase-producing Staphylococcus aureus was reported by 3% of laboratories as sensitive to penicillin and by 7% as sensitive to ampicillin. Somewhat surprisingly, a quarter of the laboratories chose to test a Lancefield A streptococcus against gentamicin; 80% of them wrongly reported it as sensitive. A carbenicillin-sensitive Pseudomonas aeruginosa was reported by 80% of laboratories as resistant, which suggests a failure to appreciate that the zone diameters for assessing susceptibility to carbenicillin are clearly stated to be different for pseudomonas and enterobacteria (Lennette et al. 1974) It was of particular interest that 35% reported a methicillin-resistant S. aureus as sensitive, and 21% reported as sensitive an ampicillin-resistant strain of Haemophilus influenzae. Organisms with these resistances are still rare in Canada and it is clear that many laboratories are not yet alert to the need for testing methods sufficiently sensitive to detect them. Finally, a comparison was made of the relative performances of different types of laboratories. The results obtained by 10 laboratories in each of 4 categories were compared for 300 tests. For university teaching hospitals, non-teaching hospitals over 100 beds, small hospitals under 100 beds, and private laboratories, the percentages of errors in all tests performed were 6, 9, 12 and 9 respectively. Tests with sulphonamides and trimethoprim were badly done by all types of laboratories, and omitting them from the calculation the percentage errors in the same order were 4, 8, 10 and 7.

Overall, the results of the first 6 months of the compulsory proficiency testing program in Ontario show that the standard of work leaves room for considerable improvement but is by no means bad. Much of the improvement could be made simply by applying knowledge we already have. The educational aspect of the program may well lead to real improvements, particularly in those laboratories with minimal supervision by microbiologically knowledgeable physicians. A comparison of the present data with results a year from now will show if this has proved to be the case.

APPROACH TO STANDARDIZATION OF AGAR DILUTION METHOD

As Canada has no nationally recommended susceptibility testing system, there is nothing to discourage the use of methods other than the disc diffusion method. In Toronto and other centres in southern Ontario an agar dilution inocula replicator method is becoming popular. At present 21 laboratories in the area are using it; 14 are hospital laboratories, 6 are private laboratories, and one is the large central provincial public health laboratory. An Ontario laboratory supply firm sells quality-controlled antibiotic containing plate media for the method as well as a patented improved version of the Steers' replicator which will inoculate round 9 cm size Petri plates. In my own laboratory the method has been in use for 4½ years and a number of advantages are apparent. For the large laboratory it is economical of time and materials; 36 bacteria can be tested on one plate and control strains are tested on the same test plates as the actual isolates. Break-points are adjustable to serum or urinary levels and MICs can be measured. Each antibiotic can be tested under optimal conditions such as incubation at reduced temperature for methicillin, reduced inoculum for sulphonamides, and thymidine deficient medium for trimethoprim. Finally, plate biochemical test media can be added to the system, either to control the purity of the inocula in the susceptibility test or as the definitive means of identifying Gram-negative rods.

Our group in the Medical Microbiology Department of University of Toronto has been working for some time to improve the standardization of the method. The first approach was to compare actual results under routine conditions in the 3 major hospitals which first used the method in Toronto; Hospital for Sick Children (Dr. Fleming), Toronto General Hospital (Dr. N.A. Hinton and Dr. E.T. Sheaff), and my own hospital. In theory these laboratories were all using the same method. The first survey compared their testing of 300 Gram-negative isolates. Discrepancies between the results of any two hospitals were around 4%. A majority of the discrepancies were observed to be in the same direction; one of the hospitals was reporting tests resistant which the other two reported sensitive. The next step in trying to resolve the cause of these differences was to reread the same plates in each hospital. This demonstrated clearly that in two of the laboratories the technologists were reading moderate but reduced growth as sensitive while the criteria for sensitivity in the third hospital was less than 5 colonies. Having standardized our method of reading end-points we carried out the same series of MIC estimations in each hospital. This time two obtained similar results never more than 2-fold steps apart, and the third, which was using Mueller-Hinton rather than the DST (Oxoid) medium used by the other two, frequently differed from them. Finally, all 3 laboratories performed the same series of tests, used the same inocula, the same media and the same criteria for reading end-points. Identical results were obtained which proved to us that we could indeed standardize the method under routine working conditions. These studies were a valuable start but we have further to go. Our current position is that we have standardized our reading of end-points, our serum-level break-points for reporting susceptibility, and the use of 3% agar (except with gentamicin) to prevent swarming of proteus. We are close to decisions on choice of media and urine-level break-points. Considerably more work is needed to settle the most suitable weight of inoculum, and to build up a collection of control bacteria with MICs close to each side of our break-points for the various antibiotics.

REFERENCES

Branch, A., Starkey, D.H. and Power, E.A. (1964), Medical Services Journal Canada, 20, 460.

Greenberg, L. and Fitzpatrick, K.M. (1958), Canadian Medical Association Journal, 79, 383.

Greenberg, L., Fitzpatrick, K.M. and Branch, A. (1957), Canadian Medical Association Journal, 76, 194.

Lennette, E.H., Spaulding, E.H. and Truant, J.P. (1974), Manual of Clinical Microbiology, Second edition, Washington, American Society for Microbiology.

ANTIBIOTIC SENSITIVITY TESTING IN AUSTRALIA AND NEW ZEALAND

S.M. Bell

Bacteriology Department, The Prince of Wales Hospital

Randwick 2031, N.S.W. Australia

The results of antibiotic sensitivity testing in practice are reviewed on the basis of information collected over a period of six years in the microbiology surveys which are conducted annually for The Royal College of Pathologists of Australia. In 1971 a simple calibrated disc method of sensitivity testing, the features of which are presented, was introduced into the surveys. It was demonstrated over the next three years that a marked improvement in the performance of sensitivity testing in practice resulted from the adoption by all laboratories of this calibrated method. The degree of precision achieved by the laboratories in the application of the uniform method was also studied and attention is drawn to its significance in determining the number of grades of sensitivity which can be reported accurately in practice. The value of collaboration between diagnostic laboratories and laboratories specialising in antibiotic sensitivity testing is discussed and emphasis is given to the need to establish reference centres for antibiotic sensitivity testing.

Antibiotic sensitivity testing has been examined in clinical laboratory practice in Australia and New Zealand since 1968, as a part of the annual microbiology surveys of laboratory proficiency conducted for The Royal College of Pathologists of Australia. In the three years between 1971 and 1973 these surveys were used to study in more detail the results of this test in practice and this report deals mainly with the results observed during this period. Participation in the microbiology surveys is voluntary and each year about 100 laboratories of vastly different interests and size take part. The three broad categories of laboratories who participate are shown overleaf.

% of total

Hospital or University Microbiology Departments   25
Hospital or Health Department General Pathology Laboratories 47
Private General Pathology Laboratories   28

Bacteriology departments represent only a quarter of the total whilst the majority are either government or private laboratories providing a general pathology service. It is emphasized therefore, that most of the laboratories who carry out antibiotic sensitivity tests in these two countries do not specialise in bacteriology but are staffed or supervised by people whose main interest may lie in other branches of pathology.

The first three microbiology surveys revealed inaccuracies in the results of antibiotic sensitivity testing similar to those demonstrated in practice elsewhere (2, 5). There was an overall error of from 5% to 10% in the results of sensitivity testing and some tests such as the detection of penicillin resistance in staphylococci and demonstration of sensitivity to sulphonamide in gram negatives were subject to considerable error. It was also obvious by 1971 that simply drawing laboratories' attention to their errors did little to improve the accuracy of sensitivity testing in practice. Therefore a three years study was undertaken to determine if the adoption by all laboratories of a uniform calibrated method would improve the results of sensitivity testing in practice.

THE UNIFORM CALIBRATED METHOD

The method introduced into the survey was based on one used in our laboratory since 1962 and some years were spent before 1971 in modifying the method to make it suitable for diagnostic laboratories and to eliminate, as far as possible, the causes of the common and serious errors of sensitivity testing previously observed in practice.

A detailed description of the method is not appropriate to this report as the method is based largely on that of Kirby-Bauer (3) and Ericsson (7) in that it is a single high potency disc diffusion technique which was calibrated to quantitative sensitivities. However, the method is unique in two ways; the first is that it specifies the use of the newer sensitivity media (Sensitest, Oxoid Ltd., or WSTA, Wellcome Reagents Ltd.) which are relatively free of sulphonamide inhibitors, thus a reproducible and simply prepared heavy inoculum can be employed to advantage with all antibiotics. The main feature of the method is that it reports the results of sensitivity into two grades only, that is either sensitive or resistant, and for this reason it is tentatively called the CDS test (Calibrated Dichotomous Sensitivity Test).

SENSITIVITY TESTING OF STAPHYLOCOCCUS AUREAUS

An appraisal of the value of the adoption of the CDS method as a uniform technique in practice was carried out with strains of Staphylococcus aureus in 1971 and 1973. Prior to the surveys the sensitivity of all strains was confirmed independently, using quantitative techniques, by two laboratories who specialise in antibiotic sensitivity testing. In 1971 the results observed when laboratories adopted the uniform technique were compared with those observed with non-uniform methods in the following way: First all laboratories were requested to use their own methods of antibiotic sensitivity testing to report the sensitivity of six strains of Staphylococcus aureus to five antibiotics, namely penicillin, tetra- cycline, erythromycin, chloramphenicol and methicillin. Later in 1971 the same six strains, each labelled differently, were again sent to participants who, in addition, received a description and all materials necessary for carrying out the CDS test. The laborat- ories were asked to record the zone size observed with each anti- biotic and report the sensitivity of each strain according to the method supplied. In 1973 all laboratories carried out sensitivity testing of a further four strains of Staphylococcus aureus to the same five antibiotics and in this year the laboratories again used the materials supplied and the uniform CDS method of sensitivity testing.

The overall improvement in the results of sensitivity testing which resulted from the adoption of the uniform method was clearly demonstrated; the percentage error with all tests was reduced from 10% observed with non-uniform methods to 1.4% when all laboratories followed the CDS method in 1971. This improvement observed with all antibiotics was continued in 1973 when 99.4% of all tests performed were correct.

As the CDS test recognises only two grades of sensitivity its use naturally corrected a common mistake made with non-uniform methods, which was to report clearly resistant strains as having intermediate sensitivity. With non-uniform techniques there were 233 reports where resistance to the antibiotic was not detected and in 47% of these the sensitivity was recorded as intermediate. A substantial proportion of laboratories incorrectly reported as intermediate penicillin-resistant (40% of errors) or methicillin-resistant (24% of errors) strains of staphylococci, although it is well recognised that for all practical purposes this organism is either clearly sensitive or resistant to these antibiotics and the term "intermediate" cannot be applied in these circumstances.

A comparison of the results observed with each antibiotic when laboratories used their own methods in 1971 and the CDS method in 1971 and 1973 is shown in Tables 1(a), 1(b) and 2.

Strain Number	Percentage of Incorrect Reports				
	Penicillin	Tetracycline	Chloram- phenicol	Erythromycin	Methicillin
1	(S) 2	(R) 14	(S) 3	(S) 1	(S) 2
2	(R) 0	(R) 2	(R) -	(R) 27	(R) 30
3	(R) 17	(S) 2	(S) 6	(S) 1	(S) 5
4	(R) 12	(R) 3	(S) 3	(R) 36	(S) 6
5	(R) 27	(S) 1	(S) 2	(S) 4	(S) 4
6	(R) 5	(R) 5	(S) 10	(R) 0	(R) 64

(S) = Sensitive strain   (R) = Resistant strain

TABLE 1(a) : Results of sensitivity testing by laboratories using their own methods with six strains of staphylococci (1971 Microbiology Survey).

Strain Number	Percentage of Incorrect Reports				
	Penicillin	Tetracycline	Chloram- phenicol	Erythromycin	Methicillin
1	2	0	1	2	1
2	0	0	0	0	1
3	0	0	0	0	1
4	1	0	0	0	8
5	1	1	0	1	1
6	1	0	1	0	25

TABLE 1(b) : Results of sensitivity testing of the same six strains of staphylococci by the CDS method (1971 Microbiology Survey).

Strain	Percentage of Incorrect Reports				
	Penicillin	Tetracycline	Chloram-phenicol	Erythromycin	Methicillin
A	(S) 0	(S) 0	(S) 0	(S) 0	(S) 0
B	(R) 0	(S) 0	(S) 0	(S) 0	(S) 0
C	(R) 0	(R) 1	(S) 0	(S) 0	(R) 7
D	(R) 0	(R) 2	(S) 1	(R) 1	(S) 0

(S) = Sensitive strain   (R) = Resistant strain

TABLE 2 : Results of sensitivity testing by laboratories of four
strains of staphylococci using the CDS method (1973
Microbiology Survey).

A significant number of laboratories failed to detect penicillin
resistance with their own methods and this error, which was as high as
27% with one strain in 1971 was reduced to 1% or less with the adoption
of the uniform method. The improved result was maintained in 1973
when in this year al laboratories tested without error by the uniform
method one penicillin-sensitive and three resistant strains of Staphylococcus aureus. A similar result was observed with erythromycin
where the average error of 30% observed with the two resistant strains
when tested by non-uniform methods in 1971 was eliminated in that year
when the laboratories used the CDS method. The results of methicillin
sensitivity testing are of particular interest in that they hielded
valuable information regarding the application of the CDS test in
practice. Two methicillin-resistant strains were included in the 1971
survey; with one strain resistance was relatively easily demonstrated
by the CDS test and the 30% error observed with non-uniform methods
was eliminated almost entirely. Demonstration of resistance in the
other strain was much more difficult and when laboratories used non-
uniform methods 64% of reports were incorrect. Although the use of
the CDS method resulted in a marked improvement in the results with
this strain 25% of the laboratories still failed to detect the
resistance of the strain to methicillin. It was apparent from the
results and the participants' comments that the method of subculture
of the test strains used by some laboratories could have led to a
reduction in the inoculum size sufficient to yield a false result when
this strain was tested against methicillin. In 1973 on the basis of
this information which explained some but not all of the errors with
the 1971 strain the wording of the method was made more detailed in
regard to the subculture of the test strains. Seven laboratories
only in 1973 failed to detect resistance in the single strain of the
methicillin-resistant staphylococcus submitted in that year whilst
all laboratories correctly demonstrated methicillin-sensitivity in
the three sensitive strains.

Inoculum size Dilutions of CDS inoculum (10^7 organisms per ml)	Annular Radius of Inhibition (mm)		
	Incubator Temperature		
	$31^\circ \pm$ IC	$39^\circ \pm$ IC	$41^\circ \pm$ IC
Undiluted	0	4.7	7.5
Diluted 1/4	0	5.2	8.4
Diluted 1/16	0	6.0	9.0
Diluted 1/32	0	5.7	8.8

TABLE 3 : Effect of variations in inoculum size and incubator temperature on the zone of inhibition with a methicillin-resistant strain (1973 Microbiology Survey) of Staphylococcus aureus.

Subsequent experiments revealed the probable source of error with the resistant strain and the results of these experiments are shown in Table 3. Methicillin disc sensitivity tests were carried out on the 1973 survey strian at different temperatures using twofold dilutions of the inoculum specified in the CDS method. It was determined from the results with other antibiotics which were also inoculum sensitive that none of the seven laboratories used an inoculum lighter than a thirty-twofold dilution of that specified in the CDS test. When the methicillin-resistant strain was tested against methicillin there was no significant difference between the zone sizes observed with the original heavy inoculum and dilutions as high as thirty-twofold. However, there was a marked increase in zone size with an increase in the temperature of incubation, that is, this strain showed the Annear effect (1) and the results demonstrated that all seven laboratories who reported the sensitivity incorrectly (zone size $\geq$ 6mm annular radius) almost certainly carried out the test at a temperature well above 37°C.

SENSITIVITY TESTING OF E. COLI

In 1972 a comparison was made of the results obtained with non-uniform methods and the CDS method in determining the antibiotic sensitivity of E. coli to eight antibiotics; but in this year comparison was made in a different way to that used in 1971. Eighty-six laboratories used their own methods to test six strains of E. coli to eight antibiotics and the results observed with this group are shown in Table 4.

Antibiotic	Percentage of Incorrect Reports					
	Strain 1	Strain 2	Strain 3	Strain 4	Strain 5	Strain 6
Ampicillin	(S) 15	(S) 6	(R) 2	(R) 1	(S) 15	(S) 9
Tetracycline	(S) 4	(S) 4	(R) 1	(R) 2	(S) 2	(R) 9
Sulphonamide	(S) 17	(S) 22	(R) 1	(R) 0	(R) 1	(R) 2
Chloramphenicol	(S) 2	(S) 2	(R) 10	(R) 1	(S) 1	(S) 1
Kanamycin	(S) 1	(S) 2	(S) 4	(S) 1	(S) 1	(S) 0
Cephalothin	(S) 6	(S) 6	(R) 46	(R) 23	(S) 8	(S) 3
Nalidixic Acid	(S) 1	(S) 2	(S) 2	(R) 1	(S) 3	(S) 0
Nitrofurantoin	(S) 0	(S) 1	(S) 7	(S) 3	(S) 9	(S) 0

(S) = Sensitive strain   (R) = Resistant strain

TABLE 4: Results of sensitivity testing by laboratories using their own methods with six strains of E. coli (1972 Microbiology Survey).

There was an overall error of 5.4% with all tests and only 19% of laboratories successfully tested the six strains to all antibiotics. The least accurate results were seen with the two cephalothin-resistant strains where 61 of the 172 tests were incorrect. There was also a 20% error indemonstrating sulphonamide sensitivity in two strains and an 11% error in the results of testing the four ampicillin-sensitive strains to this antibiotic.

At the same time a second group of 24 laboratories similar in type to the other group carried out the same tests on these six strains of E. coli using the uniform method. The CDS test had been success-fully calibrated with seven of the antibiotics, that is it was possible to divide the strains of gram negative specied into two distinct groups of sensitivity on the basis of the zone size observed with the disc test. An example of the results of this calibration with ampicillin is shown in Figure 1. However, successful calibration was not possible with cephalothin (see Figure 2) where the zones of resistant, intermediate and sensitive strains merged and attempts to improve the correlation between MIC and zone size by variation of the inoculum, changes in the media or alteration of the antibiotic content of the disc were all unsuccessful.

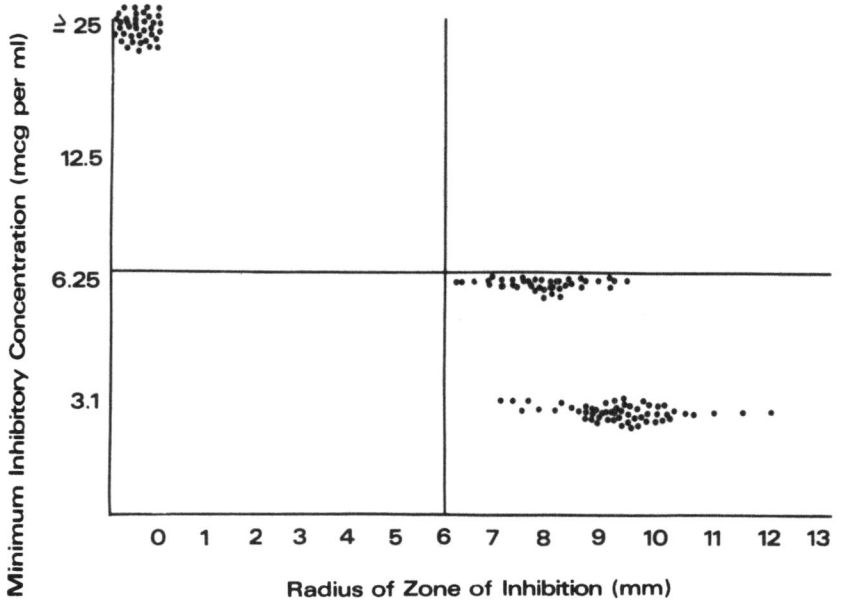

FIGURE 1: An example of successful calibration of the CDS test to
MIC values with 200 strains of E. coli tested against ampicillin.
All sensitive strains (MIC 6.25 mg/ml or less) yielded zones with
an annular radius of more than 6 mm.

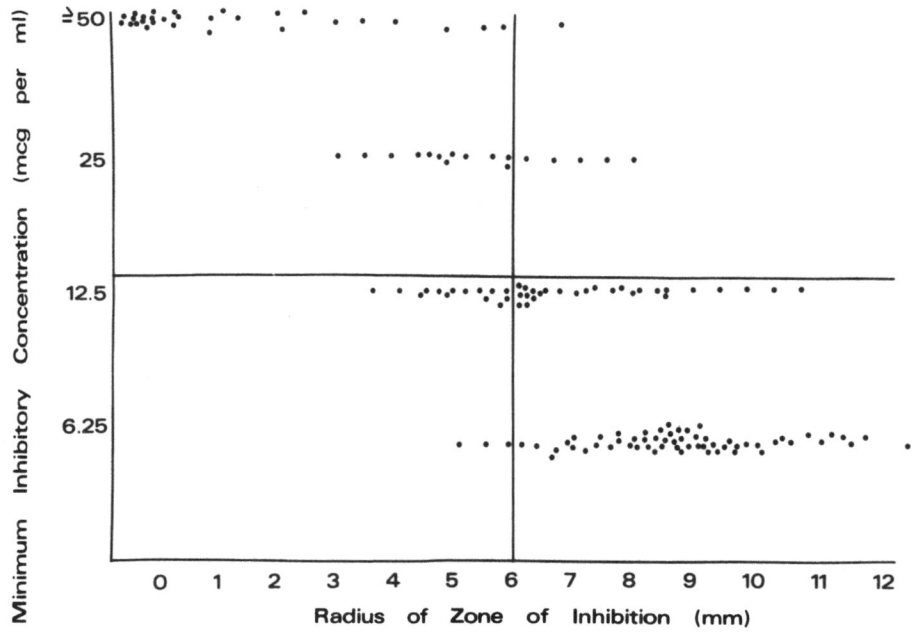

FIGURE 2: Results of calibration tests with cephalothin; showing a
lack of a clear distinction between the inhibitory zones of resistant, intermediate and sensitive strains.

Thus in this case the CDS test could not be calibrated to quantitative sensitivity and by definition, therefore should not be used to test cephalothin. Nevertheless, the laboratories were requested to attempt to test the strains to this antibiotic by the CDS method and in addition, to repeat the test after the introduction of a single modification of the method by diluting the inoculum to yield a semi-confluent growth of the organism on the sensitivity plate.

An almost perfect result was recorded by the 24 laboratories when they used the CDS method to test the seven antibiotics where satisfactory calibration had been achieved and only one error, which was shown to be clerical in nature, was observed with these antibodies. However, there was a 6% error with the two cephalothin-resistant strains when the laboratories attempted to test this antibiotic with the uncalibrated method, and further, the single modification of the method yielded a 60% error with one of the resistant strains which was similar to that observed in the group using non-uniform techniques.

THE PRECISION ACHIEVED WITH A UNIFORM METHOD IN PRACTICE

The microbiology surveys were also used to determine the variation in measurements of similar inhibitory zones recorded by laboratories with all tests when the CDS method was used. Two representative examples of the distribution of the measurements reported by the laboratories in each of the three years are shown in Figure 3.

With senstivie strains (as in Figure 3) all correct measurements for each test fell above the separation point and measurements were distributed in what was usually a symmetrical normal type distribution. The range of measurements was approximately the same in each of the three years, that is measurements fell within a 5 or 6 mm range (or a standard deviation of 1.2 to 1.5 mm). The extent of the variation from the mean did not appear to be related to the size of the zone of inhibition or to the antibiotic tested. With the resistant strains there was a variety of distributions but where an inhibitory zone was present around the antibiotic disc it was associated with a range of measurements and an example of one such distributions is shown in Figure 3. The measurements were generally scattered in a fashion resembling some part of a normal distribution curve and were spread over a range of 4 or 5 mm which was little different to the range observed with sensitive strains. It is possible that other methods of disc sensitivity testing could yield less variation in measurements in a similar population of laboratories to that observed with the CDS test in the microbiology surveys, but up to the present this had not been demonstrated. However each aspect of the CDS test was specifically designed in order that reproducibility did not depend on the possession by the operator of a highly specialised skill in bacteriological techniques. Thus it would be reasonable to expect that methods of sensitivity testing which are not so designed would be unlikely to yield a lesser variation in the measurements of inhibitory zones than the 5mm range observed with this group of laboratories.

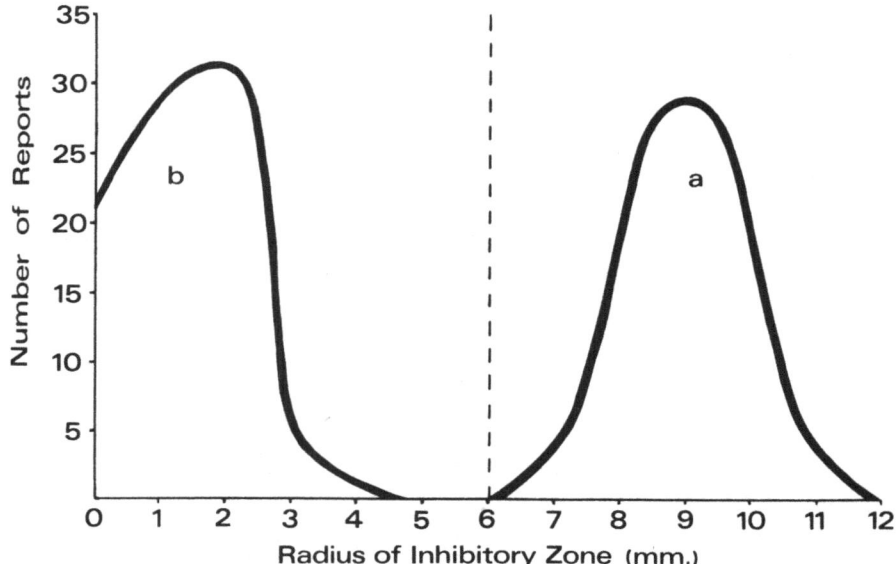

FIGURE 3: Typical examples of the distribution of measurements made
by participants in the microbiology surveys using the CDS method to
test (a) sensitive strains and (b) resistant strains.

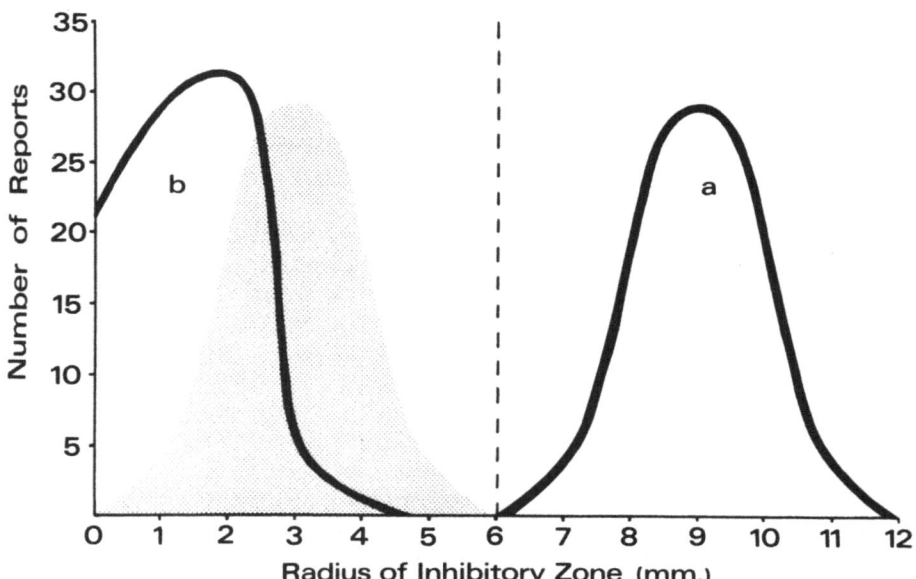

FIGURE 4: Expected distribution of measurements of a strain of
"intermediate sensitivity" superimposed on the observed distribution
of measurements shown in Figure 3. The marked overlap between measurements of resistant and intermediate zones is demonstrated.

DISCUSSION

The results of these studies demonstrated that at least with the two specied examined the common and serious errors of sensitivity testing in practice were eliminated almost entirely by the adoption of a calibrated method of sensitivity testing which divides sensitivity into only two categories. It is now generally accepted that disc tests should retlate to MIC values determined by quantitative means and the need for disc methods to be so calibrated was confirmed in the study with all antibiotics. In particular, the results with ceph-alothin demonstrated that although a method may be uniform, if it cannot be calibrated to quantitative sensitivities, it will yield inaccurate results.

The attitude of a restriction of reports of sensitivity testing to the two grades only of sensitive and resistant superficially appears to be against the current trend in antibiotic sensitivity testing. It is emphasized however, that this refers to the applica-tion of the disc test under conditions which prevail in laboratory practice in Australia and New Zealand. It is not suggested that a calibrated disc diffusion technique cannot successfully grade sensitivities into several categories in the hands of a skilled operator; however when a disc diffusion test is applied in practice the number of grades of sensitivity which can be accurately reported by a group of laboratories is determined by the precision with which the laboratories can reproduce the measurements of the zone sizes stipulated for each category.

In Figure 4 a hypothetical example of the distribution of zone sizes which would be recorded with an organism of intermediate sensitivity by the laboratories studied has been superimposed on the distribution of measurements observed in the microbiology surveys. The measurements of zones of inhibition in the intermediate category could be expected to be subject to a similar variation to that observed in the other two categories. In the example shown in Figure 4 there is considerable overlap between resistant and intermediate zones but the degree of overlap will depend on the separation point determined for intermediate strains. Nevertheless it is obvious that wherever this point is significant overlap into one or the other of the categories of sensitivity.

The obvious advantage in practice of restricting the division of sensitivity into only two grades is that it considerably simpli-flies the test and the common and serious error of reporting resistant strains as having intermediate sensitivity is eliminated entirely, which was demonstrated in the survey of antibiotic tests of staphylo-cocci. The validity of this attitude in practice is further supported by the rarity of strains of common pathogens which fall into the cate-gory of intermediate sensitivity. In the calibration of the CDS test to quantitative results, several hundred strains of different species were tested and less than 0.5% of strains were of intermediate sensitivity to any of the antibiotics examined. Similar observations were made by those who calibrated high potency disc tests in the past and Bauer (3), Petersdorf (9), Turck (10), and Kirby (8) have each drawn attention to the bimodal distribution of the antibiotic sensitivity of common pathogens. Thus the need to grade strains beyond sensitive or resistant seldom arises in practice and there is a considerable advantage in using a method of sensitivity testing which avoids the errors resulting from attempts to further define sensitivity.

The surveys also demonstrated the value of collaboration between clinical laboratories and laboratories interested in antibiotic sensitivity testing and these observations support the recommendations contained in the Report of the International Collaborative Study of Antibiotic Sensitivity Testing for the establishment of national or regional reference centres (7). Some aspects of the CDS test were refined as a direct result of the information derived from the surveys and a greater appreciation was obtained of the requirements demanded of a method of sensitivity testing which was to be applied by a large number of laboratories with vastly different skills and interests. Thus the microbiology surveys afforded a unique opportunity for a field appraisal of a method of sensitivity testing by the laboratories for whom the method was developed.

REFERENCES

1. Annear, D.I. (1968). The effect of temperature on resistance of Staphylococcus aureus to methicillin and some other antibiotics. Med. J. Australia, 1, 444.

2. Association of Clinical Pathologists (1965). Report on antibiotic sensitivity test trial organized by the Bacteriology Committee of the Association of Clinical Pathologists. J. clin. Path., 18, 1.

3. Bauer, A.W.? Perry, D.M. & Kirby, W.M.M. (1959). Single-disk antibiotic-sensitivity testing of staphylococci. Arch. Int. Med., 104, 208.

4. Bauer, A.W., Kirby, W.M.M., Sherris, J.C. & Turck, M. (1966). Antibiotic susceptibility testing by a standardized single disk method. Amer. J. Clin. Path., 45, 493.

5. College of Pathologists of Australia (1968). A survey of antibiotic sensitivity testing. Med. J. Australia, 2, 171.

6.   Ericsson, H., Tunevall, G. & Wickman, K. (1960). The paper disc method for determination of bacterial sensitivity to antibiotics. Scandinav. J. Clin & Lab. Investigation, 12, 414.

7.   Ericsson, H.M. & Sherris, J.C. (1971). Antibiotic sensitivity testing. Acta Pathol. et Microbiol. Scand., 217 (suppl).

8.   Kirby, W.M.M., Yoshihara, G.M., Sundsted, K.S. & Warren, J.H. (1957). Clinical usefulness of a single disc method for antibiotic sensitivity testing. Antibiotics Ann., 1956-1957, p. 892.

9.   Petersdorf, R.G. & Sherris, J.C. (1965). Methods and significance of in vitro testing of bacterial sensitivity to drugs. Amer. J. Med., 39, 766.

10. Truck, M., Lindemeyer, R.I. & Petersdorf, R.G. (1963). Comparison of single-disc and tube-dilution techniques in determining antibiotic sensitivities of gram-negative pathogens. Ann. Intern. Med., 58, 56.

PROBLEMS OF STANDARDIZATION OF MEDIA

H. NEUSSEL

University Institute of Medical
Microbiology, Gesamthochschule
Essen, Germany

Standardized media are needed for meaningful in vitro quantitative interpretation of susceptibility tests. However, in vitro
results with standardized methods and defined media can clinically
only be regarded as a guideline for dosis regimen if the in vitro
test approaches the conditions in vivo.

Unfortunately, during the first two decades of chemotherapy
laboratories were not widely involved in standardization. There
was a widespread opinion that it would be impossible to standardize
culture media containing natural ingredients. Growth of common
clinical pathogens is supported in commercial media by crude components.

Mueller Hinton medium, based on a simple formula, has been
shown during the last ten years to give satisfactory reproducibility with batches prepared by different manufacturers in the
United States. Nevertheless, with some antibiotics problems may
occur because this medium was not originally intended for the testing of bacterial susceptibility against chemotherapeutic agents.
In Europe, where Mueller Hinton medium is not generally accepted,
manufacturers were concerned to overcome the difficulties associated
with the Mueller Hinton formulation, using semi-defined nutrient
components. Antibiotic Sensitivity Medium from AB Biodisk and
Isotonic Sensitest Medium from Oxoid are examples of modern media,
developed specially for susceptibility testing.

Acid preparations of casein were proposed in 1941 by MUELLER
and HINTON for a medium determined for the primary isolation of the
gonococcus and the meningococcus. Casein hydrolysate is deficient
in cystine and tryptophane, but when supplemented, it can replace

33

meat peptones in media and is a very constant product, useful for standardized procedures. The high salt content of casein hydrolysate - about 35% of the dry powder consists of sodium chloride - must be taken into consideration if reproducibility of test results is demanded.

Special attention of the microbiologist is necessary with media which contain meat extracts. Mueller Hinton medium from different sources use different types of meat extracts which vary, according to the quality of meat, the length of time and the temperature during extraction. Liebig considered that 34 parts of trimmed meat should yield one part of extract. In modern commercial practice, meat extract may be a by-product of the manufacture of corned beef, which has a shorter period of immersion and uses approximately 50 parts of meat. The end product is not the same, but it exerts equivalent growth effects with the majority of organisms. Thiamin, which is an important vitamin for the growth of Staphylococcus aureus is lacking in meat extracts, being broken down during the manufacturing process.

Replacement of meat extract is possible by USP-specified-peptones from meat, available as Thiotone from BBL, Peptamin from Difco and Peptone P from Oxoid. These peptones, originally recommended to support the growth of streptococci, act as a good buffer system and prevent major changes of pH in media. If moisture ingress is not prevented, microbial growth can occur in peptones during storage. Such microbial contamination produces a high content of thymidine in the medium and markedly affects the in vitro results with cotrimoxazole. In animals thymidine is not present in sufficiently high concentrations to interfere with the activity of trimethoprim. According to BUSHBY, media used for susceptibility tests of trimethoprim should not contain more than 0.01 µg/ml of thymidine.

Yeast extract, prepared according to the specifications of the USP, is a suitable additive to test media based on casein hydrolysate. It is a peptone-like substance derived from cells of Saccharomyces after plasmolysis. Yeast extract is basically a mixture of amino-acids and peptides, water soluble vitamins and carbohydrates. It is important to realise that hop resins in brewing yeasts are inhibitory to the growth of bacteria. However, extracts prepared from bakers' yeast are free from such additives and are a useful component in semi-defined media.

Starch, criticized by GARROD and WATERWORTH as an unstable source of carbohydrates, can be replaced in media by a defined content of dextrose, unless it is needed to neutralize inhibitors similar to fatty acids which were shown in 1946 by LEY and MUELLER to be extractable from agar. Care must be taken that the supplementation of media with dextrose does not exceed a level, where primary good enhancement of growth is associated with a marked pH shift to the acid side.

Inorganic salts are essential for bacteria, and cations especially affect the growth of micro-organisms. If media with a low content of calcium and magnesium are used, Pseudomonas strains may appear more sensitive against aminoglycosides than they are in the presence of physiological concentrations of both electrolytes.

The quality of the agar is very important for a successful formulation of a medium for susceptibility tests. A satisfactory agar preparation must be free from the inhibitors mentioned above and mineral impurities must be minimized. If the formula of a test medium is changed to contain a more purified agar, the diminution of mineral content in the final composition of the medium must be carefully considered. As an example, Spanish agar contains, according to the analyses of BRIDSON and BRECKER, 0.16% of magnesium and normally 12 g per litre are used to solidify a medium. A concentration of 19.2 µg/ml of magnesium - as discussed later on, nearly the total amount of the physiological concentration - is thus added with the agar. If Oxoid agar No. 1 is taken for gelling of the medium, only 0.9 µg/ml of magnesium are added, and the broth should contain a minimum of 19.1 µg/ml of magnesium if a physiological concentration is to be achieved.

The in vitro activity of some chemotherapeutic agents is pH sensitive. JACKSON decreased the pH of the medium used for MIC-studies with gentamicin from 7.8 to 5.6 and demonstrated that MIC-values increased 8 to 32 fold for different species of Gram-negative bacteria. THORNSBERRY compared zones of inhibition of Staphylococcus aureus and E. coli over a range from 8.5 to 6.0. The most marked differences were demonstrated with tetracycline, lincomycin and erythromycin. Tetracycline zones were larger in the more acid medium, whereas the opposite result was seen for lincomycin and erythromycin. The final pH in solid media is not reached before gelling. If the pH value is adjusted in complex media at a high temperature, a later shift occurs. For commercial media the producer should provide a pH in the range of 7.2 to 7.4.

An important difficulty for standardization of media involves the Maillard reaction, where carbohydrates may complex with amino-acids, peptides and proteins to form melanoidins. This reaction causes essential amino-acids to be altered so that they are not available for bacterial metabolism. A standardized medium should always yield a relatively stable endproduct after autoclaving which gives statistically reproducible results when controlled with reference strains.

In a paper presented at the 8th International Congress of Chemotherapy in Athens, we demonstrated marked deviations of the

TABLE 1

ZONE DIAMETER (MM) OF GENTAMICIN WITH
P. AERUGINOSA (14 CLINICAL ISOLATES)

Medium	10 μg – Disc		
	Mean	SD	Range
MH-2	26.8	2.2	22.0 – 30.0
MH-R	21.9	2.7	18.0 – 28.0
ASM	19.0	2.6	14.5 – 26.0
MH-1	17.0	3.7	9.5 – 19.5
ISM	13.0	5.0	6.0 – 28.0

MIC values with ICS-reference strains of gentamicin, tetracycline
and cotrimoxazole, comparing Mueller Hinton medium and newly
developed Isotonic Sensitest medium. Antibiotic Sensitivity Medium
was not available at this time, and we did not compare different
Mueller Hinton media.

In Table 1, zones of 14 clinical isolates of P. aeruginosa are
compared with 10 μg-discs of gentamicin using five different media.

TABLE 2

INTERPRETATION OF MIC – RESULTS OF GENTAMICIN (μg/ml)
AGAINST 14 CLINICAL ISOLATES OF P. AERUGINOSA

Medium	Number of strains			
	Susceptible $\leqslant$ 1.0	Intermediate 2.0-4.0	8.0	Resistant $\geqslant$ 16.0
MH-2	13	1	0	0
MH-R	13	1	0	0
ASM	7	7	0	0
MH-1	1	12	0	1
ISM	1	2	8	3

TABLE 3

MIC-VALUES OF GENTAMICIN (μg/ml) WITH
P. AERUGINOSA REFERENCE STRAINS

Medium	ICS - Strain CIP 5838	Boston - Strain ATCC 27853
MH-2	0.5	0.5
MH-R	0.5	0.5
ASM	1.0	1.0
MH-1	4.0	4.0
ISM	4.0	8.0

We found in a recent study a high degree of variation in the mean values of the inhibition zones. Mueller Hinton agar from the Pasteur Institute (MH-2) showed a mean of 26.8 mm, whereas the mean was 21.9 mm with Mueller Hinton agar from BBL (MH-R) and 17.0 mm with Mueller Hinton agar from Difco (MH-1). The corresponding zones with Antibiotic Sensitivity Medium (ASM) were 19.0 mm, and with Isotonic Sensitest Medium (ISM) 13.0 mm.

In Table 2, when MIC-results were compared using an agar dilution test with an inoculum, which contained about 10^4 bacteria, 13 clinical isolates were sensitive with the Pasteur Institute Mueller Hinton agar (MH-2) and the BBL Mueller Hinton agar (MH-R), only one strain being in the intermediate category with both media. The 13 sensitive isolates were all inhibited by 1 μg/ml of gentamicin. Results with Antibiotic Sensitivity Medium and with Mueller Hinton medium from Difco (MH-1) indicated that the majority of the strains were in the intermediate range with MIC-values of 2 μg/ml and 4 μg/ml. With Isotonic Sensitest medium (ISM) the peak of MIC-values were at 8 μg/ml, three strains were resistant, two strains with MIC-values of 16 μg/ml and one strain with 32 μg/ml.

Table 3 shows that, as we expected, two reference strains of P. aeruginosa (CIP 5838 and ATCC 27838) showed parallel deviations in MIC-values, closely corresponding to the variations in results seen with the clinical isolates of P. aeruginosa.

RELLER, SCHOENKNECHT, KENNY and SHERRIS discussed the problem of physiological Ca^{++} and Mg^{++} content of media and proposed a uniform content of 20 - 35 μg/ml of magnesium and of 50 - 100 μg/ml of calcium for Mueller Hinton broth and for Mueller Hinton agar. The proposed concentrations give adequate tolerance limits for commercial media and correspond approximately to the concentrations of normal human plasma samples which contain according to MUNDAY and MAHY 20.3 μg/ml of magnesium and 104.4 μg/ml of calcium, 80.5% of Mg^{++} and 51.7% of Ca^{++} being unbound and present in the ultra-filtrate.

From the findings of HAMEISTER and WAHLIG with gentamicin, who compared the effect of varying concentrations of calcium and magnesium using E. coli and P. aeruginosa strains, it can be concluded that the effect of low calcium and magnesium concentrations, which causes larger zones of inhibition and decreased MIC-values with gentamicin, is species specific to Pseudomonas.

D'AMATO, THORNSBERRY, BAKER and KIRVEN tested a large number of pseudomonads and determined MIC-values for tetracycline, gentamicin, polymyxin B, and carbenicillin in Mueller Hinton broth supplemented with physiological concentrations of calcium and magnesium. Decrease of activity was seen with tetracycline, gentamicin and polymyxin B, causing major changes of interpretative susceptibility of most Pseudomonas species. P. maltophilia appeared sensitive against gentamicin with the unsupplemented Mueller Hinton medium, but was classified as resistant if the supplemented medium was used. With carbenicillin the majority of Pseudomonas species showed agreement of results, with only some minor deviations.

For the Boston reference strain D'AMATO reported the MIC-value of 8 μg/ml which corresponds to the MIC-value determined for this strain with Isotonic Sensitest Medium in our laboratory. The Boston strain of intermediate susceptibility seems to be a very useful indicator of the breakpoint for susceptibility of Pseudomonas aeruginosa to gentamicin independent of the test method used, including the STOKES' method.

Standardization raises the question whether Mueller Hinton medium should be replaced by the more newly developed media. WRETLIND, NORD and WADSTROM compared Mueller Hinton agar from Difco and Antibiotic Sensitivity Medium from AB Biodisk and concluded that Mueller Hinton agar was unsuitable for the testing of sulphonamides, whereas all other antibiotics with the agar dilution method showed agreement, mostly within two dilution steps. However, BACH, FINLAND, GOLD and WILCOX were able to demonstrate with a thymidine free Mueller Hinton agar from Difco that this modified medium was optimal for testing sulphamethoxazole singly or in combination.

We can summarise that there is no strong argument against the continued use of Mueller Hinton medium; minor modification of the formula would seem sufficient to provide reproducible biological results. To create a totally physiological medium is quite impossible with only semi-defined components. If we demand of the manufacturer standardization of product specifications which avoid possible manipulations due to differences in the composition of media, we are on the way towards reliable and rational test results.

REFERENCES

BACH, M.C., FINLAND, M. and GOLD, O. (1973) Susceptibility of recently isolated pathogenic bacteria to trimethoprim and sulpha-methoxazole, separately and combined. J. infect. Dis. 128, 508

BRIDSON, E.Y. and BRECKER, A. (1970) Design and formulation of microbial culture media. In Methods in Microbiology. Ed. Norris and Ribbons. Acad. Press, Vol. 3A, 229-295

BUSHBY, S.R.M. (1973) Sensitivity Testing with trimethoprim/ sulphamethoxazole Med. J. Aust. Special Suppl. 1, 10-18

D'AMATO, R.F.,THORNSBERRY, C., BAKER, C.N. and KIRVEN, L.A. (1975) Effect of calcium and magnesium ions on the susceptibility of pseudomonas species to tetracycline, gentamicin, polymyxin B, and carbenicillin. Antimicrob. Agents Chemother. 1, 596-600

GARROD, L.P. and WATERWORTH, P.M. (1971) A study of antibiotic sensitivity testing with proposals for simple uniform methods. J. clin. Path. 24, 779-789

HAMEISTER, V.W. and WAHLIG, H. (1971) Der Einfluss von Mg++ und Ca++ – Ionen auf die Wirksamkeit von Gentamycin gegen Pseudomonas aeruginosa im Agar diffusionstest. Arzneimittel-Forsch. 21, 1658 – 1660

JACKSON, G.G. (1967) Laboratory and clinical investigation of gentamicin. Gentamicin, First International Symposium, Paris, 72-73.

LEY, H.L. and MUELLER, J.H. (1946) On the isolation from agar of an inhibitor for Neisseria gonorrhoeae. J. Bact. 52, 453-460

MUELLER, J.H. and HINTON, J. (1941) A protein-free medium for primary isolation of the gonococcus and meningococcus. Proc. Soc. exptl. Biol. Med. 48, 330-333

MUNDAY, K.A. and MAHY, B.W.J. (1964) Determination of ultra-filtrable calcium and magnesium on small quantities of plasma. Clinica chim. Acta 10, 144-151

RELLER, L.B., SCHOENKNECHT, F.D., KENNY, M.A. and SHERRIS, J.C. (1974) Antibiotic susceptibility testing of pseudomonas aeruginosa: selection of a control strain and criteria for magnesium and calcium content in media. J. infect. Dis. 130, 454-463

STOKES, E.J. (1968) Clinical Pathology, 3rd ed., Arnold, London

THORNSBERRY, C. (1974) In Current techniques for antibiotic
susceptibility testing. Ed. A. Balows. Charles C. Thomas,
Springfield, Illinois

WRETLIND, B., NORD, C.E. and WADSTROEM, T. (1974) In vitro
sensitivity of isolates of Pseudomonas aeruginosa to carbenicillin,
gentamicin, tobramycin, and some other antibiotics. Scand. J.
infect. Dis. 6, 49-52

EFFECTS OF MEDIUM ON THE RESULTS OF
ANTIMICROBIAL SENSITIVITY TESTING

J. Bou Casals

Department of Bacteriology, A/S Rosco

Taastrup, Denmark

During the last decade several papers have been published about the influence of different components of the
medium on the results of sensitivity testing of single antimicrobials, or single bacterial strains. The problem of
the composition of the medium has not been treated as a
whole, but rather as isolated items. Let us start with the
agar. Agar is not a well-defined substance. It is very
rarely composed exclusively of a neutral polysaccharide:
agarose. In most cases it contains bound sulphate groups
OSO_3^- which are able to bind particularly divalent cations
such as Ca^{++} and Mg^{++}. The content of cations and sulphate
groups of the different agars varies from manufacturer to
manufacturer and probably between the different lots of
the same product (Barry and Effinger 1974).

Concerning the binding of antimicrobials to agar there
are several studies that show that particularly the aminoglycosides (gentamicin and neomycin most, followed by kanamycin and less streptomycin) are strongly bound to agar and
the same applies for the polymyxins (Hanus et al. 1967).
The binding of aminoglycosides and polymyxins to agar can
be reduced by adding to the medium 0.1 M of different salts
like sodium chloride, sodium acetate, sodium phosphate,
etc.; i.e. a concentration of sodium chloride corresponding to about 0.6% (El Nakeeb and Yousef 1970).

In 1969 Garrod and Waterworth showed that content of
Mg^{++} in agar was of importance in the sensitivity testing
of Pseudomonas strains with gentamicin. The MIC of gentamicin against Pseudomonas was higher, the higher the con-

tent of Mg^{++} in the agar used. When determining the MIC
values in serum and urine, the authors found higher MIC
values than when using media with a very low magnesium
content, and they concluded that the medium for sensitivity testing should contain some amount of magnesium in order to have conditions comparable to those in vivo. We are
of the opinion that the amount of magnesium in the medium
must be comparable to that in serum.

When, during the process of sensitivity testing, we
apply a tablet or paper disc containing gentamicin on the
surface of an agar medium, some interactions take place.
Gentamicin is bound to the sulphate groups of the agar, but
the salts included in the medium (mainly monovalent ions,
which give it a certain ionic strength), break down some of
the bindings between gentamicin and agar. Mg^{++} and to a
lesser extent Ca^{++} (coming from the agar, but also from
other ingredients of the medium, such as beef and yeast
extracts) act competitively with gentamicin for the vital
sites of action in the bacterial cells of Pseudomonas.
Mg^{++} and Ca^{++} have not that effect on enterobacteria. In
other words: when increasing to a certain extent the ionic
strength of the medium by the addition of salts, the inhibition zones of gentamicin with Pseudomonas will become
larger because some of the bonds between gentamicin and a-
gar are broken down and more free gentamicin is available
for diffusion.

The same phenomenon is seen with enterobacteria, but
if the addition of salt to the medium is too large, it
will act competitively with gentamicin for the vital sites
of action in the bacterial cells of enterobacteria and we
will see a reduction in zone size. With antibiotics that
are less bound to agar like kanamycin and streptomycin the
antagonistic effect of sodium chloride (or other salts)
may compensate for the reversal of binding to agar and the
result might be a slight reduction in the size of inhibition zone or no change at all when the ionic strength of
the medium is moderately increased.

The polymyxins act similarly to gentamicin and are
very strongly bound to agar. An increase in ionic strength
will therefore bring about larger inhibition zones, both
with Pseudomonas and enterobacteria.

Concerning the tetracyclines and the relationship between the medium content of divalent cations and complexing substances like phosphate, citrate, etc. several studies have been published (Brenner and Sherris 1972). Also
in this case, we mean that the amount of magnesium and

calcium in the medium must be comparable to that in serum. Some amount of buffer (such as phosphate) is also desirable in order to avoid changes of the pH value during the autoclavation process.

It is well-known that a large content of dextrose in the medium will result in misleading large inhibition zones of nitrofurantoin discs with Proteus mirabilis strains, mainly because the fermentation of dextrose brings about a reduction in the pH value of the medium increasing the activity of nitrofurantoin (Stokes 1965). Most media have now a dextrose content between 0.1 and 0.3%, which must be considered acceptable.

It is also known that the presence of p-amino benzoic acid (p-ABA) and thymidine results in a reduction or total elimination of the inhibition zones around sulfa and trimethoprim discs (Waterworth 1969). p-ABA influences only the sulfa-zone while thymidine influences both the sulfa and trimethoprim inhibition zones. If the content of these antagonists in the medium is not too large they can be neutralized by the addition of horse blood to the medium.

EXPERIMENTAL RESULTS.

We have been working with a rather simple agar medium containing only 1% agar, 0.12% yeast, 0.25% casein hydrolysate, glucose 0.35%, potassium chloride, sodium phosphate, and 5% defibrinated horse blood. The medium contains only small amounts of these not well-defined materials such as yeast extracts, casein hydrolysates, beef extracts, which are common in most media and to a great extent contribute to making the media non-reproducible from lot to lot because of variations in ionic strength, content of divalent cations, content of antagonists, etc.. In order to see, how small changes in the medium may result in variations in the inhibition zones of particular antibiotics with particular strains, we made the following studies:

1) Substitution of Agar (Japanese) with Oxoid Agar No. 1 or with Agarose. Oxoid agar No. 1 contained about $\frac{1}{2}$ of the sulphate groups and about 1/8 of Ca^{++} and Mg^{++} of the Japanese agar.

All aminoglycoside antibiotics and the polymyxins showed an increase of the inhibition zone of 1-3 mm with gram-negative bacilli. The same effect could be achieved by increasing the ionic strength of the medium containing Japanese agar by adding extra 0.2% sodium chloride. The

phenomenon can be explained by a lower binding of aminoglycosides to the agar both when a) an agar with lower
content of sulphate groups such as Oxoid No. 1 is used and
b) when the ionic strength of the medium is increased by
means of which some of the bonds are broken down.

When we used agarose (a neutral polysaccharide practically free from sulphate groups and divalent ions) instead of the Japanese agar (table I) there was still larger increase of the inhibition zones of Pseudomonas and of
Staphylococcus aureus with gentamicin, but not of Streptococcus faecalis. The use of agarose permitted a better separation of strains sensitive to gentamicin (Pseudomonas
and Staphylococcus aureus) from the resistant strains,
such as Strept. faecalis. The same phenomenon was seen
with other aminoglycosides and polymyxins, but the variation in size of the inhibition zones was more moderate.

2) Reduction of Sodium Phosphate Content from 0.8%
to 0.4%. There was a reduction in the zone size of tetracycline of about 2 mm with Pseudomonas strains and enterobacteria. When increasing the ionic strength by the addition of extra 0.2% NaCl, we observed again an increase in
the zones of inhibition of gram-negative rods with gentamicin and polymyxins. With kanamycin and streptomycin we
saw unchanged or reduced zones of inhibition with increasing ionic strength.

The medium had a magnesium content of 1.6 mg% from
which there was 0.6 mg% coming from the agar and 1.0 mg%

TABLE I.   Inhibition zones of Gentamicin Neo-Sensitabs
(tablet) on media solidified with two different agars

Strain	Agar type	Inhibition zones in mm
Pseud. aeruginosa 1974/68	Japanese	28.0
	Agarose	36.8
Pseud. aeruginosa 1266/68	Japanese	30.0
	Agarose	37.0
Streptococcus faecalis	Japanese	28.0
	Agarose	26.8
Spaphyloc. aureus 209P	Japanese	34.0
	Agarose	39.0

from the other components of the medium, mainly casein
hydrolysate and yeast extract. The addition of extra 1.0
mg% magnesium (making a total of 2.6 mg%) as magnesium
chloride together with the mentioned reduction in phosphate and addition of extra 0.2% NaCl resulted (compared
with the original medium) in a larger pigment production
with Pseudomonas strains, as expected. Besides, there was
no reduction in the zone size of gentamicin with Pseudomonas. On the contrary, because of the increase in ionic
strength, there was an increase in zone size both with
Pseudomonas and enterobacteria, but not with Streptococcus
faecalis.

Polymyxins showed also larger inhibition zones with
gram-negative rods.

3) Addition of Thymidine corresponding to 0.2 mcg/ml.
The medium used contains a low amount of antagonists which
are neutralized by the addition of 5% defibrinated horse
blood.

The meaning with this test was to show the variation
of the inhibition zones around sulfa and trimethoprim
discs/tablets in 4 media containing increasing amounts of

TABLE II.   Inhibition zones of Trimethoprim and Sulfa
(discs and tablets) against Klebsiella pneumoniae on media containing increasing amounts of antagonists   a)

Media	Trime-thoprim disc 1.25 mcg	Trime-thoprim tablet 25 mcg	Sulphame-thoxazole disc 23.75 mcg	Sulpha-methizole tablet 4 mg
Blood agar (BA)	17	25	23	33
BA (+ 0.2 mcg/ml thymidine)	17	25	23	33
A (- blood)	6	(20)	(13)	32
A (- blood + 0.2 mcg/ml thymidine)	6	9	6	31

a) Diametres were measured in millimetres. Discs measured
6 mm and tablets 9 mm; therefore a zone reading of 6 mm
(discs) or 9 mm (tablets) indicates absence of zone of inhibition. Figures in brackets indicate some growth within
the zone of inhibition.

thymidine. The 4 media are: blood agar with the composition mentioned above, BA added of 0.2 mcg/ml thymidine, the same medium without the addition of blood, and the medium without blood but with extra 0.2 mcg/ml thymidine (table II).

Because of the larger content of antimicrobials in the tablets, the inhibition zones around them are less influenced by sulfa and trimethoprim antagonists than is the case with paper discs.

References

Barry, A.L. and L.J. Effinger, 1974. Am.J.Clin.Path., 62: 113-117.

Brenner, V.C. and J.C. Sherris, 1972. Antimicrob. Agents Chemother. 1: 116-122.

El Nakeeb, M.A. and R.T. Yousef, 1970. Arzneim. Forsch. (Drug Res.), 20: 103-107.

Garrod, L.P. and P.M. Waterworth, 1969. J.Clin.Path., 22: 534-538.

Hanus, F.J., J.G. Sands, and E.O Bennett, 1967. Appl. Microb., 15: 31-34.

Stokes, E.J., 1965. J.Clin.Path., 18: 1-5.

Waterworth, P.M., 1969. Postgrad.Med.J., 45: Suppl. 21-29.

INFLUENCE OF FOUR COMMERCIAL SENSITIVITY MEDIA

ON IN VITRO ACTIVITY OF SEVERAL ANTIBIOTICS

G.Th.J. Fabius and R.P. Mouton

Division of Clinical Bacteriology, Department of

Medicine, University Hospital, Utrecht

SUMMARY

MIC's and inhibition zones of six antibiotics were determined
simultaneously on four commercially available sensitivity test media, by means of standardized procedures. Multiple strains of
several bacterial genera were used. Two media proved to be unsuitable for tetracycline and aminoglycoside testing respectively; on
one of them, most E. coli strains would be interpreted as being
resistant to tetracycline; on the other, most gramnegative rods
were marginally sensitive or resistant to the aminoglycosides.These
data and other details on differences between the media investigated are discussed in the light of the requirements with regard to
performance.

INTRODUCTION

If disc sensitivity tests are to be interpreted correctly we should
be informed on the relationship between inhibition zone diameters
and MIC values obtained on the same medium. The position of a
regressionline reflecting this relationship is determined by the
antibiotic, the medium and the bacterial species. Details of this
method have been described by Ericsson and Sherris (1971). For
agardiffusion and agardilution methods alike, the composition of
the medium is perhaps the most important factor. This applies
primarily to agardilution tests since the interpretation of diffusion tests (with the aid of regressionlines) depends on correct
MIC determinations. Theoretically a sensitivity test medium should
yield MIC values approximating those to be expected in vivo. A
practical approach to this ideal cannot be realized. Yet it was

47

thought worthwhile to register and evaluate differences between
some sensitivity test media. We confined ourselves mainly to the
aminoglycosides and tetracycline since the activity of these
antibiotics is affected most by the composition of the medium.
Except for DST medium, which is used for routine purposes in our
laboratory, the choice of sensitivity test media was determined
by their availability and their suitability for testing of cotrimoxazole. Müller-Hinton media were not included because of their
varying composition.

MATERIAL AND METHODS

Agardilutiontest Twofold dilutions of each of six antibiotics
(kanamycin, gentamicin, tobramycin, sisomycin, tetracycline and
ampicillin) were simultaneously prepared in four brands of sensitivity agar (DST, Sensitest, Isotonic Sensitest agar- Oxoid;
ASMPDM- BIO). All the media were used within 30 h, ampicillin media
within 6 h. In order to obtain a wide range of MIC values of the
antibiotics to be tested, a selection of bacterial strains was
made. They were grouped according to genus or species (E. coli,
Klebsiella, Pseudomonas aeruginosa, Staphylococcus areus and
Enterococcus). The number of strains per group varied from 18 to 40.
Inocula were prepared by diluting 20 h broth cultures (Brain Heart
Infusion, Oxoid) to 10^6 cfu/ml with the aid of an extinctiometer.
Inoculation was performed according to the principle of Steers et
al. (1959), and yielded approximately 10^3 organisms per spot.
The plates were read after 20 h incubation at 37 C.
Agardiffusion method Bacterial strains, inocula and brands
of agar were the same as for the agardilution method. Media of
4 mm depth were dried for 1 h at 37 C before use. Inoculation was
done by swabbing. 6 mm sensitivity discs were obtained from BIO
(Stockholm) except for tobramycin and sisomycin discs, which were
laboratory made. All the discs contained 30 μg of antibiotic except
for ampicillin discs which contained 10 μg. After incubation the
discs were placed on the agar symmetrically. After 20 h incubation
at 37 C, inhibition zone diameters were read by means of calipers.
Reproducibility tests A check was made on possible discrepancies resulting from inaccurate techniques, particularly disc-
loading. To this end replicate agardiffusion and agardilution tests
with 4-5 strains per genus were performed in threefold or fourfold
on separate occasions.
Determination of Ca^{++} and Mg^{++} concentration After destroying
the dry media by means of the perchloric acid method (Whitby and
Lang, 1969) Ca^{++} and Mg^{++} concentrations were determined according
to the principle of atomic absorption.

RESULTS

The results of the different bacterial genera were grouped separately, regardless of the method used. We cannot go into detail with

regard to the necessity of separate regressionlines for different
genera. Suffice it here to say that regressionlines of different
genera rarely proved to be identical. Fig. 1 illustrates this
for gentamicin sensitivity tests on the Sensitest medium.
The results of the agardilution tests have to be limited here to a
few of the numerous results obtained. Fig. 2 shows high MIC values
of tetracycline versus E. coli on Isotonic medium. The majority of
MIC's on ASM is also higher than the critical concentrations for
tetracycline. Fig. 3 is typical of the problems which are encountered with Isotonic medium: high MIC's of gentamicin versus
Pseudomonas aeruginosa, most of them not compatible with sensitivity. Fig. 4 gives an example of high MIC's of kanamycin on ASM. Most
strains have MIC values of 8 g/ml or more.
Table 1 sums up all the comparative tests.
Another approach was to establish whether one medium, more than the
other media, showed a wider variation of inhibition zone diameters

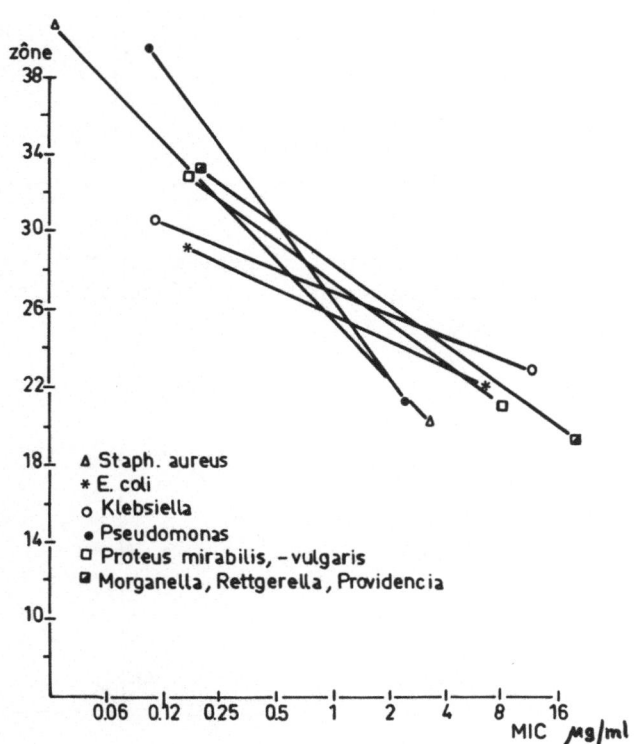

Fig. 1. Regressionlines of gentamicin on Sensitest medium for 6
        bacterial species or species groups (16-26 strains/species
        or group).

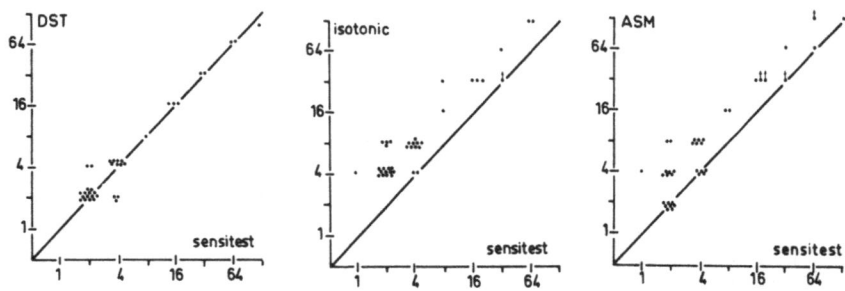

Fig. 2 Comparison of MIC's (µg/ml) of tetracycline for E. coli, as
        determined on four different media.

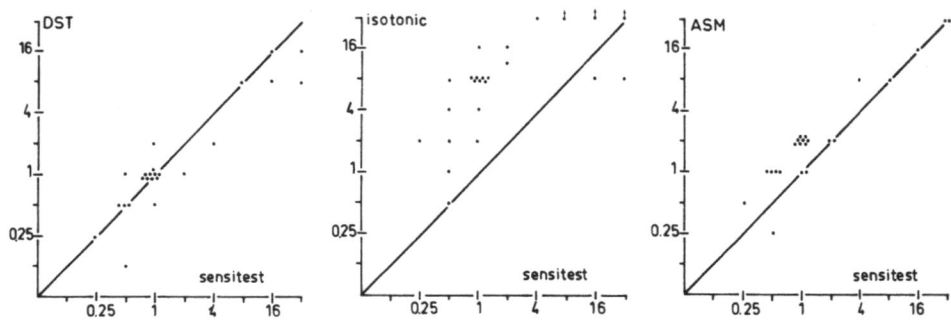

Fig. 3 Comparison of MIC's (µg/ml) of gentamicin for Pseudomonas
        aeruginosa as determined on four different media.

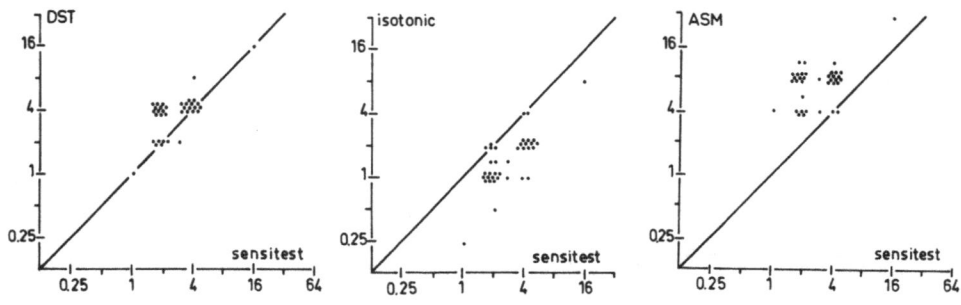

Fig. 4 Comparison of MIC's (µg/ml) of kanamycin for E. coli, as
        determined on four different media.

Table I   Effect of medium   on MIC, in comparison with Sensitest
          medium

Antibiotic	Species	DST	Isotonic	ASM
Ampicillin	E. coli	0	0	0
	Enterococ	0	0	-
	Proteus mir.	0	0	-
Tetracycline	Staph. aur.	0	(+)	0
	Enterococ	0	+	0
	E. coli	0	+	+
	Klebsiella	0	+	0
	Morganella	0	+	0
	Pseudomonas	0	+	+
Kanamycin	Staph. aur.	-	-	0
	E. coli	0	-	+
	Klebsiella	0	-	+
	Proteus mir.	+	0	+
	Morganella	0	0	+
Gentamicin	Staph. aur.	0	0	+
	E. coli	0	-	+
	Klebsiella	0	0	+
	Proteus mir.	+	0	+
	Morganella	0	0	+
	Pseudomonas	0	++	+
Tobramycin	Staph. aur.	(-)	0	+
	E. coli	0	-	++
	Klebsiella	0	(-)	++
	Proteus mir.	(+)	0	++
	Morganella	0	0	++
	Pseudomonas	(-)	+	++
Sisomicin	Staph. aur.	(-)	-	++
	E. coli	(+)	0	++
	Klebsiella	0	0	++
	Proteus mir.	+	0	++
	Morganella	0	0	++
	Pseudomonas	(-)	+	++

0   MIC equal on Sensitest, + higher MIC (2x), ++ higher MIC (4x),
-   lower MIC (2x), (+) about 50% of strains higher MIC (2x),
(-) about 50% of strains lower MIC (2x)

in repeated tests with the same strain and in strains with the same
MIC. Our data do not allow final conclusions on this point, but
some differences between media were noted in sensitivity testing
for tetracycline. Statistical analysis showed that the variance
of the diffusion test results of tetracycline on DST and Sensitest was generally lower than on Isotonic medium and on ASM.
However, the differences were not statistically significant. From
fig. 5 (tetracycline/E. coli) it is evident that the means of the
inhibition zone diameters as related to a given MIC do not allow
the drawing of a regressionline for the ASM medium.
In view of the relevance of Mg^{++} and Ca^{++} content of media for
testing tetracycline and gentamicin susceptibility, the concentrations of these bivalent kations were determined in the four media.
Table 2 lists the results of this analysis.

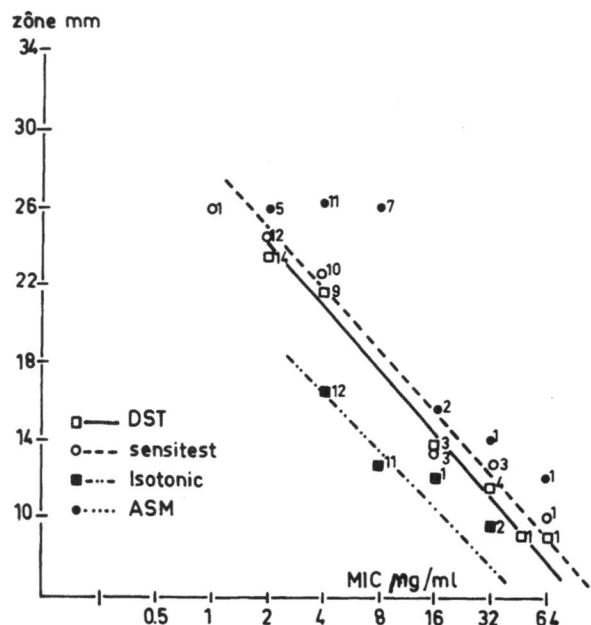

Fig. 5. Means of inhibition zone diameters as related to given
        MIC's of tetracycline for E. coli, determined on four
        different media. Except for ASM, the regressionlines are
        drawn. The numbers indicate the numbers of strains with
        the same MIC.

DISCUSSION

A proper evaluation of sensitivity test media is complicated by the
lack of accepted criteria. The introduction of the Isotonic Sensitest Medium by Oxoid was a novelty since an attempt was made to

imitate the physiological situation with this medium (Neussel and Linzemeier, 1973). Unfortunately the results cast some doubt upon

Table 2. Ca^{++} and Mg^{++} concentrations of four prepared media and of normal human plasma

Medium	Ca^{++}		Mg^{++}	
	mmol/l	ppm	mmol/l	ppm
ASM	0.79	32	0.96	23
DST	0.08	3.2	1.2	29
Isotonic	2.32	93	2.06	50
Sensitest	0.16	6.4	1.28	31
Human plasma	2.3	98	0.89	21.7

the validity of this approach. Particularly, the high MIC's of gentamicin for Pseudomonas are improbable (fig. 3). Several authors (Garrod and Waterworth, 1969; Reller et al., 1974) have pointed out that Ca^{++} and Mg^{++} content of the medium may affect these MIC's. Reller et al.(1974) concluded that there is an optimum concentration of calcium ions of 50-100 ppm and of magnesium ions of 20-35 ppm. The high MIC values of tetracycline, and of gentamicin to Pseudomonas, on Isotonic medium (fig. 3), are compatible with a high Mg^{++} and/or Ca^{++} content of this medium. We found the Mg^{++} content of this medium to be 50 ppm, which is higher than the concentration in human plasma. Also the Ca^{++} content was the highest of all the media, although at a physiological level. The bivalent kation content of the ASM medium does not explain the comparatively high MIC values found with most genera, for all the aminoglycosides. The cause of these high values is not clear. Except for higher MIC values of the aminoglycosides and Proteus mirabilis strains, no essential differences were found between DST and Sensitest agar.
Attractive as the use of more or less physiological media may be, the results of sensitivity tests should be primarily compatible with in vivo results. If this correlation is difficult to prove, a comparison with widely accepted critical concentrations indicating limits of sensitivity, may allow some conclusions. The MIC values of tetracycline versus E. coli and of gentamicin versus Pseudomonas aeruginosa on Isotonic Medium, are predominantly higher than the critical concentration. In other words most strains seem to be resistant, which means that this medium will often yield misleading results. Likewise, aminoglycoside sensitivity as determined on ASM medium becomes too rare an event to be compatible with clinical experience. We realize that the problem of finding the best medium for sensitivity testing has not been solved by this investigation. Reviewing our results, it is tempting to conclude that Sensitest Medium is the most reliable, also being suitable for cotrimoxazole

testing. However, there is no proof that the MIC values obtained on
Sensitest Medium reflect those in vivo. The lack of standardization
of bivalent kation content of this medium is another argument
to be careful with our conclusions. We may only hope that the media
producers will not rest and will continue to improve the available
products.

ACKNOWLEDGEMENTS

We are grateful to Dr. J.A. Faber for the statistical evaluation
of the results, to Dr. J. de Wael for the analysis of Ca- and Mg-
ion concentrations of the media, and to Oxoid Ltd. for the generous
supply of Isotonic Sensitest Medium and for the information on their
products.

REFERENCES

Ericsson, H.M. and Sherris, J.C. (1971) Acta Pathol. Microbiol.
      Scand. (B) 215 Suppl.
Garrod, L.P. and Waterworth, P.M. (1969) J. Clin. Pathol. 22, 534.
Neussel, H. and Linzemeier, G. (1973) 8 th Intern. Congr. Chemother.
      Athens (A-11).
Reller, L.B., Schoenknecht, F.D., Kenny, M.A. and Sherris, J.C. (1974)
      J. Infect. Dis. 130, 454.
Steers, E., Foltz, E.L., Graves, B.S. and Rider, J. (1959) Antibiot.
      Chemother. 9, 307.
Whitby, L.G. and Lang, D. (1960) J. Clin. Invest. 39, 854.

A SPOT PLATE METHOD FOR ANTIBIOTIC-BACTERIAL KILLING RATES

S. H. Zinner, R. B. Provonchee and K. S. Elias

Roger Williams General Hospital and Brown University

Providence, Rhode Island, U.S.A.

The large amount of material and the multiple pipettings involved in the standard pour-plate method used to derive antibiotic induced bacterial killing curves prompted studies of a method utilizing a spot plate technique. This method produces similar _in vitro_ results and allows for rapid sampling, ease of colony counting, a considerably shortened incubation period and the ability to test several bacterial strains concurrently.

MATERIALS AND METHODS

Pour Plate Method

Ten strains of _Escherichia coli_, incubated in a shaking water bath at 37°C and standardized by optical density measurements, were diluted to final concentrations of 3 to 6 x 10^4 organisms/ml. Amikacin at a final concentration of 0.75 µg/ml in one set of experiments and 1.5 µg/ml in a second series was added to the reaction tubes.

At each sampling time appropriate dilutions were made and duplicate 1 ml samples were mixed in petri dishes with 9 ml of trypticase soy agar at 50°C. Colonies were counted after overnight incubation at 37°C.

Spot Plate Method

A 0.2 ml sample of the antibiotic-bacterial mixture from the pour plate reaction tubes was placed in the wells of a sterile microtiter plate, fitted with a 5 mm magnetic stirring bar.

55

To sample from each well, a plunger was constructed to hold a
5 µl micropipet. The plunger allows for the complete delivery of
the sample onto antibiotic free nutrient agar plate with minimal
splattering. A separate micropipet was used for each sample.
Samples were made at 0, 30, 60, 90, 120 and 150 minutes of incubation of the bacterial-antibiotic mixture. The wells were mixed
vigorously on a magnetic stirrer before sampling. A single petri
dish can accommodate up to 21 spot samples.

The inoculated agar plates are allowed to dry and each spot
is overlaid with an additional drop of cooled sterile agar to prevent spreading of the surface colonies. These plates are incubated at 37°C for 4 or 5 hours until the microcolonies are ready for
counting.

A microfiche viewer was modified so that the film holding
tray was replaced with a plastic tray that accommodates a round
petri dish. Each spot is placed under the magnifying lens and a
25x magnification is projected onto the ground-glass screen where
the microcolonies can be distinguished easily. A felt marking pen
is connected to an electronic counter which automatically tabulates
the number of colonies marked on the screen. The spots can be
counted by more than one observer, and the plates remain countable
for several days if stored at 4°C.

Statistical Studies

A block design was used to compare the variability between
the spot plate method and the pour plate method with respect to
bacterial enumeration. Four dilutions were prepared from an overnight growth of one strain of E. coli, and four readings were made
by each method.

Secondly, to compare the acceptable counting ranges for the
two methods, 17 or 18 replicate samplings were made from a range
of dilutions of a log phase culture of a single strain of E. coli.

Finally, killing curves using duplicate pour plates and triplicate spot plates were derived for 10 strains of E. coli with two
concentrations of Amikacin (0.75 µg/ml and 1.5 µg/ml). A paired
T test was used to compare the results obtained with the two
methods.

RESULTS

As seen in Table 1, analysis of variance fails to reveal any
significant difference either in the variation due to replications
within each method or in the variation between the spot plate and
pour plate methods. In addition, and not seen in the table, there

was no significant difference in results obtained independently by two observers.

In Table 2 the mean counts obtained from 17 or 18 replicate samplings over a range of low to high bacterial counts are compared for each method. Although the spot plate in this series tends to produce slightly lower counts, the coefficients of variation are similar for both methods. Up to 300 counts per spot can be counted easily with the spot plate method.

The results of timed bacterial killing studies are plotted in Figure 1 for both methods at the two antibiotic concentrations. Similar curves are produced with both methods, and there is no significant difference between the mean percent survival at any sampling time.

DISCUSSION

The spot plate method described herein provides a rapid technique for bacterial enumeration with several advantages over the standard pour plate procedure. Firstly, the results are available

TABLE 1

ONE WAY ANALYSIS OF VARIANCE TABLE COMPARING REPLICATION ERROR INHERENT IN THE TWO METHODS

Spot Plate	Degrees of Freedom	Sum of Squares	Mean Square	F
Between Replications	3	41.25	13.75	0.310 NS
Within Replications	12	532.50	44.38	
	15	573.75		
Pour Plate				
Between Replications	3	69.19	23.06	0.535 NS
Within Replications	12	517.75	43.15	
	15	586.94		

Comparison of Within Mean Square from the Two Methods Yields:

$$\frac{44.38}{43.15} = 1.029 \quad F_{12,12}{}^{NS}$$

TABLE 2

MEAN COUNTS OVER A RANGE OF BACTERIAL CONCENTRATIONS
WITH BOTH METHODS

Spot Plate	n	Mean Counts	Standard Deviation	Coefficient of Variation
1	18	46.55	8.79	18.88
2	18	86.55	10.96	12.66
3	18	171.05	17.39	10.16
4	18	293.61	25.80	8.78
Pour Plate				
1	17	51.11	7.45	14.59
2	17	103.47	9.96	9.62
3	17	196.94	19.16	9.73
4	17	389.24	34.72	8.92

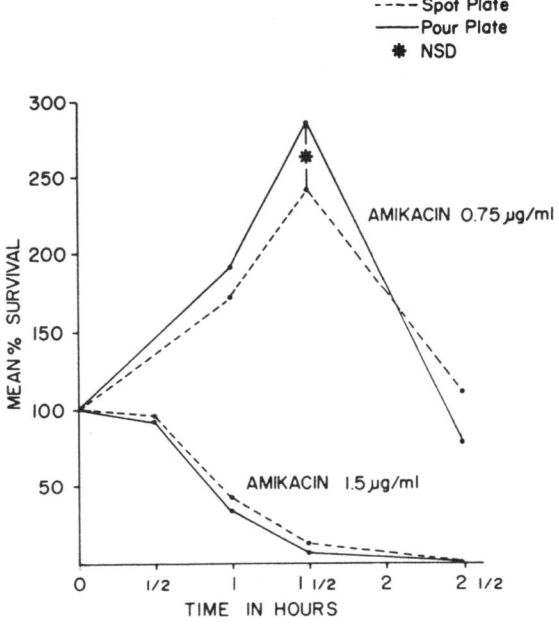

Figure 1.   Effect of AMIKACIN on Ten Strains of Escherichia coli.

for counting within 4-5 hours (for all Gram-negative bacilli tested as well as Staphylococcus aureus). Secondly, up to 21 organisms can be studied on a single agar plate resulting in considerable reduction in the number of petri dishes and in the amount of material needed. Thirdly, the microcolonies remain countable for several days and can be counted by several observers.

The data presented suggest that the variability of counts from dilutions of bacterial suspensions does not differ for the spot plate and standard methods. The generally accepted range of 30 to 300 colonies per plate for reasonable counting accuracy applies well to this method. A minimal concentration of 1×10^4 organisms per ml is necessary to use the 5 µl sample in the spot plate method. More dilute bacterial suspensions can be counted accurately by utilizing a 10 µl sample or greater.

In summary, the spot plate procedure is a useful alternative to the standard pour plate for deriving bacterial killing curves.

Usefulness of Commercially Available Media

to MIC-Determinations of Trimethoprim

B.van Klingeren and A.Rutgers

National Institute of Public Health

Postbox 1, Bilthoven, The Netherlands

Since trimethoprim and cotrimoxazole came into use several authors have pointed out the presence of antagonists to TMP in most commercially prepared media. In 1971 Koch and Burchall showed that thymidine was the most important TMP-antagonist in those media. Amyes and Smith (1974) recently compared several media, among others Oxoid Diagnostic Sensitivity Test Agar and Wellcotest Agar; they observed that DST supported the growth of thymineless mutants; the suggestion that this medium contained thymine and/or thymidine was confirmed by sensitivity-testing indicating that DST was unsatisfactory for TMP-sensitivity-testing; they also showed that Wellcotest Agar contains a uridinelike compound and that this prevents the utilisation of thymine (not of thymidine) by thymineless mutants.

When the results of Amyes and Smith were published we were comparing five commercially available media that are supposed to be free or practically free of TMP-antagonists for their suitability for MIC-determinations of TMP. These media were Diagnostic Sensitivity Test Agar (Oxoid), Sensitest Agar (Oxoid), Wellcotest Agar (Wellcome) and Antibiotic Sensitivity Medium (A.B.Biodisk). As antagonist-free control medium we used a minimal medium supplemented with 0.2 % glucose and 0.1 % casamino-acids.

Two-fold dilutions of TMP and cotrimoxazole - ratio TMP : SMX = 1 : 20 - were prepared in these media and poured in petridishes. Suspensions in saline (ca 10^5 c.f.u./ml) of recently isolated strains of E.coli, Salm.typhimurium, Staph.aureus and Streptococcus faecalis were inoculated on the dosed media by means of a Steers replicator. After overnight incubation at 37 $^\circ$C minimal inhibitory concentrations were read.

I should like to show the results of the MIC-determinations with TMP in the different media in the next slides. The first

Figure 1   Inhibition by trimethoprim and cotrimoxazole

Organism	Medium	Trimethoprim in µg/ml								Cotrimoxazole in µg/ml*)							
		0.03	0.06	0.12	0.25	0.5	1	2	4	0.015	0.03	0.06	0.12	0.25	0.5	1	2
E.coli 20 strains	MM	●	●	O	O	-				●	O	-					
	ASM	●	●	O	O	-				●	●	O	-				
	Wellcotest	●	●	O	O	-				●	●	O	-				
	Isot.Sens.	●	●	●	O	O	-			●	●	●	O	O	-		
	Sensitest	●	●	●	O	O	O	O	-	●	●	O	O	O	-		
	DST	●	●	●	O	O	O	O	O	●	●	O	O	O	O	O	-
Salm. typhi- murium 21 strains	MM	●	O	O	-					O	-						
	ASM	●	●	O	-					●	O	-					
	Wellcotest	●	●	O	-					●	O	-					
	Isot.Sens.	●	●	O	O	-				●	O	O	-				
	Sensitest	●	O	O	-					●	O	-					
	DST	●	O	O	O	O	O	O	O	●	O	O	O	O	O	O	-
Staph. aureus 20 strains	ASM	●	●	●	●	-				●	O	-					
	Wellcotest	●	●	●	●	-				●	O	-					
	Isot.Sens.	●	●	●	O	-				●	O	-					
	Sensitest	●	●	●	●	O	O	O	-	●	O	O	O	O	-		
	DST	●	●	●	O	O	O	O	O	●	O	O	O	O	O	O	-
Strep. faecalis 21 strains	ASM	●	●	O	-					●	O	O	-				
	Wellcotest	●	●	O	-					●	O	O	-				
	Isot.Sens.	●	●	-						O	-						
	Sensitest	●	●	●	O	O	O	-		●	O	O	O	-			
	DST	●	O	O	O	O	-			●	●	O	O	O	-		

● = normal growth
O = incomplete inhibition
- = complete inhibition

*) TMP of the 1:20 combination of TMP and SMX

Figure 2   Growth of thy⁻ mutant 500 of Salm.typhimurium

| Medium | thymine conc. µg/ml | | | | | | | | | | | | | | |
| | without desoxyadenosine | | | | | | | | | | + 25 µg/ml d.a. | | | | |
	0	1	2	4	8	16	32	64	128	256	0	0.12	0.25	0.5	1
MM	-	0	●								-	0	●		
DST	0	0	0	●							0	0	0	0	●
Sensitest	-	-	-	0	●						0	0	0	●	
Isot.Sens.	-	-	-	-	-	-	-	-	0	●	-	-	0	0	●
Wellcotest	-	-	-	-	-	-	-	0	0	●	-	-	0	0	●
ASM	-	-	-	-	-	-	-	0	0	●	-	-	0	0	●

● = normal growth
0 = incomplete inhibition
- = complete inhibition

one shows the inhibition by TMP of 10 strains of E.coli and 10
strains of Staph.aureus on Wellcotest Agar. You can see that MIC's
of 0.25 to 0.5 µg/ml can be read rather easily. The next 2 slides
show the same experiment on DST and Sensitest, also with MIC's of
about 0.25 to 0.5 µg/ml on both media. ASM and Isotonic Sensitest
gave the same picture. On MM too MIC's of about 0.5 µg/ml were
found with E.coli and Salm.typhimurium, indicating that all media
tested are suitable for quantitative MIC-determinations by this
method.

However, we found that DST and to a lesser extent Sensitest
contain small amounts of antagonists to TMP. This was indicated
by a very faint growth on media containing often more than 16
µg/ml TMP. This incomplete inhibition was hard to show in photo-
graphs, and so I present the results in the next table (fig. 1).
From this table you can read MIC's of TMP and cotrimoxazole by
looking for the points where the black dots become open circles.
As already mentioned all 5 commercially available media tested
are suitable, approximately the same MIC's being found per test-
organism.

More than two open circles per medium and organism indicate
the presence of small amounts of antagonist, probably thymidine
and/or thymine. Hence we concluded that especially DST and to a
lesser extent Sensitest contain these antagonists.

To get information about the thymine and/or thymidine concentration in these media, we investigated whether thymineless
mutants of Salm.typhimurium could grow on media without and with
increasing concentrations of thymine or thymidine.

All of the seven thymineless mutants we tested grew optimally
on all media when 1 to 2 µg/ml thymidine was added. Very faint
growth on plates without additions was only seen on DST, indicating that this medium contained some thymine and/or thymidine.
On the other media growth was visible on 0.03 µg/ml thymidine;
on Sensitest usually one two-fold dilution earlier.

Assuming that the antagonist is thymidine one can estimate
that DST contains about 0.03 µg/ml and Sensitest about 0.01 µg/ml
of this substance. The fact that amounts of thymidine of this
order of magnitude can inhibit the action of TMP is illustrated
on the next two slides; the first one shows a sub-optimal but
clearly visible antagonism of the action of 1 µg/ml trimethoprim
by 0.1 µg/ml of thymidine on Wellcotest. The next slide shows this
effect on Sensitest. The fact that the antagonism of 0.1 µg/ml
thymidine is somewhat stronger on Sensitest than on Wellcotest
is an other indication that the former contains a small amount of
the antagonist.

I assumed that thymidine is the antagonist; why should not
it be thymine. I think that is very unlikely, because our own
findings and those of Then (1974) show that at least 5-10 µg/ml
of thymine is needed for antagonizing TMP in gram negative
bacteria. Our experiments with thy⁻ mutants (fig. 2) demonstrate
that all media contained less than 0.5-1 µg/ml thymine. This

slide also shows that especially Isotonic Sensitest, Wellcotest
and ASM contain significant amounts of a uridinelike compound,
that inhibits the utilisation of thymine. Its effect could be
overcome by adding 25 µg/ml of desoxyadenosine, an inducer of
thymidine phosphorylase. I want to remark here that the phenomena
seen in this and other experiments gave us the strong impression
that Wellcotest and ASM are identical.

Coming to a conclusion we have to answer the question whether
the presence of very low concentrations of antagonist render media
useless or unsatisfactory for TMP sensitivity testing. We are
inclined to conclude that thymidine levels of not more than 0.03
µg/ml are acceptable when agar dilution methods are used. It is
likely that more problems will arise when broth dilution methods
are carried out. Difficulties also may arise in agardiffusion
assays. The last slide illustrates this: the inhibition zones of
this strain of Staph.aureus on Sensitest are less sharp than on
Wellcotest due to faint growth in the zones.

In general therefore it is advisable to use a medium which
is free of antagonist, in TMP and cotrimoxazole sensitivity
testing.

References

Amyes, S.G.B. and I.T.Smith. Trimethoprim-sensitivity testing and
        thymineless mutants.
        J.Med.Microbiol. 7 (1974) 143-153.

Koch, A.E. and J.J.Burchall. Reversal of the antimicrobial activi-
        ty of trimethoprim by thymidine in commercially prepared
        media.
        Appl.Microbiol. 22 (1971) 812-817.

Then, R. Mechanismus der bakteriziden Wirkung von Folatantago-
        nisten.
        Zbl.Bakt.Hyg., I.Abt.Orig.A 228 (1974) 273-277.

THYMIDINE AND THE ASSESSMENT OF CO-TRIMOXAZOLE ACTION

IN LIQUID MEDIA

R. Then

Department of Experimental Medicine
F. Hoffman-La, Roche & Co. Ltd.
Basle, Switzerland

SUMMARY: Thymidine and thymine contents in human blood and urine seem to be too low to interfere with the bactericidal activity of co-trimoxazole, (sulphamethoxazole/trimethoprim), observed in vitro in thymidine-free media. Most of the commercially available liquid media contain high thymidine concentrations which prevent a bactericidal action and are not suitable for testing purposes. Although the addition of 5% lysed blood converts the thymidine in those media very effectively into thymine, many media remain unsatisfactory since the relatively high thymine concentrations generated also antagonize a bactericidal action.

The conditions for accurate testing of co-trimoxazole on agar plates have been described sufficiently (Waterworth 1969, Bushby 1973). The mainly interfering substance is thymidine, which prevents accurate MIC-readings and antagonizes a bactericidal action very effectively.

In this respect it was of interest to check the action of co-trimoxazole in those fluids where it acts during therapy, viz. blood and urine. It has recently been shown that E. coli strains are effectively destroyed in human blood and urine by this drug (Then and Angehrn 1974). Thymine - and in much lower concentration thymidine - prevent this destruction. Gram positive strains respond in the same way, as it was demonstrated for Staph. aureus.

The thymine and thymidine levels in these fluids seem to be sufficiently low not to interfere with the bactericidal action obser-

ved in vitro in suitable media. This was further confirmed by
following up the growth kinetics of E. coli 15T⁻ in these fluids
(Then and Angehrn 1975). This thymine-auxotroph strain did not
survive after transfer into blood and urine and underwent rapid
"thymineless death".

From these experiments it seems reasonable to use thymidine-free
media for testing purposes, not only because of technical reasons,
e.g. to obtain low and reproducible MICs, but also to get the
bactericidal action, observed in blood and urine.

About twenty commercially available media were investigated for
their suitability for testing co-trimoxazole, as well as the single
components. Some of the results are shown in Fig. 1.
E. coli 15T⁻ grew well in most of the media, as e.g. in Nutrient
Broth No. 2 (Oxoid). In a few media this strain started to die

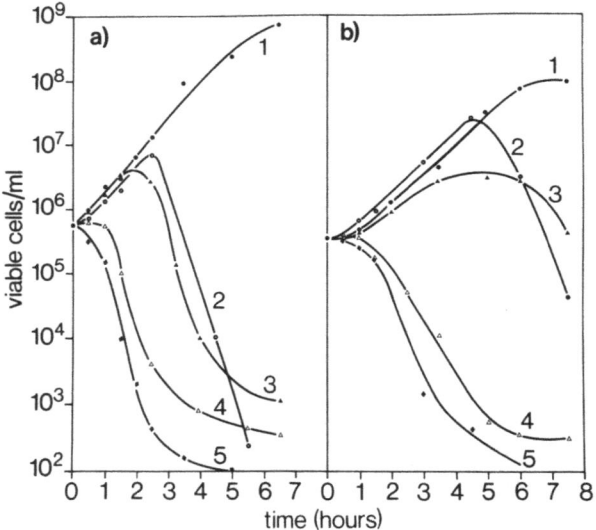

Fig. 1: a) Growth of E. coli 15T⁻ in different media.
         b) Effect of trimethoprim (2 μg/ml) on E. coli B in the
            same media as in a). 1 = Nutrient Broth No. 2 (Oxoid),
            2 = Sensitivity Test Broth (Oxoid), 3 = Isotonic Sen-
            sitest Broth (Oxoid), 4 = SR-Medium Base (Difco),
            1 : 1 diluted, 5 = Folic Acid Assay Medium (Difco),
            1 : 1 diluted.

after a certain lag, thus indicating a limiting thymidine content. The only medium found suitable for testing co-trimoxazole, and which did not contain any thymidine was SR-Medium Base (Difco), where E. coli 15T⁻ died rapidly without lag. This is also true for some media, used for the microbiological determination of folic or folinic acid (No. 5 in Fig. 1), but these media contain p-aminobenzoic acid. The results obtained with E. coli 15T⁻ were paralleled by the findings observed for the bactericidal action of trimethoprim on E. coli B in these media (Fig. 1, b). A rapid bactericidal effect takes place only in thymidine-free media. In the presence of limiting thymidine cell destruction occurs after a lag, depending on the thymidine concentration. In many media no bactericidal effect could be demonstrated, neither on E. coli nor on Staph. aureus, due to elevated thymidine levels.

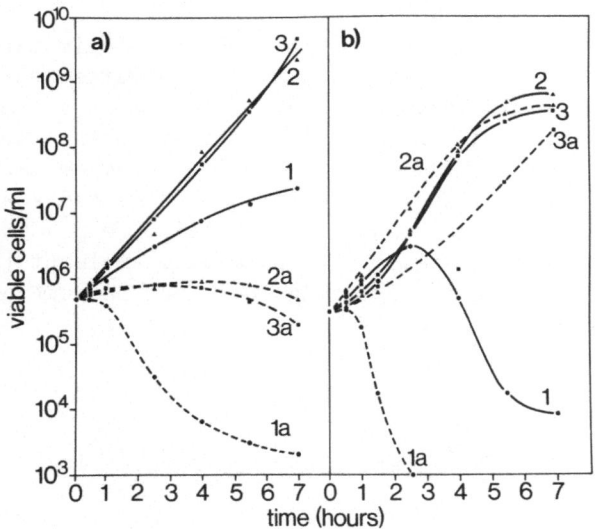

Fig. 2: Influence of 5% lysed horse blood (after overnight incubation) on a) the effect of trimethoprim (2 μg/ml) on E. coli B in different media and b) the growth behaviour of E. coli 15T⁻ in the same media. The blood containing media were heated for 30 min. to 56°C before inoculation. 1 = Sensitivity Test Broth (Oxoid), 1a = 1 plus 5% lysed horse blood. 2 = Nutrient Broth No. 2 (Oxoid). 2a = 2 plus 5% lysed horse blood. 3 = Brain Heart Infusion (Difco), 3a = 3 plus 5% lysed horse blood.

It seems of interest to mention that in media with a limited amount
of thymidine the time lag between the addition of the drug and the
destruction of bacteria is not only dependent on the thymidine concentration, but also on the drug concentration. This was demonstrated in Sensitivity Test Broth (Oxoid). Whereas 2 µg/ml of trimethoprim caused the cell death of E. coli B after a lag of about four
hours, 20 µg/ml trimethoprim or a combination of sulphamethoxazole/
trimethoprim (100/10 µg/ml) did not kill this strain over the observed time of eight hours. The increased drug concentration led
to a drastic prolongation of the generation time, which is known to
occur via the inhibition of protein synthesis. This results in a
slower exhaustion of the thymidine present - and thus preventing a
bactericidal effect for a longer time.

The effect of 5% lysed horse blood, which recently was shown to
contain thymidine phosphorylase (Ferone et al. 1975), on some of
the media was investigated. Representative results are shown in
Fig. 2.

The inhibitory effect of trimethoprim or of co-trimoxazole could
be enhanced in many of the media tested. It turned out that the
addition of 5% lysed horse blood rapidly leads to a complete break
down of thymidine in all media. In contrast to the improved bacteriostatic action observed in the blood-treated media, a bactericidal action, however, took place only in those media which were
shown to contain limited amounts of thymidine (e.g. Sensitivity
Test Broth (Oxoid) in Fig. 2). Many media, at least those containing more than 5 µg/ml thymidine could not be sufficiently improved for demonstrating bactericidal activities.

References:

Bushby, S.R.M. (1973), J. Inf. Dis., 128 Suppl., 442.

Ferone, R., Bushby, S.R.M., Burchall, J.J., Moore, W.D. and
Smith, D. (1975), Antimicrob. Ag. Chemother., 7, 91.

Then, R. and Angehrn, P. (1974), Biochem. Pharmacol., 23, 2977.

Then, R. and Angehrn, P. (1975), Biochem. Pharmacol., 24, 1003.

Waterworth, P. (1969), Postgrad. Med. J., Suppl. Vol. 45, 21.

ANTIBACTERIAL SUSCEPTIBILITY TESTING OF ANAEROBES

KUNITOMO WATANABE,KEIU NINOMIYA,IZUMI MOCHIZUKI,
TOSHIO MIWA,HIROMU IMAMURA,SHUNRO KOBATA,KAZUE
UENO AND SHOICHIRO SUZUKI
Department of Bacteriology,Gifu University
School of Medicine
Gifu,Japan

There are a lot of ploblems associated with susceptibility testing of anaerobes which are not encountered in
the testing of aerobes and facultative anaerobes. Anaerobiosis itself,medium composition and carbon dioxide concentration in the atmosphere may all influence the test
results. In this study,we examined influence of these variants and established a standardized agar dilution test.

1) Influence of test agar media on agar dilution test re-
    sults
    Susceptibility of 20 strains against 2 cephalospori-
nes,cephaloridine and ceftezole,were determined by using
5 kinds of agar media and the mode(or the median) was determined. G A M agar,Brain heart infusion agar,Liver Veal
agar,Brucella agar and Columbia agar were employed. These
test agars except G A M agar were used for 5 % blood agar
plates. The extent of deviation from the modes was shown
in Table 1.
    About 30 % of the strains tested deviated from the
modes by more than 2 dilution steps. Most of these strains
were rapid growing anaerobes,such as C.perfringens,B.frag-
ilis and F.varium. Results of 70 % of strains fell within
± 1 dilution step from the modes.

2) Influence of anaerobiosis on agar dilution test results
    The steel wool copper sulfate method usually employed
in our laboratory was compared with the GasPak method.
    MIC's of pivampicillin,a new derivative of penicillin,
to 20 strains obtained by the steel wool method were almost the same as those obtained by the GasPak method.

Table 1.Influence of test agar media on MIC

Strain	Cephaloridine							Ceftezole						
	-3	-2	-1	M*	+1	+2	+3	-3	-2	-1	M*	+1	+2	+3
1				5							5			
2			3	2					1	3	1			
3			4		1				2	3				
4			4	1					1	3	1			
5			4	1							4	1		
6			3	2				1	1	3				
7			4		1			1	1	3				
8			5					1	1	2	1			
9		1	4							1	3	1		
10		1	2	2							2	1	2	
11		1	3	1							3		2	
12		2	3							1	4			
13			5							1	4			
14		1	4							1	4			
15		1	3	1							4	1		
16		1	3	1							3	1	1	
17	1	1	2		1				2	3				
18		1	3	1						1	4			
19			4	1							4	1		
20	2	1	1		1				1	2	1	1		

*M; the mode(or the median)
Results below the mode are given a minus sign
and those above a plus sign.Thus +2 indicates
a MIC of 2 dilution steps above the mode.

But with lincomycin,the steel wool method tended to give
somewhat higher MIC's than the GasPak method. (Table 2.)

3) Influence of CO_2 concentration in jars on dilution test
   results
       Influence of CO_2 concentration in jars on MIC of piv-
ampicillin,lincomycin and thiamphenicol was examined. CO_2
led to marked differences in the activity of pivampicillin
and lincomycin due to resulting difference in the pH of
the medium. But MIC of thiamphenicol was not influenced by
CO_2 concentration in jars. Among anaerobic bacteria,almost
all strains of gram negative rods and one strain of gram
negative cocci,A.fermentans were markedly influenced.

4) Reproducibility of agar dilution test

       Eight different kinds of methods for determinating
MIC were prepared as in Table 3. MIC's of seven strains
were determined five times by each method.   Pst.anaerobi-
us,E.lentum,B.fragilis,P.acnes,V.parvula,F.nucleatum   and
P.asaccharolyticus were used.

Table 2. Relationship of MIC's by steel wool method
to those by GasPak method

method Antibiotic	Steel wool < GasPak	Steel wool = GasPak	Steel wool > GasPak
Pivampicillin	8*	11	1
Lincomycin	0	7	15#

*8: 8 strain #: 7 out of 15 were more than 2 dilution
steps.

Table 3. Eight different methods for determinating
MIC

Method	Inoculum	Inoculating method	Incubation time
No.1	24 h culture	loop	24 h
2	24	device	24
3	6	loop	24
4	6	device	24
5	24	loop	48
6	24	device	48
7	6	loop	48
8	6	device	48

Extent of deviation from the mode(or the median) was
determined for all methods and one of the results was
shown in Table 4.

All of the eight methods were fairly reproducible. The
methods with a loop were more reproducible than those with
a replicating device. For inoculum, a 6 hrs culture were
appropriate for rapid growing anaerobes but not for slow
growing anaerobes. For incubation time, a 24 hrs incubation was sufficient for rapid growings but not for slow
growings. V.parvula,F.nucleatum and P.acnes were slow growing anaerobes.

Table 4. Distribution of MIC's by Method No.4 in
relation to the mode

Strain	Agar dilution steps						
	-3	-2	-1	M	+1	+2	+3
1.Pst.anaerobius				4	1		
2.E.lentum			2	3			
3.B.fragilis				3	2		
4.P.acnes				2	2		
5.V.parvula			2	2		1	
6.F.nucleatum				3	2		
7.P.asaccharolyticus				4	1		

Table 5. Variability of readings of MIC

| Strain | Reader | Inoculum | |
		6 h culture	24 h culture
1	A	3.13*	6.25
	B	3.13	6.25
	C	3.13	200
2	A	3.13	6.25
	B	3.13	6.25-12.5
	C	1.56-3.13	12.5-200
3	A	1.56	1.56-6.25
	B	1.56	1.56-3.13
	C	0.78-1.56	100 -200
4	A	0.19-0.78	1.56
	B	0.39	1.56
	C	0.39-0.78	1.56-6.25
5	A	1.56	1.56
	B	0.78-1.56	1.56
	C	0.39-0.78	0.78-3.13
6	A	0.78-1.56	6.25
	B	1.56-3.13	12.5
	C	0.39-1.56	200
7	A	1.56	6.25
	B	1.56	1.56-3.13
	C	0.78-1.56	100

*MIC(ug/ml) Two replicates were used for this test.
MIC's of < 100 μg/ml were considered as 200 μg/ml.

5) Reproducibility of the reading of results among three
   workers
   Three workers(A,B and C) read the end-point of growth
on the same susceptibility plates. Two replicates were
used for this test.(Table 5)
   Using a 24 hrs culture for inoculum,the readings by
A and B were almost the same,whereas those by C showed
marked deviation from A and B. Using a 6 hrs culture for
inoculum,the readings by A,B and C were almost the same.

6) Correlation between agar dilution MIC's and inhibition
   zone diameters
   For clinical use,single disc diffusion test was also
examined. Single disc diffusion test was performed as follows; The inoculum was prepared in the same manner as for
the agar dilution test and diluted to the turbidity of a
No.1 McFarland standard solution. G A M plates poured to
a depth of 3 to 4 mm were inoculated by means of a cotton
swab and antibiotic discs were applied. Measurements of
the zone diameter were made from the front of the plate
with sliding calipers.
   Inhibition zone diameters of C.perfringens,B.fragilis

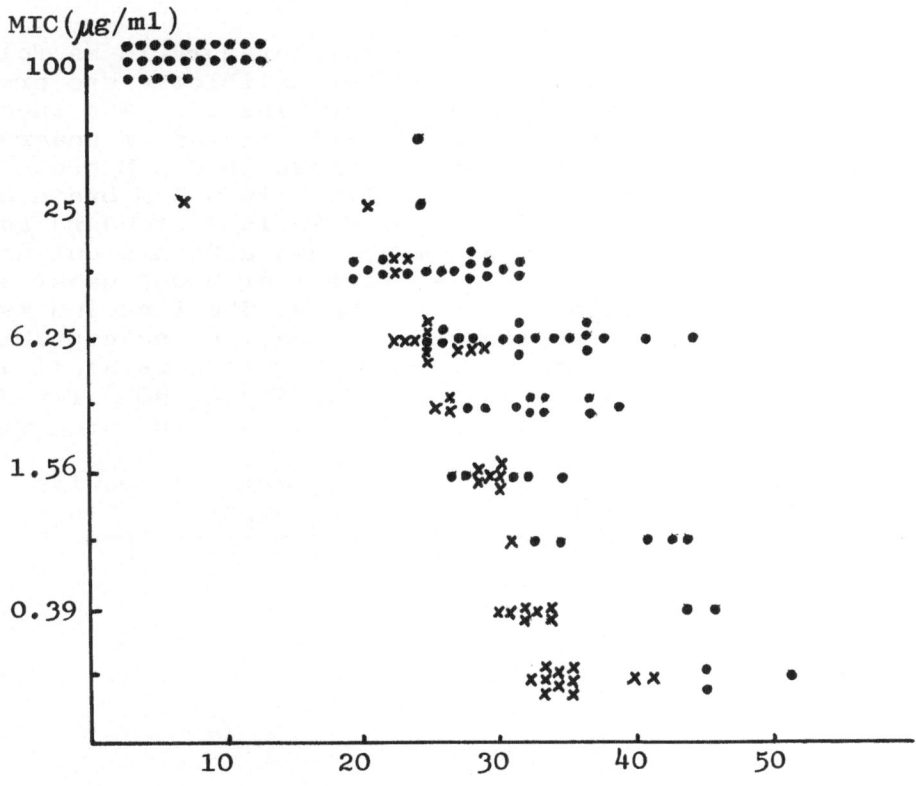

Inhibition zone diameter(mm)
Figure 1. Regression plot of zone diameters versus
MIC's for lincomycin(30 μg disc)
. B.fragilis 85 strains, x C.perfringens 45 strains

F.varium and anaerobic cocci were measured after 24 hrs.
Discs used were lincomycin(30μg),clindamycin(30μg), tetra-
cycline(200μg),cephaloridine(30μg),aminobenzylpenicillin
(30μg),chloramphenicol(100μg) etc. The strains tested were
85 strains of B.fragilis,45 strains of C.perfringens and
60 strains of anaerobic cocci.

    With B.fragilis and C.perfringens,inhibition zone
diameters and MIC's had a considerably good correlation to
each other for lincomycin and tetracycline. But with anaerobic cocci good results were not obtained. 24 hrs incubation was not appropriate for anaerobic cocci.

    As shown in Figure 1., a great deal of overlapping of
zone diameters among strains classed as susceptible,inter-
mediate and resistant was noticed.

Summary

The agar dilution method in our laboratory is as follows; Serial two-fold dilutions of the antibiotic are prepared and incorporated into G A M agar(Nissui). The inoculum is prepared as follows; Almost all strains of anaerobes except slow growing strains are grown in G A M broth (Nissui)for about 6 hrs. A 6 hrs culture in G A M broth has the turbidity of a half of a No. 1 McFarland standard solution(10^5-10^6 viable cells per ml). When a 24 hrs culture is used,it is diluted in Ueno's diluent or 0.05% yeast extract water to the same turbidity above. The inoculum is applied by means of a replicating device. The susceptibility plates are incubated at about 37 C in jars(steel wool copper sulfate method,atmosphere CO_2 10%,N_2 90%) for 24 hrs. MIC is read as the highest dilution of the drug yielding no growth.

In the absence of agreed reference methods,results from different laboratories cannot be compared with confidence. We are looking forward to establish international agreed reference methods.

SENSITIVITY TESTING OF MIXED INFECTIONS

M. Taufer and J. Zangger

Dept. of Exp.Cell Res. and Oncology
Inst. of Pathology,University Graz
A 8036 Graz, Austria

Summary

In a high percentage of the clinical patient's samples being
tested for antibiotic sensitivity, we are confronted with mixed
infections. To prove approxemately the germ relation how it
is given at the infection region we use primary cultures for
the first sensibility testing. To become aquainted with the
behaviour of the mixed cultures of different relation to each
other, we produced artificial mixed cultures (from these isolated germs) and tested the resistance. To give the therapist
guiding directions -we mean however- the sensibility testing
in primary cultures with mixed infections comes nearest "in
vivo" conditions. Referring to this our results will be discussed on examples from the practice.

Measurement of the sensitivity of bacteria to antibiotics
and chemotherapeutics in specimens with polymcrobial infections
is problematical now as before.There are many different con-
ceptions and we do not know a recommendation for a standard-
method. So we think the problem should be discussed by this
international forum.

The chief point of interrogation is the choice of inoculum. A survey undertaken 1970 in the United Kingdom (Castle
and Elstub 1971) showed the following facts of choice of inoculum: Tests employing pure cultures were done by 53% of all
hospitals. 17% prefer the direct plating method in which the
specimen is used as the inoculum and 30% use either direct
plating method or subculture according to the nature of the
specimen. The argumentation for the different choice of inoculum

are manifold but no argument is concerned in the specimens of
concurrent infections. Corresponding to the study of CASTLE
and ELSTUB some laboratories use the direct plating method to
obtain the results earlier. Other laboratories which employ
pure cultures do so, because they are convinced that this method only is capable to make a categorization of sensitivity.
Not to understand are the explanations of laboratories using
both -direct plating and subcultures. Some make direct plating
of urines and subcultures of other specimens,other laboratories
use the direct plating of all specimens except urines.
So far a short overview about antibiotic sensitivity testing in
routine laboratories of many hospitals. But now to our chosen
problem " the right antibiotic sensitivity testing of concurrent infections" .

     In a high percentage of our own bacterialogical samples
we find two or more species of bacteria. In urines par example
we have mixed cultures in 7,2%. In comparison to a study made
in 100 american hospitals (Gosslin Hospital Pathology Audit,
1971) the percentage of concurrent infections of the urinary
tract is 5,8%. On the overage we observe mixed infections in
17,4% of our whole material.

     We will give you now a short description of test methods
we use: In every case microscopy of a coloured smear will be
taken. Macroscopical clear urines will be centrifuged before.
As microscopical control shows several species of bacteria, the
specimen then is used as the inoculum in a direct plating method
to test antibiotic sensitivity. In a second step we are iso-
lating the diverse bacteria in subcultures. From clinical samples with only one species of microbes first will be taken a
culture with well separated colonies. One up to ten of these
colonies - corresponding the nature of the bacterium - will
be diluted in broth and then seeded on the culture plate for
testing antibiotic sensitivity.

     Let us give you an example from our practice. In this
special case we got an aspirated secret from the trachea. By
microscopical examination we found a compositum of Gram-negative
short sticks resp.small Gram-positive Cocci. In sensitivity
testing of the primary culture, we could very well differencia-
te the single kinds of bacteria - as it is shown in figure 1.
The mucous growing on the right side of the agar plate was
identified as Klebsiella, inside the inhibition zone of Streptomycin (S 25) and Kanamycin (K 30) we found Staphylococcus
Aureus and - on the photography to be seen not so very clearly
and marked by an arrow - single colonies of Streptococcus
faecalis. With reference to this example we want to say
emphatically that by different sensitivity of single kinds of
bacteria in mixed cultures, it is also possible in a multitude
of the cases to identify themselves.

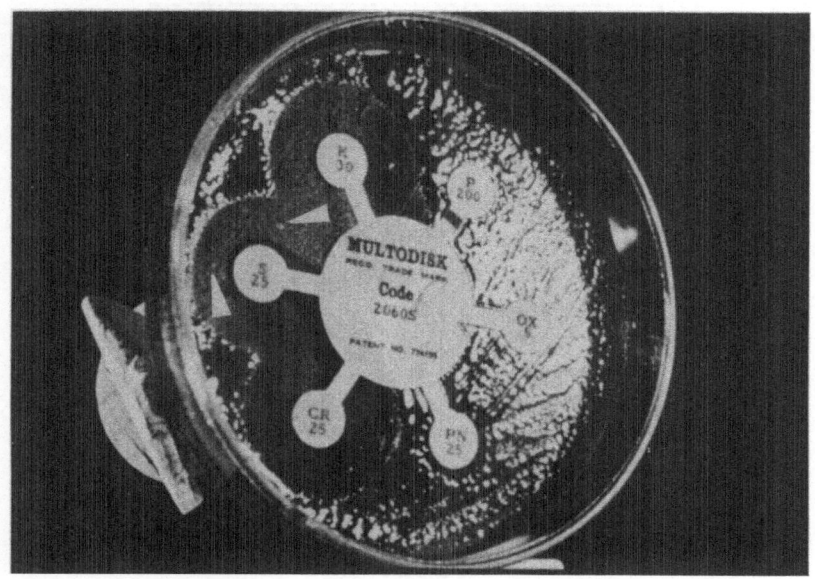

Figure 1

Direct plating culture of an aspirated secret from the trachea.
(Explanation see text.)

On this passage let us briefly say one sentence for using
test stars named "multodisk". Four years ago at the 7th International Congress of Chemotherapy in Prag (Zangger 1971), we
condemned the multodisk but now we are forced to use it because
the " Sen-test" of Evans Medical Ltd. we used before, is not
produced any longer. Nevertheless, we want to accentuate that
six different antibiotics at one test star are the maximum to
avoid wrong statements.

Table 1 will give you a concentrated overview about the
sensitivity-testing of the isolated germs in the mixed culture
examined before.

This is the result we may give to the therapist. The de-
cision wether and which of the bacteria being proved is pathogen or which of them is mainly responsible for the kind of illness, the therapist has to make himself.

Furthermore to help the clinician and to become aquainted
with the behaviour of concurrent infections, respectively of
mixed cultures in different relations to each other at the
region of infection, we produced artificial polymicrobial cultures. The different behaviour and growth in diverse broths and

Antibiotic	Sensitive	Resistent
Penicillin G	+ ×	▢
Ampicillin	+	▢ ×
Oxacillin	+	▢ ×
Kanamycin	▢ ×	+
Erythromycin	×	▢ +
Cephaloridine	▢ +	×
Gentamycin	▢ + ×	
Streptomycin	▢	+ ×
Tetracycline		▢ + ×
Chloramphenicol	+ ×	▢
Sulphonamides		▢ + ×

▢   Klebsiella

×   Strept.faec.

+   Staph.aur.

Table 1

Sensitivity-testing of the isolated germs in the mixed culture.

agar-plates of different consistence and the observation of
mutual interaction of the single species,let us draw conclusions from the reactions of bacteria " in corpore ".

What is the closing challenge we may postulate for helping
to make the best in testing concurrent infections ?
All specimens sent to any bacteriological routine laboratory
must be examined microscopically at first. Direct plating culture is to demand in any case of mixed bacteria found in the
smear. In most of the cases after antibiotic testing it is
posible to get informations about different species and behaviour of the infection in question. Furtheron you may test
selected germs at subcultures of their specific sensitivity to
antibiotics. If the microbiologist is going this way and there
is a real cooperation with the clinician, so we hope, they may
do the best to help the patient which is the most important in
our opinion.

References: Castle,A.R. and Elstub J. (1971), Journ.Clin.
Path., 24,773. Pfizer Corporation, Personal Communication.
Zangger J., (1971), Proc. VIIth Intern.Congr. Chemotherapy 1971

A DIFFUSION DISC SUSCEPTIBILITY TEST FOR 5-FLUOROCYTOSINE

C. Utz and S. Shadomy

Departments of Medicine (Infectious Disease) and
Microbiology, Medical College of Virginia, Virginia
Commonwealth University, Richmond, Virginia, U.S.A.

SUMMARY

A diffusion disc test for testing with 5-Fluorocytosine (5-FC)
was described. A commercial 1 ug and an experimental 10 ug disc
were evaluated using Yeast Morphology Agar supplemented with 2.5
ug/ml of thiamine at pH 5.0. Zones of inhibition were correlated
with MIC values obtained with a modification of the ICS agar dilution procedure using the same agar.

Excellent correlation was obtained between MIC values and zones
of inhibition produced by both discs. However, the 10 ug disc
proved superior to the 1 ug disc in prediction of susceptibility of
pathogenic yeasts, particularly with Cryptococcus neoformans.

INTRODUCTION

The feasibility of diffusion disc susceptibility testing with
5-fluorocytosine (5-FC) and yeast-like organisms already has been
demonstrated. Marks and Eickhoff (1970) first showed the usefulness of a 1 ug disc test with Candida albicans and Scholer and
Polak (1973) more recently described a procedure employing a
standardised 1 ug disc together with modified yeast morphology agar.
Neither procedure has been subjected to critical evaluation to permit use in the clinical laboratory in the United States. This
report describes a disc test procedure evaluated within the physical
limitations of the standardised Food and Drug Administration disc
test (1971).

MATERIALS AND METHODS

Two discs were evaluated: a commercial 1 ug disc provided by
Hoffman-La Roche, Basle, Switzerland, and an experimental 10 ug
disc prepared in our laboratory. Plates of Yeast Morphology Agar,
or YMA, supplemented with 2.5 ug/ml of thiamine and adjusted to
a pH of 5.0 as recommended by Scholer and Polak (1973) were poured
to a depth of 4.00 mm. Yeasts were grown on Sabouraud's agar
after which they were harvested, suspended in saline and adjusted
to a transmission of 94 to 97%. Plates were inoculated in the
fashion described for the FDA disc test and incubated without pre-
diffusion after application of the discs at 30°C for 48 hours.
Following incubation, zones of inhibition were measured to the
nearest 0.1 mm.

The International Collaborative Study agar dilution procedure
described by Ericsson and Sherris (1971) was used to determine
minimal inhibitory concentrations of 5-FC. The test medium was
supplemented YMA. Concentrations of 5-FC ranged from 0.008 to
256 ug/ml. Inocula containing approximately 10^4 cells were applied
with a replica inoculator. Incubation was at 30°C for 7 days.
MIC endpoints were read after 24 and 72 hours incubation and again
after 7 days. Data to be reported here were based upon readings
made after 72 hours of incubation.

216 yeasts were tested. These included 27 isolates of Torulopsis glabrata, 58 of Candida albicans, 53 of Candida species
other than Candida albicans, and 78 of Cryptococcus neoformans.
All identifications were based upon morphological characteristics
and biochemical reactions.

Regression analyses and related statistical studies employed
the least squares method and the estimating equation; drug concentrations were expressed as base 2 log values.

RESULTS

New data regarding the activity of 5-FC against yeast-like
organisms were obtained. Most isolates of C.neoformans were susceptible to 5-FC (Table 1). Taking an MIC of 16 ug/ml as the
upper limit of probable clinical susceptibility, 95% of the 78
isolates were susceptible and 4% were totally resistant. This
finding is essentially identical to our earlier report of 97% of
77 isolates being susceptible to 12.5 ug/ml or less (Shadomy et
al, 1969).

T.glabrata proved to be highly susceptible to 5-FC. The majority of isolates, 85%, were susceptible to less than 1 ug/ml; 3
isolates were inhibited at concentrations 1 and 16 ug/ml while

Table 1. Susceptibility of 216 Isolates of Pathogenic and Commensalistic Yeasts to 5-FC as Measured by Agar Dilution Technique

	Cumulative Percent Susceptible								
Species	Concentrations of 5-Fluorocytosine (µg/ml)*								
	0.25	0.5	1.0	2.0	4.0	8.0	16.0	>16.0	>128
Cryptococcus neoformans	28	63	91	95	95	95	95	95	100
Candida albicans	43	62	67	72	74	74	74	/8	100
Candida species (other than C. albicans)	30	53	59	74	74	76	75	85	100
Torulopsis glabrata	20	85	92	92	92	92	96	96	100

*As determined by 72 hour incubation

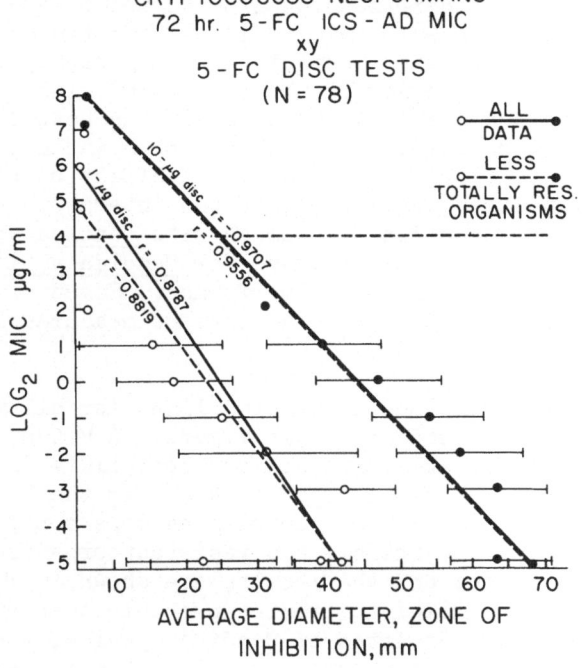

Figure 1. Relationship between minimal inhibitory concentration of 5-fluorocytosine (5-FC) and zones of inhibition obtained with 1- and 10-µg 5-FC discs and 78 isolates of Cryptococcus neoformans

only one was totally resistant. We previously reported that
approximately 50% of clinical isolates of C.albicans may be resistant to 5-FC (Shadomy, 1970). This finding,based on a relatively
small number, 15, has been disputed. Data shown in Table 1 are
derived from a much larger number and may be more representative
for this species at least as it occurs clinically in America.
Although nearly 70% of the 58 isolates were susceptible to 1 ug/ml
or less of 5-FC, 23% were resistant. Thus, it is apparent that
resistance to the drug is, in fact, a major problem with C.albicans.
A similar pattern was seen in isolates of Candida species other
than C.albicans. Fifty percent of this group were inhibited by
0.05 to 1.0 ug or less. But, again 23% were resistant.

Excellent correlation was demonstrated when 72 hr MIC end-
points and paired average 48 hr zone size values for C.neoformans
were subjected to regression analysis. Regression lines are shown
for both discs in Fig.1. The best correlation was obtained with
the 10 ug disc. 9 of 72 isolates susceptible by agar dilution
testing failed to give measureable zones of inhibition with the
1 ug disc.

While apparently good correlation was obtained for Torulopsis
glabrata, the calculated regression lines did not agree well with
plotted data pairs (Fig.2). This reflects both the small number
of organisms tested and the clustering of many highly susceptible
organisms at the lower region of the regression lines. Good correlation was obtained for C.albicans; again the best correlation
was with the 10 ug disc (Fig.3). Exclusion or inclusion of data
for totally resistant organisms had little effect on the slopes
of the regression lines, but did shift the intercepts several
millimeters. Regression lines obtained with Candida species other
than C.albicans were similar to those for Candida albicans (Fig.4).
Again the 10 ug disc was the best performer. Seven of 41 isolates
susceptible by agar dilution testing gave no measureable zones
with the 1 ug disc.

Fig.5 shows the combined regression lines for all yeasts.
Correlates can be obtained from this figure. A MIC of 16 ug/ml,
the upper limit of probable clinical susceptibility in our dilution scheme, correlates with zones of 14 mm for the 1 ug disc and
26 mm for the 10 ug disc. These correlates were applied to the 48
hr zone readings for susceptible and resistant organisms as determined by agar dilution, and the results are shown in Table 2. The
1 ug disc would have failed to predict probable susceptibility
with nearly 25% of the isolates of Candida species, about 15% of
the isolates of C.neoformans and about 5% of the isolates of
Candida albicans and Torulopsis glabrata. In contrast, the 10 ug
disc would have failed with 5% or less of any of the groups. The
1 ug disc was slightly better in predicting probable resistance.

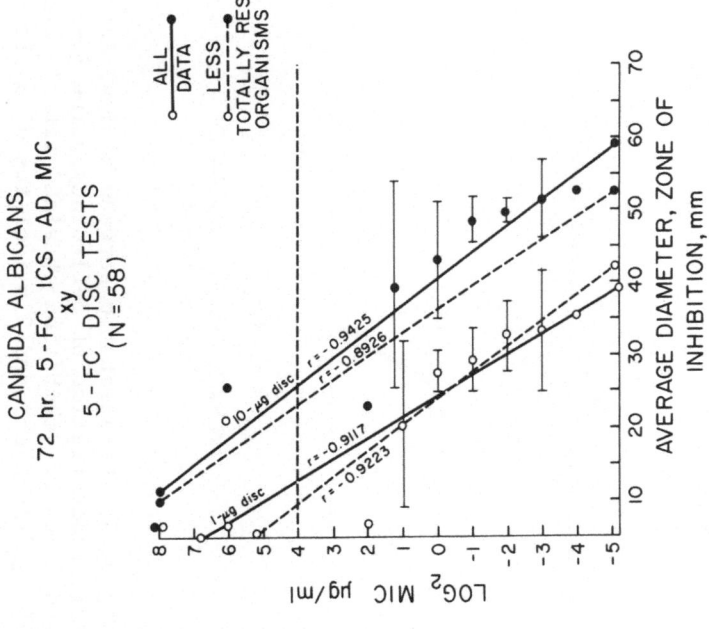

Figure 3. Relationship between minimal inhibitory concentration of 5-fluorocytosine (5-FC) and zones of inhibition obtained with 1- and 10-µg 5-FC discs and 58 isolates of _Candida albicans_.

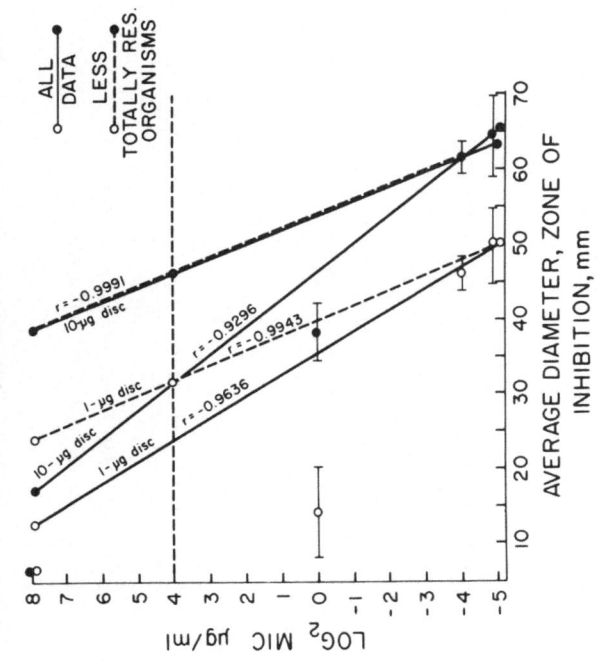

Figure 2. Relationship between minimal inhibitory concentration of 5-fluorocytosine (5-FC) and zones of inhibition obtained with 1- and 10-µg 5-FC discs and 27 isolates of _Torulopsis glabrata_.

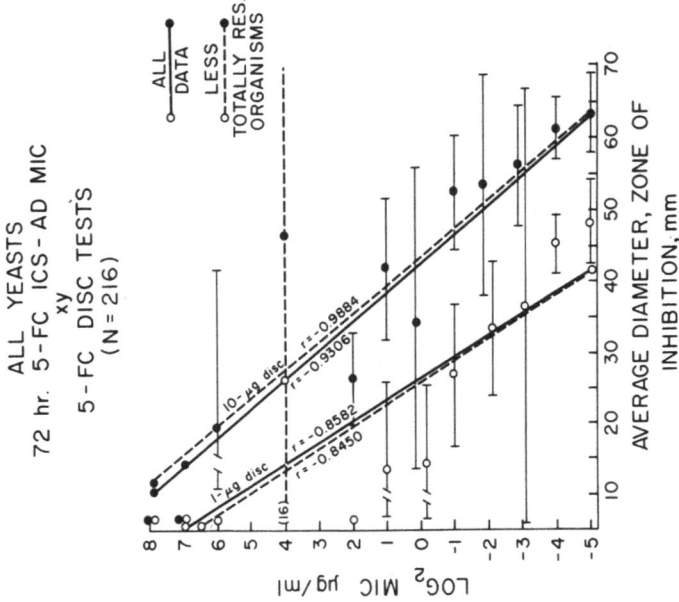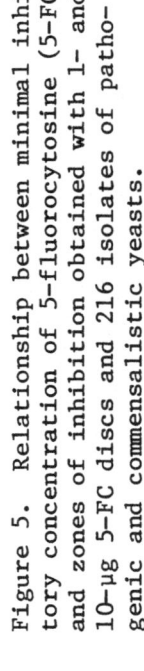

Figure 5. Relationship between minimal inhibitory concentration of 5-fluorocytosine (5-FC) and zones of inhibition obtained with 1- and 10-μg 5-FC discs and 216 isolates of pathogenic and commensalistic yeasts.

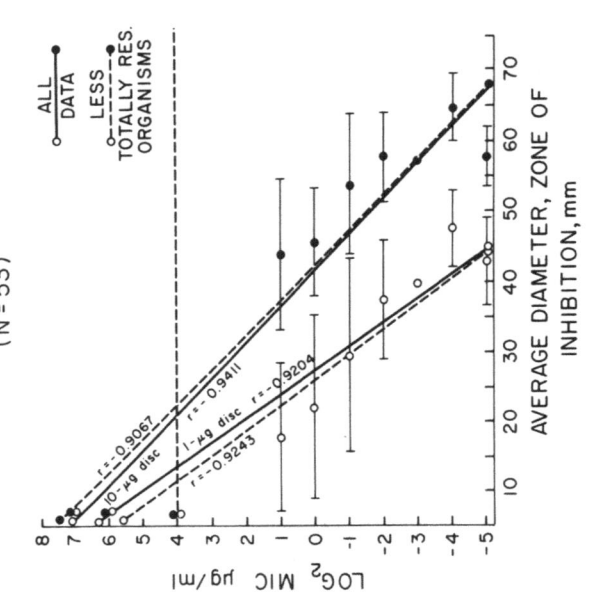

Figure 4. Relationship between minimal inhibitory concentration of 5-fluorocytosine (5-FC) and zones of inhibition obtained with 1- and 10-μg 5-FC discs and 53 isolates of Candida species other than C. albicans.

TABLE 2

RESULTS OF SUSCEPTIBILITY TESTING WITH
5-FLUOROCYTOSINE DISCS

		Susceptible by Agar Dilution			Resistant by Agar Dilution	
		Suscept.by 1 ug disc %	Suscept.by 10 ug disc		Resist.by 1 ug disc %	Resist.by 10 ug disc
	(N)			(N)		
T.glabrata	(26)	96	100	(1)	100	100
C.species	(41)	76	98	(13)	100	92
C.albicans	(43)	93	95	(15)	100	93
C.neoformans	(75)	84	97	(4)	100	100

DISCUSSION

The correlates presented here represent the results of analyses of nearly 1,000 data pairs. As has been shown, correlation
between measureable zones of inhibition with both the 1 and 10 ug
discs and minimal inhibitory concentrations for 5-FC for most
isolates of yeast-like organisms is good. Thus, disc testing with
this drug is feasible and should be capable of yielding clinically
reliable results. If such testing is done within the framework
of the FDA disc test procedure, the correlates presented here should
prove usefuly. Our data favour the use of the 10 ug disc rather
than the 1 ug disc.

REFERENCES

1. Dept. Health, Education and Welfare, Food and Drug Admini-
       stration (USA). (1971) Fed.Reg., 36, 6899.

2. Ericsson, H.M. and Sherris, J.C. (1971) Acta Pathol.Microbiol.
       Scand. Suppl., 217, 1.

3. Marks, M.I.and Eickhoff, T.C. (1971) Antimicrob.Ag.Chemother.,
       1970, 491.

4. Scholer, H.J. and Polak, A. (1973) Symposium International de
       Mycologie Medicale, Bucharest, September 20th - 22nd.

5. Shadomy, S., Shadomy, H.J., McCay, J.A. and Utz, J.P. (1969)
       Antimicrob.Ag.Chemother., 1963, 452.

6. Shadomy, S. (1970) Infection and Immunity, 2, 484.

THE SUSCEPTIBILITY OF CLOSTRIDIA FROM THE ANTARCTIC SOIL TO ANTIBIOTICS

TOSHIO MIWA, IZUMI MOCHIZUKI, KUNITOMO WATANABE, SHUNRO KOBATA, HIROMU IMAMURA, KEIU NINOMIYA, KAZUE UENO AND SHOICHIRO SUZUKI

Department of Bacteriology, Gifu University School of Medicine,   Gifu-city, 500 Japan

Summary

From the Antarctic soil, a total of 193 strains of clostridia were isolated and identified. Of them were assigned to 11 species; i.e., C.perfringens, C.bifermentans and C.sordellii were isolated frequently.

The Antarctic strains were almost the same susceptibility with the control(Japan) strains to Penicillin-G, Cephaloridine, Clindamycin and Lincomycin.

To Tetracyclines, the Antarctic strains were all sensitive(0.19 µg/ml or less), but the control strains had about 30 % resistant strains(50-3.13 µg/ml).

Introduction

One of the authors(T. Miwa) had been the Antarctica for bacteriological research and stayed at the Japanese Syowa Station from 1972 to 1973 as a member of the 13th Japanese Antarctic Research Expedition.

In this study, we explored the susceptibility of clostridia isolated from the Antarctic soil to 7 antibiotics.

Soil specimens

Most soil specimens were obtained from 10-20 cm under the surface of the ground at places about 300 km of the Syowa Station, including the places where has been scarcely contaminated by human beings and animals (i.e., moraine, permafrost and bottom mud of lake).

Prcedures of isolation

Soil specimens were cultured with two kind enrichment media(Bacto Cooked Meat Medium and GAM semisolid medium). After incubation for 1-10 days, the cultures were streaked onto egg yolk CW agar and GAM agar medium. A steel wool copper sulfate was used with anaerobic jar in enviroment of N_2 and CO_2 gas at 37 C for 24 hrs. The biochemical tests and identification were made according to the VPI manual, Bergey's manual and our own manual[1].

Isolated clostridia

From the Antarctic soil, a total of 193 strains of clostridia were isolated and assigned to 11 species as shown in Table I. The distribution of clostridia were summarized as follows;

1. C.sordellii and C.paraperfringens, which were very rarely from the soil in other continents, especially, in Japan were never found from soil, were isolated frequently from the Antarctic soil.
2. Distribution of aerobes were less than clostridia in the Antarctic soil.
3. Heat resistant strains could not isolated from the Antarctic soil at 80 C for 10 min. or more.
4. In surprisingly, from the places where were scarcely contaminated , were found to contain many clostidia.

We reported already on this data in Japan Society Microbiology [2][3][4].

Table 1. CLOSTRIDIA ISOLATED from the ANTARCTIC SOIL

Species	Number of strains	Toxigenicity
C.perfringens	50 (26 %)	+
C.bifermentans	44 (23)	−
C.sordellii	41 (21)	−
C.sporogenes	6	−
C.plagarum	5	−
C.paraperfringens	4	−
C.septicum	1	+
C.tertium	1	−
C.cadaveris	1	−
C.butyricum	1	−
C.felsineum	1	−
Unidentified strains	38	−
Total	193	

The susceptibility of clostridia to antibiotics

We tested the susceptibility of the Antarctic strains to 7 antibiotics and compared with the control strains.

As tested clostridia were C.perfringens, C.bifermentans and C.sordelii isolated from the Antarctic soil (65 Antarctic strains) and from soil in Japan, clinical specimens and labeled strains (58 control strains). Inoculum was adjusted to viable cell counts of 10^{5-6}/ml. The tested plate was spot-inoculated with a inoculating device on GAM agar and incubated anaerobically at 37 C for 24 hrs [5].

Table 2 shows the minimum inhibitory concentration (MIC) values of C.perfringens from the Antarctic and the control strains to Penicillin-G, Cephaloridine, Clindamycin and Lincomycin. To 4 antibiotics, the Antarctic strains were almost the same susceptibility with the control strains. Penicillin-G was active, Cephaloridine was less active, Clindamycin was active and Lincomycin also, but a half strains of both groups to a lesser degree.

Table 2. The SUSCEPTIBILITY of C.PERFRINGENS ISOLATED from the SOIL in the ANTARCTICA and JAPAN to ANTIBIOTICS

MIC (μg/ml)	PC-G A.	PC-G J.	CER A.	CER J.	CLDM A.	CLDM J.	LCM A.	LCM J.
100 ≦								
50								
25								
12.5							o	● ●
6.25							oooo	●●●●●●
3.13			ooooooooooooo	●			ooo	●
1.56			oooooo	●●●●●●●●	o	●	ooooo	●
0.78	o		ooooo	●●●●●●●●●●	oooooo	●	o	
0.39	ooo	●		● ●	oo	●●●●●●	ooo	●●● ●●●
0.19 ≧	oooooooooooooooooo	●●●●●●●●●●	o		oooooooooo	●●●●●●●●●	ooooooooo	●●●

```
 * A. : Antarctic strain,  25 strains
   J. : control strain ( soil in Japan), 20 strains

** PC-G : Penicillin-G        CLDM : Clindamycin
   CER  : Cephaloridine       LCM  : Lincomycin
```

Table 3 shows the susceptibility of C.perfringens from the Antarctic and the control strains to Tetracycline, Oxytetracycline and Doxycycline.   The susceptibility of both groups were clearly differentiated to 3 antibiotics.
        The Antarctic strains were all sensitive (0.19 µg/ml or less).   On the other hand, about 30 % of the control strains were resistant(50-3.13 µg/ml).

        For another strains (C.bifermentans and C.sordellii), both groups were almost the same susceptibility to Penicillin-G, Cephaloridine and Clindamycin.   To Lincomycin, the Antarctic strains had a half strains resistance(6.25 -1.56 µg/ml), but the control strains were all resistant (12.5-1.56 µg/ml).   To tetracyclines, about 30 % of the control strains were lesser than the susceptibility (0.19 µg/ml or less) of the Antarctic strains just as like C.perfringens.

Table 3. The SUSCEPTIBILITY of C.PERFRINGENS ISOLATED from the SOIL in the ANTARCTICA and JAPAN to ANTIBIOTICS

MIC (µg/ml)	A. TC	J. TC	A. OTC	J. OTC	A. DOTC	J. DOTC
100 ≦						
50		●		●●●●		
25		●		●●●		●
12.5		●▲		●●●●●▲		●●●
6.25		●●●		●		●●▲
3.13		●●●●●●				●
1.56		●				
0.78						●
0.39	○					●●●●●
0.19 ≦	(many)	(many)	(many)	(many)	(many)	(many)
Origin*	A.	J.	A.	J.	A.	J.
Drug **	TC		OTC		DOTC	

 * A. : Antarctic strain, 25 strains
    J. : control strain(soil in Japan), 37 strains and
         one strain(▲) from a clinical specimen
 ** TC : Tetracycline   DOTC : Doxycycline
    OTC : Oxytetracycline

Discussion and Conclusion
    In this study, the different susceptibility to Tetra-
cyclines are significant.
    Martin,[6] et al. and Sapico,[7] et al. confirmed with
C.perfringens the resistance developed to Tetracyclines,
while the analogues Doxycycline and Minocycline are still
active. As is evident also in this study, the resistant
strains of Doxycycline (21 %) were less than Tetracycline
(34 %) and Oxytetracycline(37 %).

    This study is an important evidence since it indica-
tes the start of an evolution of C.perfringens and other
clostridia towards resistance to Tetracyclines. In future,
this phenomenon will be seen with another antibiotics.

Reference
  1) Kosakai, N. and Suzuki, S.(1968) : Anaerobes and Anae-
     robic infection, p.19-135, Igaku Shoin, Tokyo.
  2) Miwa, T., et al.(1974) : Clostridia isolated from the
     Antarctic soil , Reports of the 4th anaerobic infection
     research meeting, Esai, Tokyo, 4, 50-52.
  3) Miwa, T.,et al.(1975) : Distribution of aerobes and
     anaerobes isolated from the Antarctic soil, Reports
     of the 5th anaerobic infection research meeting, Esai,
     Tokyo, 5 (in print).
  4) Miwa, T.(1975) : Clostridia in soil of the Antarctica,
     Japan J. Med. Sci. Biol., 28 (in print).
  5) Miwa, T., et al.(1975) : Susceptibility of Clostridium
     perfringens isolated from the Antarctic soil against
     antibacterial agents, Medicine and Biology, 91, 455-
     460.
  6) Martin, W.J., et al. (1972) : In vitro antimicrobial
     susceptibility of anaerobic bacteria isolated from
     clinical specimens, Antimicr. Agents Chemoth., 1,
     148-158.
  7) Sapico, F.L., et al.(1972) : Standardized antimicro-
     bial disc susceptibility of Clostridium perfringens
     to nine antibiotics, Antimicr. Agents Chemoth., 2,
     320-325.

BRIEF ANTIBIOTIC EXPOSURE AND EFFECT ON BACTERIAL GROWTH

P.J. McDonald*, W.A. Craig, C.M. Kunin

Department of Medicine, University of Wisconsin and
Veterans Administration Hospital, Madison,
Wisconsin, U.S.A.
*Flinders University School of Medicine, Bedford Park,
 South Australia 5042

SUMMARY

The effects of Staph.aureus and E.coli of 0.5 to 4 hrs antibiotic treatment have been examined. A period of growth suppression after removal of antibiotic from broth cultures was docu-
mented with penicillin, ampicillin, cephalothin, erythromycin,
tetracycline, and clindamycin. This post-antibiotic effect was
related to time of treatment with the penicillins, erythromycin
and clindamycin.

Increasing penicillin concentration beyond .05 mcg/ml failed
to prolong post-antibiotic suppression whereas a dose-related
effect was observed with erythromycin and clindamycin. Persistent
effect of gentamicin could not be demonstrated.

INTRODUCTION

Animal infections can be successfully treated with penicillin
dosage regimens which do not achieve effective levels of drug in
tissue for the whole of the dosage interval (Eagle et al, 1953).
Continuous antimicrobial activity resulting from intermittent
exposure to antibiotic has been attributed to the phenomenon of
post-antibiotic growth suppression (Eagle, 1949; Parker and Luse,
1948). This phenomenon refers to a period of bacteriostasis
observed after Penicillin-G is inactivated or removed from cultures to which drug has been added for 15-60 minutes (Parker and
Marsh, 1946). The present study documents and analyses some
factors contributing to post-antibiotic suppression with a
variety of antibiotics.

METHODS

Organisms examined were E.coli A.T.C.C.25922 and Staph.aureus
A.T.C.C. 6538P. Both strains have standard biochemical properties
and are sensitive to all antibiotics studied. In each experiment,
organisms in the phase of logarithmic growth were added to tryptic
soy broth (T.S.B., Difco Laboratories) containing the required
amount of antibiotic. Cultures were disposed in 20 ml aliquots in
centrifuge tubes, and bacterial concentration was 10^4 organisms/ml.

After 0.5 to 4 hours exposure time, bacteria were separated
from antibiotic by centrifugation twice at 15,000 r.p.m. for 10
minutes. Eighteen mls of supernatant were removed after each
centrifugation, and the 20 ml volumes reconstituted with fresh
T.S.B.

Viable bacterial counts were performed hourly during exposure,
and every 1 - $1\frac{1}{2}$ hours thereafter until either turbidity was
marked, or cultures were observed to remain clear over 24 hrs.
In each experiment, a control culture was added to antibiotic-free
medium, and examined in the same way as the antibiotic-treated
culture.

Drugs used were penicillin-G and ampicillin from Bristol
Laboratories, Syracuse, N.Y.; cephalothin and erythromycin from
Eli Lilly Pty. Ltd., Indiannapolis, Ind.; clindamycin from Upjohn
Pty. Ltd., Kalamazoo, Mich.; tetracycline from Lederle division
of American Cyanamid, Pearl River, N.Y.; and gentamicin from
Schering Corp., Kenilworth, N.J. Estimations of minimal inhibi-
tion concentration (M.I.C.) were performed according to the method
described by Washington and Barry (1974).

RESULTS

The effects on E.coli of 2 hours treatment with five times
the M.I.C. of ampicillin are shown in Fig.1. After removal of
antibiotic there was a period of bacteriostasis before regrowth
occurred. A similar effect was observed with penicillin-G and
Staph.aureus (Fig.2). Normal logarithmic growth of both organisms
had always resumed by the time the treated culture increased in
viable count by one $\log_{10}$ over the count after centrifugation.

Calculations used to quantitate the effects of antibiotic
are shown in Fig. 2. These are:-

   - T_1 the time in hours for the antibiotic-treated culture
        to increase in viable count by one $\log_{10}$ above the
        original inoculum.

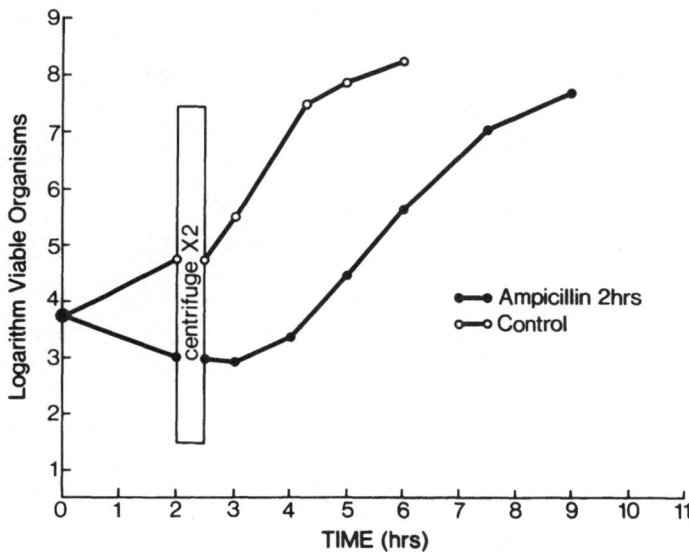

<u>Fig.1</u> The effects of E.coli of 2 hrs treatment with five times the M.I.C. of ampicillin are shown in the lower graph. Control culture not exposed to antibiotic shown in upper graph

- T_2 the time in hours for the antibiotic-treated culture to increase in viable count by one $\log_{10}$ above the count after centrifugation.

- C_1 the time in hours for the control culture to increase one $\log_{10}$ above inoculum, and

- C_2 the time in hours for the control culture to increase in viable count by one $\log_{10}$ above the count after centrifugation.

T_2 is considered to measure post-antibiotic growth suppression whereas T_1 includes the effects of antibiotic during and after treatment.

Calculations of the effects on <u>Staph.aureus</u> of five times the M.I.C. of penicillin, cephalothin, erythromycin, clindamycin, tetracycline and gentamicin are shown in Table 1. Except for gentamicin, each of the antibiotics has a T_2 value in excess of C_2, indicating a persistent effect of antibiotic after removal of

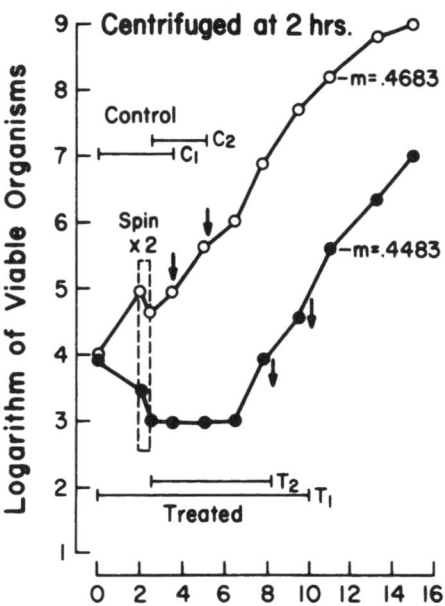

<u>Fig. 2</u> The effects on Staph.aureus of 2 hrs treatment with
five times the M.I.C. of penicillin-G are shown on
lower graph. Control culture is shown on upper graph.
T_2 indicates period of growth inhibition

<u>TABLE 1</u>

<u>EFFECTS OF STAPH.AUREUS OF 2 HRS TREATMENT
WITH A VARIETY OF ANTIBIOTICS</u>

Antibiotic	Concentration (mcg/ml)	T_1 (hrs)	T_2 (hrs)
Penicillin-G	.05	10.0	5.7
Cephalothin	0.5	8.1	4.0
Erythromycin	1.0	8.6	5.8
Clindamycin	0.5	7.7	5.2
Tetracycline	0.5	8.4	5.0
Gentamicin	2.5	9.6	2.5
Control (no antibiotic)		C_1 2.5	C_2 2.6

99% of drug from the medium. Persistence of gentamicin activity after 2 hrs treatment could not be demonstrated against either E.coli or Staph.aureus as shown in Fig.3.

    With the penicillins, erythromycin and clindamycin, increasing the length of treatment from 1 to 4 hours prolonged the phase of post-antibiotic suppression. An example of E.coli treated with ampicillin for 1, 2, 3 and 4 hrs is given in Fig.4. Post-antibiotic suppression after 3 and 4 hrs is greater than after 1 and 2 hrs. Calculations of T_1 and T_2 for increasing periods of penicillin-G (.05 mcg/ml) against Staph.aureus are shown in Table 2.

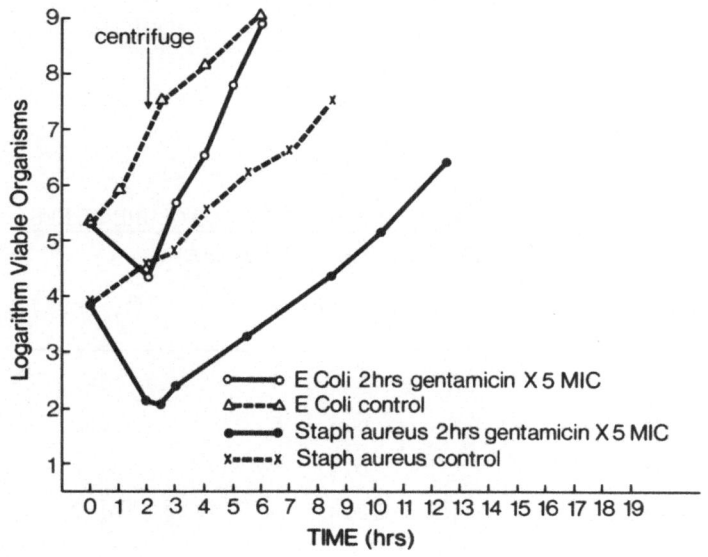

Fig.3 The effect of 2 hrs treatment with five times the M.I.C. of gentamicin is shown for E.coli on upper pair of graphs and Staph.aureus on lower pair of graphs

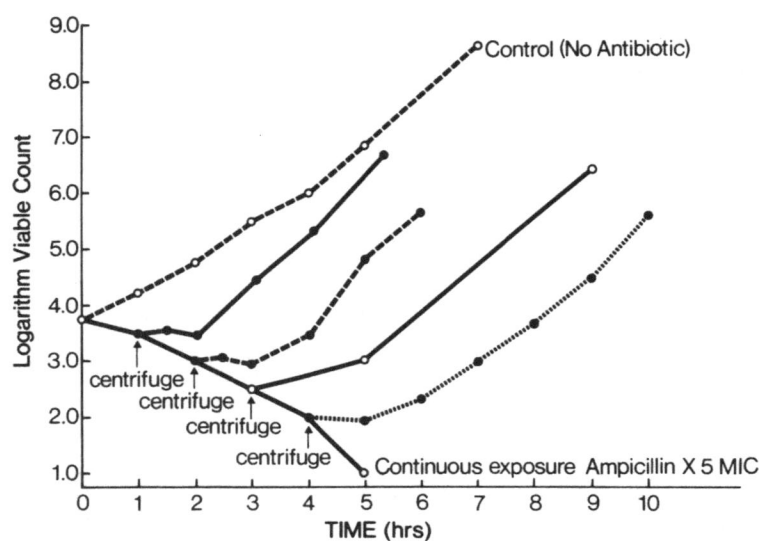

Fig. 4 The effects of E.coli of 1,2,3 and 4 hrs treatment
with ampicillin, five times M.I.C.

TABLE 2

EFFECTS ON STAPH.AUREUS OF VARYING EXPOSURE TIMES
TO PENICILLIN-G, .05 mcg/ml

Exposure	T_1 (hrs)	T_2 (hrs)
30 min	4.8	3.1
1 hr	6.3	4.2
2 hrs	8.4	4.9
4 hrs	12.4	6.0

Increasing treatment time with erythromycin, tetracycline and clindamycin was also associated with prolongation of T_1 and T_2.

The effects of concentration varied according to the group of antibiotic. Penicillin-G was increasingly active against Staph.aureus up to a threshold of .05 mcg/ml. Higher concentrations did not prolong the post-antibiotic T_2 value beyond approximately 5.5 hrs.

Concentrations of erythromycin from 0.01 mcg/ml to 1.0 mcg/ml were associated with a proportional increase in T_2 from 2.3 to 5.7 hrs for treatment of Staph.aureus for two hours. A similar concentration-dependence was observed for clindamycin and tetracycline.

DISCUSSION

These experiments have confirmed the observations of Parker and Eagle with Penicillin-G, and shown that other penicillins, cephalosporins, erythromycin, clindamycin and tetracycline also have an anti-bacterial effect which persists after organisms have been removed from antibiotic milieu. This persistent action may represent recovery phase from non-lethal damage such as interference with cell wall synthesis. Alternatively, drug may become "fixed" intracellularly and continue to exert an effect even though it cannot be detected extracellularly. The varying propensity of antibiotics to have a persistent effect most likely relates to their differing modes of action. The failure of gentamicin to product post-antibiotic suppression can be explained by the irreversible and lethal attachment of aminoglycosides to their site of action (Weisblum and Davies, 1968). The prolonged T_1 value for gentamicin shown in Table 1 is due entirely to the profound bactericidal activity during treatment, and this compensates for the lack of post-antibiotic effect.

The net result of a limited exposure to antibiotic can be calculated by applying the data described herein to pharmacokinetic information. Following a standard dose of penicillin-G, tissue concentrations are in excess of .05 mcg/ml for approximately 4 hrs (Tan et al, 1972). Using data from Table 2 an exposure of Staph.aureus to penicillin-G for 4 hrs would result in a T_1 value of approximately 12 hours. If the growth time for 1 $\log_{10}$ (2.5 hrs or C_1) is deducted from this T_1 value, then the time for which a single dose of penicillin is essentially bacteriostatic can be determined (9.5 hrs).

This type of data could be employed to determine optimal dosage intervals. With bacteriostatic agents such as erythromycin, there seems little point in reducing dosage frequency below that which takes account of effects both during and after antibiotic exposure. Frequency of dosage with bactericidal agents, however, could be manipulated to achieve a wide range of antibacterial effects. Preliminary data suggests that when bacteria have been re-exposed to antibiotic (after T_1 interval) their response is similar to that observed with initial treatment.

The purpose of this study has been to document and analyse the post-antibiotic effect. A method has been shown for determining the "total" effect on bacteria of a limited exposure to antibiotic and it is seen that these effects vary widely between the classes of antibiotic. This information can be used to resolve the clinical dilemma of the contribution of peak, trough and mean serum levels in determining successful outcome of chemotherapy.

REFERENCES

1. Eagle, H. (1949) The recovery of bacteria from the toxic effects of penicillin. J.Clin.Investigation, 28, 2, 832.

2. Eagle, H., Fleischman, R., Levy, M. (1953) "Continuous" vs "Discontinuous" therapy with penicillin; effect of interval between injections on therapeutic efficiency. New England J.Med., 248, 481.

3. Parker, R.F., Luse, S. (1948) The action of penicillin on Staphylococcus: Further observations on effect of short exposure. J.Bacteriol., 56, 75.

4. Parker, R.F., Marsh, M.C. (1946) The action of penicillin on Staphylococcus. J.Bacteriol., 51, 181.

5. Tan, J.S., Trott, A., Phair, J.P., Watanakunakorn, C. (1972) A method for measurement of antibiotics in human interstitial fluid. J.Inf.Dis., 126, 5, 492.

6. Washington, J.A., Barry, A.L. (1974) "Dilution test procedures" in Manual of Clinical Microbiology, 2nd ed. Editors Lenette, E.H., Spalding, E.H., Truant, J.P. Published by American Society of Microbiology, Washington, D.C., 410.

7. Weisblum, B., Davies, J. (1968) Antimicrobial inhibitors of the bacterial ribosome. Bact.Rev., 32, Suppl. 493.

TRIMETHOPRIM AND RIFAMPICIN : IN VITRO ACTIVITIES SEPARATELY AND IN COMBINATION

D.W. Kerry, J.M.T. Hamilton-Miller and
W. Brumfitt

The Royal Free Hospital
Pond Street, Hampstead, London NW3 2QG

Rifampicin (rif) and trimethoprim (tm) are familiar broad-spectrum oral antimicrobial agents. Both drugs owe their antibacterial activity primarily to their effect on the biosynthesis of nucleic acids. Their target sites may thus be regarded as occurring on the same metabolic pathway; sequential blockade of a metabolic pathway has been shown to result in a potentially synergistic situation. Consequently, we tested rif and tm in combination, to investigate possible antibacterial interactions.

MATERIALS AND METHODS

Each drug was tested against a total of 386 strains of common hospital pathogens recently isolated by our routine bacteriology laboratory. The MIC of the drugs was determined by inoculating 200-300 viable units of each strain onto Wellcotest Sensitivity Agar containing appropriate dilutions. MIC was taken as that concentration of the drug which inhibited growth or allowed less than 2-3 colonies to grow (99% inhibition) after overnight incubation.

To test the drugs in combination, a series of concentrations of each compound in the presence of a range of concentrations of the other was prepared. Organisms were inoculated and end-points read as above. The results were interpreted by the use of isobolograms (Sabath 1967; Kerry et al 1975). The interaction of the two drugs can be seen in the shape of the isobol; a straight line connecting the two MIC's indicates addition, a concave line implies synergy and a convex line shows antagonism. We judged synergy or antagonism to have occurred if any value of ΣFIC (Elion et al 1954) was 0.7 or less on one hand or 1.3 or more on the other, respectively.

RESULTS AND DISCUSSION

Trimethoprim may reach blood levels of approximately 3-4 μg/ml during continuous therapy (Brumfitt et al 1969). Pseudomonas aeruginosa and Bacteroides fragilis were the only two species which we found required substantially higher concentrations of tm than these for inhibition; mean MIC for these two species were 670 μg/ml and 33 μg/ml respectively. For the Proteus spp. tested, MIC were close to or only slightly greater than blood levels. Our results with this species are 2-4 times higher than those found by other authors (Reisberg et al 1967; Darrell et al 1968; Reeves et al 1969); the discrepancy may be due to methodological differences. All the other organisms tested, with the exception of a few Klebsiella aerogenes and streptococcal strains, had MIC less than 2 μg/ml and in most cases were considerably more sensitive than this.

Rifampicin is intrinsically more active, the least sensitive species being Ps.aeruginosa, but even here the maximum MIC which we found was 30 μg/ml (for one strain only). A few K.aerogenes strains also reached this figure. These were the only strains which exceeded the blood level of approximately 20 μg/ml found after a 600 mg dose of rif (Binda et al 1971). All other K.aerogenes, Escherichia coli, Enterobacter spp., Proteus spp., Salmonella typhimurium and Strept. faecalis strains have MIC values for rif ranging from 1 to 10 μg/ml. Staphylococcus aureus strains have a narrow range of MIC's around 0.02 μg/ml, and MIC against Strept. pyogenes and B.fragilis strains are spread from 0.01 to 0.1 and 0.1 to 1.0 μg/ml respectively.

Combined Activity

Table 1 gives the percentage of each species tested which showed synergism. All the streptococcal strains showed synergy, the degree of which (as expressed by the minimum observed ⨋FIC) was greater than for any other species. The Proteus spp. tested also have a high percentage of strains which exhibit synergism with this combination. Most of the other species show synergism or addition, while E.coli and Salm. typhimurium showed mainly an additive effect. Staph. aureus strains all showed some degree of antagonism, but only at very low concentrations of rif, where the MIC of tm was raised by a maximum of 2-fold.

Resistance

A relatively high proportion of rif-resistant mutants exists in any microbial population. This may lead to the rapid emergence of a rif-resistant population during therapy, or cause relapses after short-term treatment. We tested several bacterial strains and found a mutation rate to high-level rif-resistance (MIC >1 mg/ml) of between 1 in 10 million and 1 in 100 million, for Gram-negative strains, and for Gram-positive strains from 1 in 1 million to 1 in 10 million. The rate is fairly constant at a number of rif concentrations, which suggests a single-step mutation to high-level resistance.

The rif-resistant mutants retained the sensitivity to tm of the parent strain; thus it was to be expected that the outgrowth of such mutants should be prevented by the concomitant presence of sub-inhibitory levels of tm. We found that concentrations of tm ranging from 0.1 MIC upwards did indeed cause a substantial decrease in the apparent incidence of rif-resistant mutants (Table 2). The effect of up to 0.5 MIC of tm on the mutation rate of E.coli and K.aerogenes strains was not as great as the other strains, causing a 3 to 5 fold decrease. Increasing amounts of tm caused dramatic decreases in the apparent incidence of mutants in the other species tested, up to 0.5 MIC of tm causing a greater than 10 fold decrease in the rate, to a point which was not measurable (i.e. less than 1 in 10,000 million).

SUMMARY

The in vitro interaction between rifampicin and trimethoprim is favourable in terms of synergistic activity against many pathogenic bacterial species, and in suppressing the outgrowth of rifampicin-resistant mutants. We suggest that this combination warrants further investigation.

Table 1.   Strains Showing Synergy

Organism	No. Tested	%age Showing Synergy
Strept. faecalis	20	100
Strept. pyogenes	24	100
Prot. morganii	12	92
Prot. rettgeri	12	92
Prot. mirabilis	32	72
Prot. vulgaris	16	56
Pseudo. aeruginosa	20	45
Bact. fragilis	19	37
Kleb. aerogenes	40	35
Enterobacter spp.	13	23
Esch. coli	48	4
Salm. typhimurium	24	–
Staph. aureus	24	–

304

Table 2.   Effect of tm on the rate of mutation to rif-resistance.

	%age of Rif-Resistant Mutants Capable of Growing in Indicated Fraction of MIC of Tm		
Organism	0.1	0.2	0.5
Kleb. aerogenes		47	18
Esch. coli		57	36
Ent. cloacae		10	<5
Prot. rettgeri	50	38	<13
Prot. morganii	40	20	<20
Pseudo. aeruginosa	30	15	<15
Bact. fragilis	55	<2.5	
Staph. aureus		80	<2.5
Strept. faecalis		10	<1.5

REFERENCES

Binda, G., Domenichini, E., Gottardi, A., Orlandi, B., Ortelli, E., Pacini, B. & Fowst, C. 1971 Arzneimittel-Forschung, 21, 1907.

Brumfitt, W., Faiers, M.C., Pursell, R.E., Reeves, D.S. & Turnbull, A.R. 1969 Postgrad.Med.J. Suppl. 45, 56.

Darrell, J.H., Garrod, L.P. & Waterworth, P.M. 1968 J.Clin.Path., 21, 202.

Elion, G.V., Singer, S. & Hitchings, C.H. 1954 J.Biol.Chem., 208, 477.

Kerry, D.W., Hamilton-Miller, J.M.T. & Brumfitt, W. 1975 J. Antimicrob.Chemotherapy. In press.

Reeves, D.S., Faiers, M.C., Pursell, R.E. & Brumfitt, W. 1969 Brit.Med.J., 1, 541.

Reisberg, B., Hertzog, J. & Weinstein, L. 1967 Antimicrob. Agents Chemotherapy-1966, 424.

Sabath, L.D. 1968 Antimicrob. Agents Chemotherapy-1967, 210.

A^{125}I-BASED RADIOIMMUNOASSAY FOR SERUM GENTAMICIN

R.A.A. Watson*, E.J. Shaw+ and C.R.W. Edwards*

* Dept of Chemical Pathology, St. Bartholomew's Hospital

+ Dept of Bacteriology, St. Bartholomew's Hospital,
  London E.C.1.

SUMMARY: A radioimmunoassay for serum gentamicin, based on a ^{125}I labelled tracer and specific antibodies raised against a gentamicin – human serum albumin conjugate has been developed.

Gentamicin is a useful broad spectrum antibiotic which, however, can also be oto- and nephrotoxic. Thus, the availability of a reliable and rapid assay is an important adjunct to its use, especially in patients with impaired renal function.

Three groups have developed radioimmunoassays for gentamicin suitable for clinical application (Lewis et al., 1972; Mahon et al., 1973; Minshew et al., 1975). The assays employ tritrated gentamicin as tracer, which has the serious disadvantages for routine use of requiring costly liquid scintillant, vials and counting equipment, the need for prolonged counting times if error is to be kept within acceptable limits, and tedious preparation of samples for counting. These disadvantages are, of course, shared by adenylation and acetylation enzyme assays, which use ^{3}H or ^{14}C tracers. It was decided therefore, to develop a RIA based on an ^{125}I tracer.

Pure standards are readily available for most drugs; however, gentamicin is an exception, since it is a mixture of three compounds, gentamicins C_{1a}, C_1 and C_2. This problem is considered later. Nicholas reference standard, batch no. GMC-4-X-6007, was used in this study. Donkey antirabbit serum, Wellcome batch no K. 9437 was used to separate the bound and free fractions. The antibody-bound component was precipitated by centrifugation and counted.

Antisera were raised in New Zealand White rabbits by immunization with gentamicin and human serum albumin, conjugated with carbodiimide

(Khorana, 1953; Sheehan and Hlavka, 1956). Rabbits were immunized and boosted with aliquots of conjugate emulsified in Freund's complete adjuvant and administered intradermally at multiple sites at approximately monthly intervals for six months. Two rabbits gave satisfactory antisera.

Gentamicin contains no reactive groups which can be iodinated and it was therefore, first necessary to conjugate the drug to a protein to produce a complex for this purpose. Glutaraldehyde (Reichlin et al., 1968; Habeeb and Hiramoto, 1968) was used to conjugate gentamicin to lysozyme; aliquots were iodinated by the chloramine-T method (Greenwood et al., 1963) and subsequently purified by Sephadex column chromatography.

Several conjugates have now been iodinated once by this procedure and one conjugate several times. In each case, 45 to 60% of the purified tracer was bound by antibody excess, and the specific activity of the tracer was approximately 50 μCi/ug.

Since gentamicin circulates in the μg per ml range and RIA's are commonly used to measure compounds circulating in the nanogram or picogram per ml range, sensitivity was not a problem in setting up this assay.

Interference from other antibiotics is a problem with gentamicin bioassays but non of the antibiotics listed in Table 1 showed any cross-reaction in the assay even when tested at levels of up to 5mg. per ml. Thus, gentamicin can be accurately measured in the presence of any of these compounds.

TABLE 1

Non-Cross-Reacting Antibiotics

Clindamycin	Oxytetracycline
Neomycin	Cephalothin
Kanamycin	Chloramphenicol
Tobramycin	Benzylpenicillin
Lincomycin	Cloxacillin
Streptomycin	Flucloxacillin
Carbenecillin	Cephaloridine
Methicillin	

Gentamicin is a mixture of three compounds, each of which is indistinguishable in this assay from the pharmaceutical mixture. Samples can, therefore, be readily assayed for total gentamicin concentration.

Twenty-five gentamicin-free sera were assayed to check for non-specific effects which might simulate gentamicin in the assay. No such effects were found.

Doubling dilutions of a serum sample containing high endogenous levels of gentamicin gave parallel inhibition of binding to that observed in this standard curve

Thus, the material determined as gentamicin in patient samples is immunologically identical to the standard used. Samples from two patients were each assayed 20 times to determine the precision of the assay. The low sample gave a coefficient of variation of 7.9%, and the high sample of value of 4.1%.

The recovery of know samples of gentamicin made up in serum over the range 0.5--16 µg/ml was 92--110%, indicated a satisfactory recovery.   The computer-calculated line of best fit was indistinguishable from the line of equivalence with an r value of more than 99%.

The correlation between RIA results and those obtained with a well-type agar diffusion assay is shown in Figure 3. The correlation between assay results was reasonable, but the accuracy of the RIA when know amounts of gentamicin were assayed was much better than the correlation between the two assay methods. The accuracy and precision of the bioassay compared unfavourably with that of the RIA and the inaccuracy of the bioassay may well explain the spread between bioassay and RIA results.

Finally the ^{125}I gentamicin assay compares well in terms of practicality with other assay methods. Results can be obtained in under 5 hours, and this will be reduced still further. Technology is now available to automate the assay when this is justified by sample throughput. Sample capacity of even the manual RIA is high; assays of 100 or 200 samples can be easily performed. Only 15 ul, or less, of serum are required. Since the protein, rather than gentamicin itself, is iodinated, the tracer does not readily lose immunoreactivity on storage. Therefore, frequent iodinations are not required.

REFERENCES

1. Greenwood, F.C., Hunter, W.M. & Glover, J.S.
    (1963) Biochem. J. 89, 114.

2. Habeeb, A. & Hiramoto, R.
    (1968) Arch. Biochem. Biophys, 126, 16.

3. Khorana, J.G.
    (1953) Chem. Rev. 53, 145.

4. Lewis, J.E., Nelson, J.C. & Elder H.A.
    (1972) Nature N. Biol. 239, 214-216.

5. Mahon, W.A., Ezer, J. & Wilson, T.W.
    (1972) Antimicrob. Agents Chemother. 3, 585.

6. Minshew, B.H., Holmes, R.K. & Baxter, C.R.
    (1975) Antimicrob. Agents Chemother. 7, 107.

7. Reichlin, M., Schnurr, J.J. & Vance, V.K.
    (1968) Proc. Soc. Exper. Biol. Med. 128, 347.

8. Sheehan, J.C. & Hlavka, J.J.
    (1956) J. Org. Chem. 21, 439.

FLUORIMETRIC ASSAY OF TETRACYCLINE MIXTURES IN PLASMA

D. Hall

Dept. of Clinical Pharmacology, St. Bartholomew's

Hospital London EC1A 7BE, U.K.

SUMMARY: A fluorimetric technique is described for the analysis of mixtures of tetracyclines in plasma. The method is capable of accurately measuring the individual levels of each tetracycline present in the therapeutic range, to as low as 0.1 mg/L or less. In operation it is simple and inexpensive to perform, consisting of only two or three basic steps: (1) Conversion of the tetracyclines into a fluorescent form by simple acid hydrolysis, or where appropriate, by alkaline degradation, (2) intensification of the fluorescence, where necessary, by complexation with aluminium, and (3) measurement in a spectrofluorimeter.

No extractions or separations of the component tetracyclines are required, and a batch of ten samples, each containing three tetracyclines, can be assayed in as little as three hours, a procedure which cannot be performed using current microbiological methods.

The tetracycline group of antibiotics are capable, after suitable simple chemical alterations, of exhibiting fluorescent properties. Tetracyclines bearing an OH group at C_6 (this includes all of the commonly used tetracyclines, with the exceptions of minocycline and doxycycline, can be readily hydrolysed by heating in dilute acid to produce the respective anhydro-salt, (Boothe et al., 1953). This consists of an equilibrium mixture of two tautomers, due to keto-enol tautomerism at C_{11} and C_{12}, one of which is fluorescent and can be used as a basis for the measurement of the amount of tetracycline present in a sample.

Due to structural differences between the different tetracyclines, the arrangement of chemical groups around the fluorescent nucleus of the anhydro-salt are different and as a result, each exhibits its own individual spectral characteristics with the fluorescent

excitation and emission peaks of each occurring at different wavelengths. By irradiating these fluorescent structures with light at
the appropriate excitation wavelength in a spectrofluorimeter and
measuring the emitted fluorescence at the peak emission wavelength it
is possible to measure very accurately the amount of tetracycline in
a sample. As each tetracycline has its own "fingerprint" combination
of fluorescent peaks it is possible not only to measure tetracyclines
in the presence of other microbiologically active agents, but also
in the presence of other members of the same homologous series, a
procedure which cannot be achieved by current microbiological techniques without prior separation of the components.

Unfortunately, each tetracycline after undergoing acid hydrolysis
does not produce equally fluorescent anhydro-salts and whereas the
fluorescents of some members of the series, for example oxytetracycline, is sufficiently intense to permit easy measurement of low
concentrations of this antibiotic in plasma (Hall et al 1974), the
fluorescents of other members of the series, such as tetracycline, is
too weak to permit a really sensitive assay technique.

It has been found that by utilising the chelating properties of
the tetracyclines to metal ions by directly complexing the anhydro-
salts with aluminium, large increases in their intrinsic fluorescense
are produced (Hall 1975). All the tetracycline anhydro-salts respond
to this procedure to produce an intensified fluorescents, permitting
an easier and more accurate measurement of small quantities of the
tetracyclines and thereby improving assay sensitivity. Using this
simple technique it has been found possible to accurately measure
concentrations of the tetracyclines in the therapeutic range to as
low as 0.1 mg/L or less.

An alternative method of improving assay sensitivity, which can
be used for chlortetracycline is to produce the strongly fluorescent
iso-chlortetracycline salt by alkaline degradation of the chlortetracycline nucleus. The resulting assay sensitivity is then sufficiently
high to obviate the necessity for intensification of the fluorescence
by aluminium complexation.

The assay of individual tetracyclines using fluorimetry is a
relatively simple procedure, however problems can arise when
measurement is required of combinations of tetracyclines in
admixture. The fluorescence spectrum of a compound consists of an
excitation and emission curve, and although maximum fluorescence is
observed when the compound is irradiated with light at the peak
excitation wavelength, there is a narrow range of, perhaps, 20-30nm
either side of this peak value over which a fluorescent response can
still be elicited. If two structurally closely related tetracyclines
exhibit similar fluorescent characteristics so that parts of their
spectral curves overlap, then they produce "interfering" fluorescence
during the measurement of each other. If this occurs, allowance has

to be made for the simultaneous presence of the "interfering" tetracycline during estimation of the tetracycline concentrations in a mixture.

For example, it was found during a study in which plasma samples containing chlortetracycline, demethylchlortetracycline and tetracycline were to be measured, that chlortetracycline interfered with the measurement of the other two compounds. This was verified by studying the superimposed spectra of demethylchlortetracycline, chlortetracycline and tetracycline at the wavelengths used for the measurement of demethylchlortetracycline (385nm, 485 nm) and tetracycline (465nm, 555nm) respectively. These superimposed spectra showed clearly that there was a significant contribution of aluminium complexed chlortetracycline at the measurement wavelengths of the other two compounds. As there were no other interferences between the three compounds and chlortetracycline could be measured without any difficulty, the problem could be easily solved by calibrating for the contributive effect of chlortetracycline upon the remaining two tetracyclines at their measurement wavelengths. (The amount of "contributed fluorescence" by chlortetracycline was found to be a function of concentration of chlortetracycline only over the therapeutic range (0-10mg/L) and independent of concentrations of the other tetracyclines present). Consequently, after calibrating for this contribution, allowance could be made for the presence of chlortetracycline in each sample and the correct results could be calculated.

The precise method for measuring individual tetracyclines in combinations therefore depends upon the constituent tetracyclines in that mixture. Mutual interferences in measurement may or may not occur, depending upon the relative positions of the excitation and emission curves of the tetracyclines involved. Such possible interferences must be studied before each particular combination is measured.

Despite this problem of interference which can arise from combination of certain tetracyclines in a mixture, no serious interference due to the presence of other microbiologically or pharmacologically active agents has been observed. This is in part due to the limited range of such agents which can exhibit fluorescence, and because of the selectivity of the combinations of peak excitation and emission wavelengths used.

The precision of this technique was evaluated by a blind determination of a series of prepared test plasma standards containing chlortetracycline, demethylchlortetracycline and tetracycline in admixture. Six estimations of each standard were performed, and the results of the determinations, with the corresponding coefficients of variation of the results are presented in Table 1.

TABLE 1

Assay test results

Plasma standard	Added	Mean Found	%Recovery	Coefficient of variation
Chlortetracycline				
A	1.4mg/L	1.382mg/L	98.7	3.2
B	0.2	0.165	82.5	5.0
C	0.7	0.715	102.1	1.2
Demethylchlortetracycline				
A	0.3	0.313	104.3	20.3
B	1.4	1.385	98.9	5.8
C	0.7	0.69	98.6	10.1
Tetracycline				
A	0.8	0.776	97	3.7
B	0.4	0.383	95.7	2.0
C	1.6	1.512	94.5	2.1

Although it can be seen that the variation in measurement of the lowest concentrations of demethylchlortetracylcine (one of the least fluorescent of the tetracyclines) was found to be high (20.3%), in numberical terms this represents a maximum variation of only 0.06mg/L either side of the true value of 0.3mg/L, a deviation which for most purposes may be considered adequate.

To determine the correlation of this purely physico-chemical approach to tetracycline assay to the biological activity of these antibiotics, a comparison was performed using this fluorimetric method to determine plasma concentrations of samples containing a single tetracycline, oxytetracycline, and comparing the results obtained with those found using a large plate agar diffusion micro-biological assay. The results from the two methods were found to be very closely related (r = 0,98,∅=51) (Hall et al. 1974)and the method can therefore be considered to give a direct indication of tetracycline microbiological activity, as related to the amount of chemical component present.

REFERENCES

1. Boothe, J.H., Morton II, J., Petisi, J.P., Wilkinson, R.G., Williams, J.H. (1953) J. Am. Chem. Soc., 75, 4621.
2. Hall, D., O'Grady, F., Turner,P.(1974)J. Pharm.Pharmacol.,26,Su 117
3. Hall, D. (1975), J. Pharm. Pharmacol., in press.

ASSAY OF ANTIBIOTICS

WITH AGAR DIFFUSION TECHNIQUE

Anna-Stina Malmborg

Department of Clinical Microbiology

Huddinge Hospital, Huddinge, Sweden

Laboratory control of antibiotic treatment may be necessary both to ensure therapeutic concentrations, and to avoid toxic side effects in the patients. There is thus a great need in clinical practice for simple and reliable methods for the analysis of antibiotic concentrations in plasma and other body fluids. Quantitative determinations of antibiotic concentrations is often made by microbiological assay techniques and the agar diffusion method is frequently used. The antibiotic in the test sample is allowed to diffuse from a centre towards the periphery. The growth of a test strain is inhibited in a concentric zone around the centre. At the Karolinska Hospital in Stockholm, Sweden, we started many years ago to use filter paper discs as diffusion centres. The principles for the method have been known from the beginning of the antibiotic era, and different variants have been described (Jalling et al 1972, the publication contains a list of references).

The present paper evaluates the paper disc method for quantitative determination of antibiotics in body fluids like serum, plasma, sinus secretion, pleural fluid and seminal fluid. The possibilty to assay individual antibiotics during combined treatment is also investigated (Malmborg 1974).

Paper Disc Micromethod

The aim was to develop a system for studies of pharmacokinetics, especially in neonates, and for laboratory control of therapy in neonatal septicaemia. For this purpose a paper disc micromethod was worked out (Jalling et al 1972). The method allows the use of small samples, and frequent sampling. Capillary blood can be taken from fingertips by means of heparinized capillary tubes. Ten ul of plasma is withdrawn from the capillary tube by means of a micropipette, and put on paper discs (5.5 mm in diameter).

The culture media and the test strains vary with the antibiotics used. The bacteria are either flooded on the agar surface to produce a dense but not completely confluent growth, or the bacteria are seeded into the agar. At least two discs with the material to be tested are placed on the agar surface together with a series of standard discs. The standard discs are prepared from dilutions of known standard solutions of the antibiotic to be tested.

After incubation of the plate over night the inhibition zones around the discs are measured with a sliding caliper. A standard curve is plotted, and the values obtained with the patients discs are extrapolated from the curve. The diameters of the standard discs and of the patient discs may also be fed into a computer, which immediately gives the antibiotic concentration of the test samples.

Errors can be introduced into the agar diffusion method by variations in agar depth and in inoculation. With increasing agar depth the zone size decreases. A dense inoculum of the test strain gives smaller inhibition zones. The errors can be avoided if a standard series is used on each plate. The test samples and the standard series will then be equally affected.

Standards

Errors may obviously be introduce into the assay if adequate standard curves are not used (Kaplan et al 1973). it is well-known that the binding of penicillin to serum proteins varies considerably between animal species (Rolinson and Sutherland 1965). When anti-biotic concentrations are determined in human serum or plasma it is important to dissolve also the standard in human serum or plasma. Botaining adequate standards is more difficult when the concentration is measured in other body fluids and tissues. For ethical and practical reasons it is often not possible to puncture and aspirate from the foci frequently enough to obtain sufficient quantities for adequate standard curves. A careful evaluation must be made if a medium other than the specimen is used for preparing

the standard curve (Kaplan et al 1973). For example in the present
study horse serum was evaluated as a substitute for sinus mucosa
and for sinus secretion (Malmborg 1974).

     Figure 1 shows that horse serum is not a valid substitute
when assaying penicillin G and penicillin V. At large zone
diameters the calculated penicillin concentrations are 0.3 to 0.7
ug/ml higher using standard curves for horse serum compared to
curves for sinus secretion.

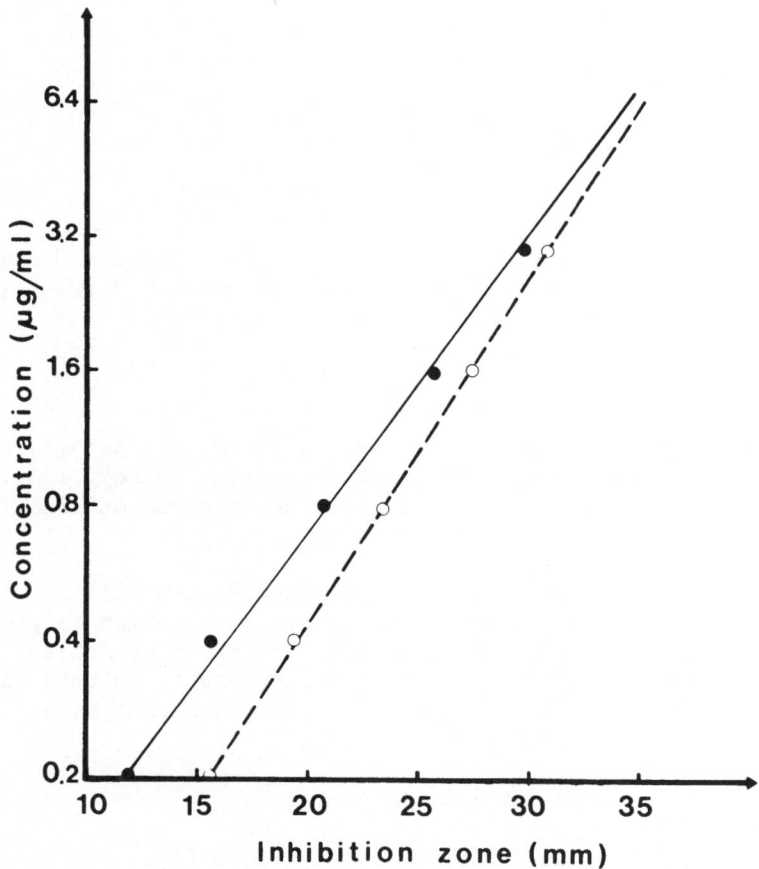

Figure 1. Standard curves for benzylpenicillin dissolved
in horse serum (•——•) and in pooled sinus secretion
(o——o).

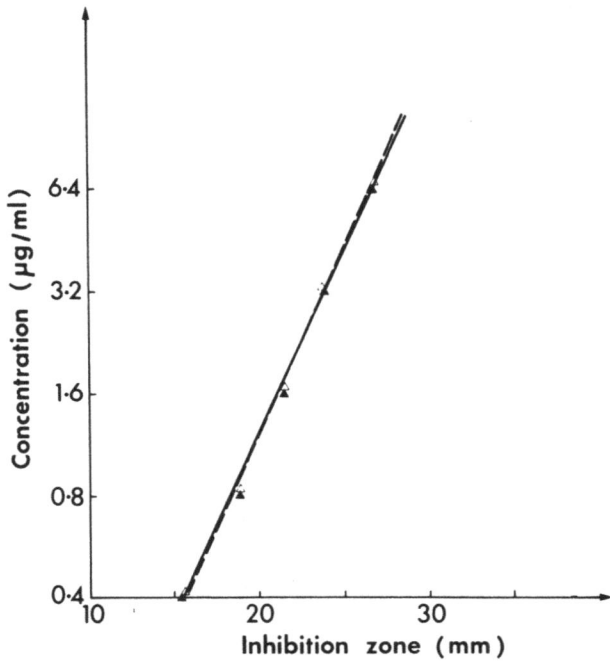

Figure 2.   Standard curves for tetracycline dissolved in horse
serum (▲——————▲) and in pooled sinus secretion (△———△).

Figure 2 shows that, in contrast to penicillin assays, horse
serum is an acceptable substitute when assaying tetracycline.
Standard series of tetracycline made in horse serum and in sinus
secretion give almost identical curves.

The reason for the difference obtained in penicillin
concentrations between horse serum and sinus secretion is probably
that serum has a lower protein content than sinus secretion.
The same error does not occur with tetracycline since both test
sample and standard are diluted 1:3 in potassium phosphate.
Thereby the protein binding decreases.

Statistical Analysis

Few statistical data for the paper disc diffusion method
have been published (Bell et al 1969). The 95 per cent confidence
interval of the standard curves has been calculated for each

antibiotic used in the present study (Malmborg 1974). The results
are acceptable for scientific and practical work. With two standard
series the accuracy of the determination is improved. For example,
using 2 standard series the confidence interval is; ampicillin $\pm$ 15%,
cloxacillin $\pm$ 8%, and rifampcin, streptomycin and tetracycline
$\pm$ 3%.

Assay of Antibiotics given in Combination

The use of antibiotics in combination is common when treating
severe infections. The assay method should therefore allow
determination of each antibiotic in the combination. Three
seperation procedures were used for the determination of the
antibiotics when two or more of the drugs were given in combination.

1. Microbiological determination with bacterial test strains
selected to be sensitive to only one of the drugs. The procedure
is well-known. But the method may fail when the antibiotics are
closely related to each other e.g. various pencillins.

2. Microbiological determination subsequent to chemical
inactivation of all drugs but one. Example of inactivators which
can be added to the culture medium: penicillinase to eliminate
penicillins, semicarbazide to eliminate streptomycin, magnesium
sulphate to eliminate tetracycline and PABA to eliminate sulphonamide.

3. Microbiological determination following separation of the
antibiotics by high voltage electrophoresis. The present work
started with separation of cloxacillin and ampicillin in plasma
(Carlström et al, 1974). Plasma samples of 10 ul are applied
to a Whatman paper, and the high voltage electrophoresis is made
during 90 minutes. After the electrophoresis the paper is placed
on an agar layer seeded with a test strain and incubated over
night. The paper is then removed, and the plate is stained to
visualize the inhibition zones. The diameter of the inhibition
zones is measured. The concentrations of the test samples are
determined from a standard curve, which is calculated from a
standard series on the same plate as the test samples (Figure 3).
Cloxacillin has a high affinity for albumin in plasma. Due to
this affinity the inhibition zones are seriously distorted after
separation by high voltage electrophoresis. This effect is
compensated for digestion of the plasma proteins by trypsin before
the electrophoresis. This separation method has recently been
made more convenient for routine work (Carlström et al 1975). The
electrophoresis is made in agarose-gel to separate the drugs before
the microbiological assay.

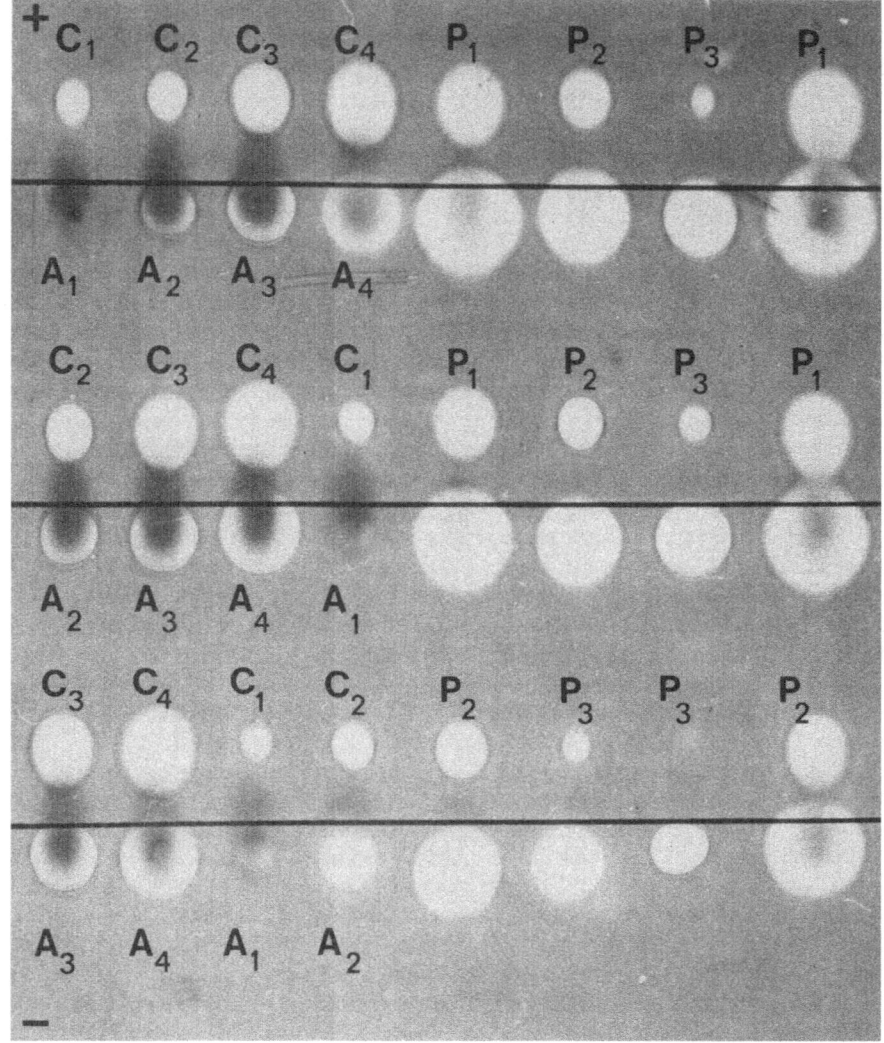

Figure 3. Inhibition zones of ampicillin and cloxacillin after
separation by high voltage electrophoresis. Samples taken after
1 (P_1), 3 (P_2), and 5 (P_3), hours after administration of the
drugs. The black horizontal lines represent the place of application.
Each sample is applied on 4 different points. (The last application
of P_3 on bottom line has failed). The inhibition zones of
ampicillin are under the lines and cloxacillin above. Standard
series: cloxacillin; C_1:8, C_2:16, C_3:32 and C_4:64 ug/ml; ampicillin;
A_1:2, A_2:4, A_3:8 and A_4:16 ug/ml. +: anode, − : cathode.

Clinical Applications

The paper disc method can be used for sufficiently frequent
controls to ensure therapeutic concentrations of antibiotics, and
to avoid toxic levels or accumulation of the drugs. The capillary
sampling technique is easy and not too disturbing for the patient.
Nevertheless, in clinical work frequent sampling is laborious
even if each sampling is easy, and frequent sampling is not
always necessary. If the concentration diminishes monoexponentially
only 2 to 3 measurements needs to be made to calculate approximately
the decline in antibiotic concentration with time.

Figure 4 shows such a "point-control" in a patient 23 days
old, treated with gentamicin. Blood sampling is made 1,3 and 5
hours following the morning dose on the second, the seventh
and the twelfth day of treatment. If the antibiotic had accumulated
the concenration should have risen step-wise. The plasma half-
life of the drug can also be calculated from three points. The 3
point-control is routinely used in some Swedish hospitals,
especially to avoid toxic plasma concentrations and accumulations
in patients treated with aminoglycosides (Boreus and Jallin 1972).

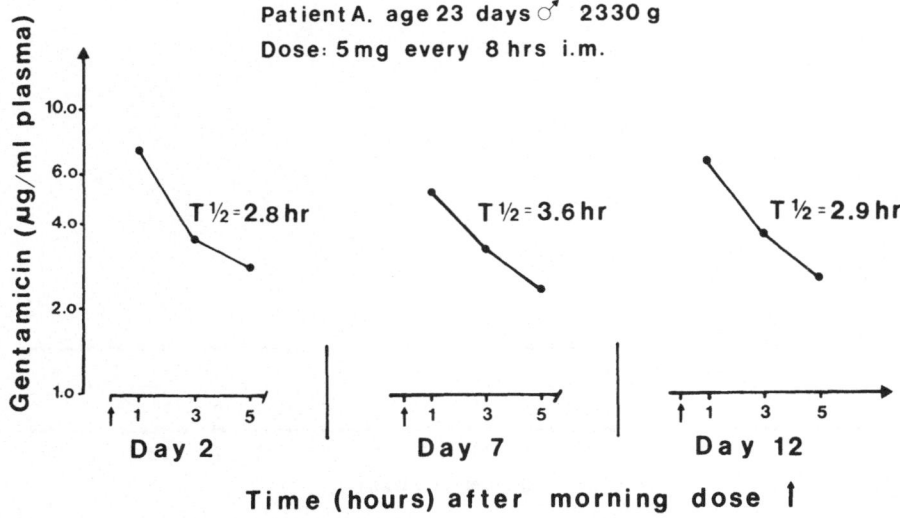

Figure 4. Plasma concentrations of gentamicin after i.m. injection.
Blood sampling 1, 3 and 5 hourse following the morning dose, 3
different days. $T_{\frac{1}{2}}$ = plasma half-life

Monitoring the antibiotic concentration in infected tissues is
less easy. For ethical and practical reasons samples sometimes
can not be taken as frequent as desirable, e.g. from maxillary
sinus. If tissue samples are easily accessable the paper disc
methods can be used for pharmacokinetic studies of drugs. The method
has been used for studying the concentration of rifampicin in
plasma and pleural fluid in patients after a single dose (Boman
and Malmborg 1974).

Figure 5 shows plasma and pleural concentrations in one
patient. The curves are representative for the whole material
(Boman and Malmborg 1974). The average maximal concentration
in the plasma samples was reached within 3 hours, and in pleural
fluid between 5 and 11 hours, after the drug was given. The
concentration reaches a plateau lasting for several hours. The
level was lower than that in plasma during the first 12 hours.
After 24 hours the level exceeded that in plasma.

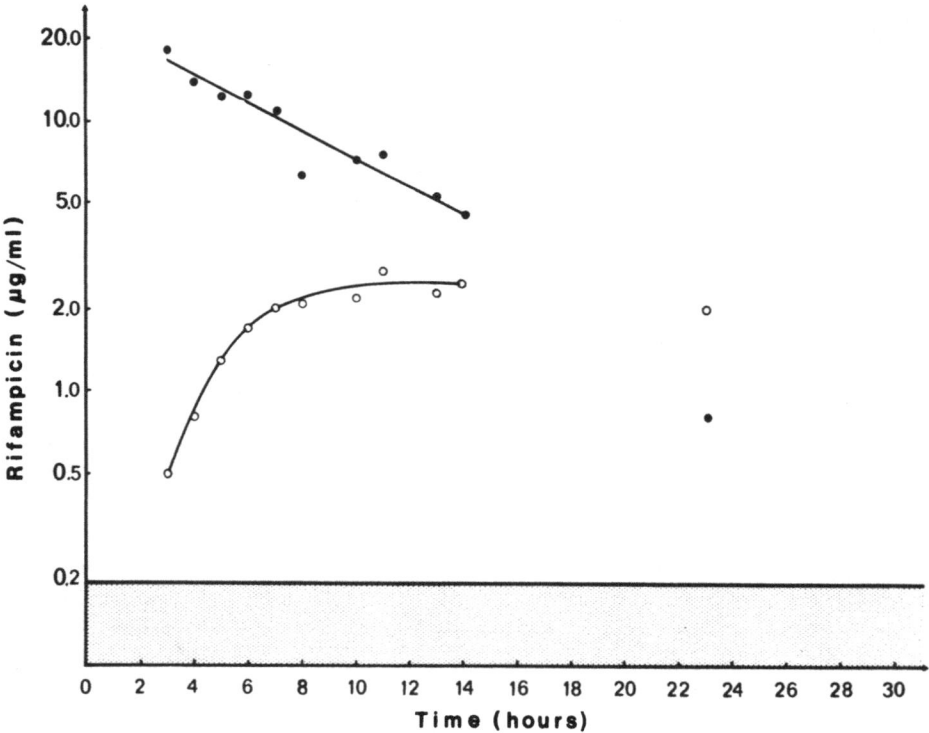

Figure 5. Time-course of rifampicin concentrations in plasma
(●——●) and pleural fluid (O——O) after single oral
dose (10 mg/kg b.w.). The shaded area represents concentrations
too low to be measured.

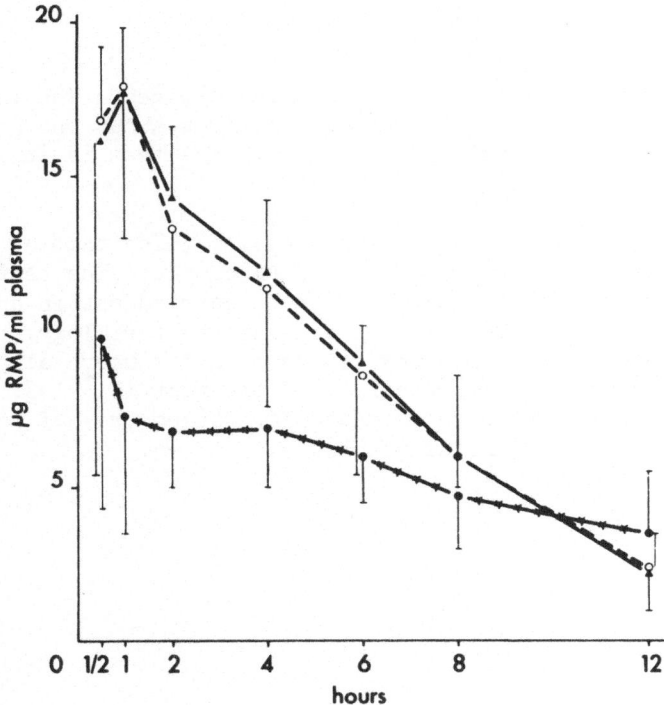

Figure 6. Plasma concentrations of rifampicin after oral solution (10 mg/kg b.w.), given alone (▲——▲), with PAS granules (●─x─x─●) or with Na-PAS tablets (Δ----Δ). Means and S.D. indicated (n=6).

Another example of the usefulness of the method is a study on the concentration of rifampicin in patients treated for tuberculosis (Boman et al 1971). Unexpectedly an interaction was found between para-aminosalicylic acid (PAS) and rifampicin. The plasma concentration og rifampicin decreased when the drug was given simultaneously with PAS. The cause for the decrease is tha the major excipient of the PAS granules, a mineral called bentonite, absorbs rifampicin rapidly and strongly (Boman et al. 1975).

The interaction is avoided by giving sodium-PAS Figure 6 shows the plasma concentrations of rifampicin given alone togehter with PAS granules, and together with sodium - PAS tablets.

Conclusions

The paper disc method has some disadvantages. The test
is rather time-consuming. Each test requires about one hour, and
the incubation period is 18 to 20 hours. The test is influenced
by other antibiotics in the samples.

There are, however, several advantages. The samples are
easy to collect and can be made on 10 ul sample. The test is
inexpensive and easy to make. It can be carried out in any
laboratory which performs routine clinical bacteriology. In
Sweden standard series of discs can be bought commercially which
facilitates the work. The accuracy of the test is $\pm$ 10%. The
paper disc method can be recommended for the control of antibiotic treatment in clincial practice.

A NEW ASSAY TECHNIQUE FOR ANTIBIOTICS

M. J. HARBER and A. W. ASSCHER

K. R. U. F. Institute of Renal Disease, Welsh National School of

Medicine, Royal Infimary, Cardiff, U. K.

SUMMARY

Endogenous ATP levels have been used as an index of bacterial growth in a rapid microbiological assay for aminoglycoside antibiotics.   The test organism is Klebsiella edwardsii var atlantae (NCTC 10896) which is resistant to penicillins and cephalosporins.   Bacterial ATP is extracted with a solution of EDTA in H_2SO_4 and measured using the firefly biolumin-escence system.   There is a close inverse relationship between bacterial ATP and serum antibiotic level.   This assay technique is potentially applicable to any group of antimicrobial agents.

INTRODUCTION

In the two surveys of the accuracy of gentamicin assays Reeves (1974) showed that approximately 80% of laboratories sampled produced results which were either poor or highly misleading.   The majority of these labor-atories (70%) used a plate diffusion assay.   A more reliable assay procedure is clearly desirable for routine use in hospital laboratories.

Several new methods have been described in recent years for rapidly assaying serum levels of aminoglycoside antibiotics (Faine and Knight, 1968; Noone et al, 1971; Lewis et al, 1972; Smith et al, 1972; Haas and Davies, 1973).   Of these the most accurate and reliable methods appear to be radioimmunoassay (Minshaw et al, 1975) and enzymatic assay techniques (Ten Krooden and Darrell, 1974; Broughall and Reeves, 1975).   Unfortun-ately these methods are beyond the scope of most routine laboratories due to

125

their requirement for expensive radiochemicals and apparatus.

Presented in this study is a technique which utilizes relatively simple
equipment for the rapid assay of antibiotics in serum.   This method is
based on the observation that estimation of endogenous adenosine tri-phos-
phate (ATP) provides a sensitive index of bacterial growth (D' Eustachio and
Johnson, 1968).   Depression of bacterial growth produced in vitro by an
antibiotic may therefore be accurately quantitated by measuring cellular
ATP levels.   Bacterial ATP may be detected by means of the firefly bioluminescence system in which light emission is measured during the oxidation
of ATP-activated firefly luciferin (McElroy and Strehler, 1949; Strehler and
Totter, 1952; St. John, 1970).

MATERIALS AND METHODS

Test Organism -   Gentamicin and Tobramycin were assayed using
Klebsiella edwardsii var atlantae (NCTC 10896).   This organism is
resistant to antibiotics such as penicillins and cephalosporins which are
commonly administered in combination with aminoglycosides.   A master
culture was maintained on slopes of Oxoid Dorset egg medium without
crystal violet.   Liquid cultures in 10 ml Oxoid nutrient broth no. 2 were
sub-cultured daily.   The inoculum was prepared by diluting an overnight
broth culture in fresh medium to E_{560} of 0.20 units which gave approximately
9×10^7 colony-forming units per ml.

Reagents -   ATP grade 1, N-2-hydroxyethylpiperazine-N^1-2-ethane-
sulphonic acid (HEPES) and firefly lantern extract (FLE) were obtained
from the Sigma London Chemical Co.   HEPES buffer was prepared by
adjusting a 100 mM solution to pH 7.5 with NaOH.   Vials containing
50 mg lyophilized FLE were reconstituted with 5 ml de-ionized water, stood
at room temperature for 1-2 h to reduce background activity, and then centrifuged before use.   Excess FLE reagent could be stored overnight at 4°C
without appreciable loss of activity.   Bacterial ATP was extracted with a
solution of 2 mM ethylenediaminetetra-acetic acid (EDTA) in 0.2 N H_2SO_4.
This reagent was prepared freshly every 2-3 days.   Serum was dispensed
using Finnpipettes (Jencons) fitted with sterilized disposable tips.   Other
reagents were dispensed from adjustable volume dispensors (Oxford Laboratories).

Instrumentation - Light emission from the bioluminescence reaction was
measured using an Amino Chem-Glow Photometer coupled to a Kontron inte-

grating recorder.   FLE (100 μl) was injected from a Hamilton repeating syringe into 200 μl sample contained in a Durham tube.   The light emission was integrated for 30 sec from the time of injection, this being more accurate than measurement of peak-height alone.

Antibiotic Standards —   Stock aqueous solutions of 400 μg gentamicin or tobramycin/ml were kept at 4°C and prepared freshly every month. Immediately prior to each assay 40 μl stock solution was diluted in 960 μl normal human serum.   This was further diluted to give a range of standards of 16, 8, 4, 2, 1 and 0 μg antibiotic/ml serum.

Assay Procedure —   Antibiotic standards and test sera were assayed in triplicate.   Fifty μl serum was added to 850 μl Oxoid nutrient broth no.2 contained in 100 x 11 mm bacteriological tubes fitted with aluminium caps. Each sample was heated at 56°C for 30 min to destroy serum antibacterial activity and then inoculated with 100 μl test organism delivered from a Hamilton repeating syringe.   Controls of normal serum and of each test serum were inoculated with 100 μl of a heat killed preparation of the test organism.   All tubes were incubated without shaking for 110 min in a waterbath at 37°C.   Tubes were withdrawn singly from the waterbath and treated immediately with 0.5 ml EDTA/H_2SO_4 reagent.   After mixing for 3-4 sec on a vortex mixer all samples were left to stand for 2 min.   The solutions were neutralized with 0.5 ml 0.2 N NaOH and brought to pH 7.5 by addition of 2 ml HEPES buffer.   The ATP content of each sample was measured in turn.

RESULTS

A linear relationship was observed between the relative integrated intensity (R11) of light emission and concentration of ATP in HEPES buffer measured using the firefly bioliminescence system (Fig 1).   Illustrated in Fig 2 are growth curves obtained by extraction of endogenous ATP from K. edwardsii var atlantae grown in serum broth containing different concentrations of gentamicin.   By plotting R11 values for a selected incubation period against antibiotic concentration a standard graph may be prepared.   A standard graph for the assay of gentamicin which represents the mean $\pm$ S.D. of two observations in normal serum and two observations in pooled uraemic serum is presented in Fig 3.   It should be noted that the relationship between R11 and antibiotic concentration is not linear but characteristically is slightly sigmoidal.

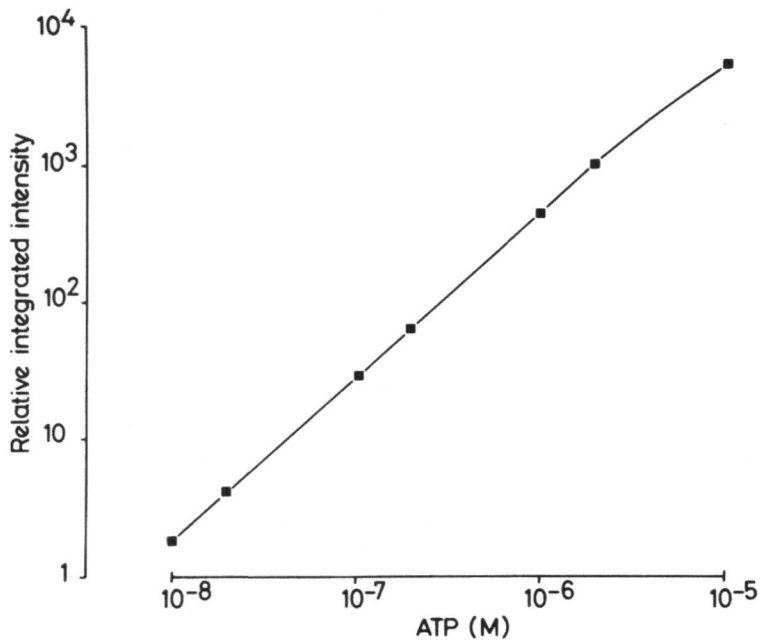

FIGURE 1 : Relationship between light emission (relative inte
grated intensity) and concentration of ATP in buffer pH 7.5

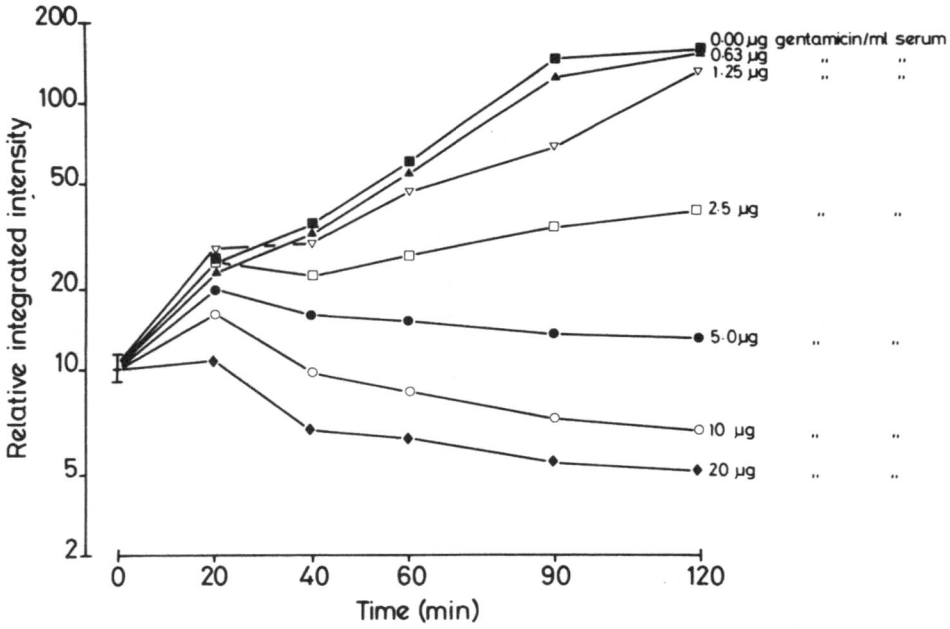

FIGURE 2 : Effect of gentamicin on the growth of K.
edwardsii var, atlantae in serum broth

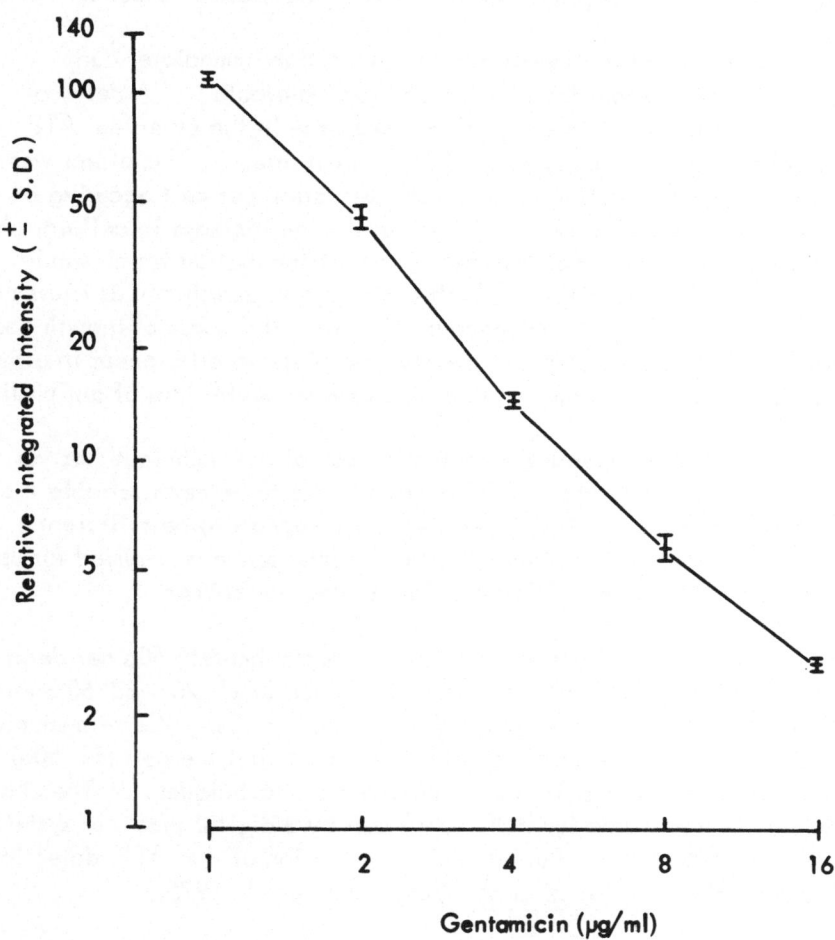

FIGURE 3: Standard graph for the
assay of serum gentamicin.

DISCUSSION

Extraction of ATP from the test organism is a critical stage in the assay procedure.   The method chosen fulfils a number of necessary criteria in that it is rapid and simple to perform, is consistently efficient, and does not pre-cipitate serum proteins or produce quenching of the bioluminescence reation.

It was found necessary to perform the extraction immediately on withdrawal of each sample from the incubation waterbath.   A delay of even 1-2 min could result in a significant decrease in the observed ATP level, particularly in cultures with a high growth rate.   This effect was considered due to a reduction in ATP concentration per cell occuring on cessation of exponential growth.   Conversely, an increase in cellular ATP might be expected to occur on commencement of incubation which would explain the initial rapid rise in R11 observed in the growth curves illustrated in Fig 2.   Variability in endogenous ATP with the phase of growth does not invalidate the assay system but merely amplifies the differences in growth level between cultures containing high and low concentrations of antibiotic.

Although a formal appraisal of the accuracy of the technique has yet to be undertaken the ATP assay in our hands appears to be more reliable than a plate diffusion method.   The system certainly appears to be sufficiently accurate for clinical use.   Only 150 µl patients' serum is required for assay and a result may be quoted within 4h of receiving a specimen.

The cost of running a gentamicin assay is approximately 60p per deter-mination which compares favourably with the range of £1.20 - £3.60 quoted for various enzyme assays (Broughall and Reeves, 1975).   Certain special-ized instrumentation is necessary for the ATP assay but the cost (£1,500) is low compared with that required for radiochemical techniques.   The chart recorder may be repleaced for little extra cost by a digital read-out system should this be preferred.   Furthermore, automation of the ATP detection method is possible (Van Dyke et al, 1969; Conn et al, 1975).

One major advantage of the method described here is that it is potentially applicable to any group of antibiotics.   An assay for cephaloridine is currently being developed.   With appropriate modifications the technique should also be suitable for rapidly measuring serum levels of vitamins such as B12 and folic acid.   The firefly system per se has already been used for detecting bacteriuria (Conn et al, 1975).

The ATP assay technique appears to offer the scope of standard microbiolog-ical assay methods combined with rapidity and greater potential accuracy. This method may be more attractive to routine hospital laboratories concerned with the assay of aminoglycoside antibiotics than the more specialized techniques which are currently available.

REFERENCES

Broughall, J.M. and Reeves, D.S. (1975),   Journal of Clinical Pathology, 28, 140.

Conn, R.B., Carache, P. and Chappelle, E.W. (1975), American Journal of Clinical Pathology, 63, 493.

D'Eustachio, A.J. and Johnson, D.R. (1968), Federation Proceedings, 27, 761.

Faine, S. and Knight, D.C. (1968), Lancet, 2, 375.

Haas, M.J. and Davies, J. (1973), Antimicrobial Agents and Chemotherapy, 4, 497.

Lewis, J.E., Nelson, J.C. and Elder, H.A. (1972), Nature New Biology, 239, 214.

McElroy, W.D. and Strehler, B.L. (1949), Archives of Biochemistry, 22, 420.

Minshew, B.H., Holmes, R.K. and Baxter, C.R. (1975), Antimicrobial Agents and Chemotherapy, 7, 107.

Noone, P. Pattison, J.R. and Samson, D. (1971), Lancet, 2, 16.

Reeves, D.S. (1974), Postgraduate Medical Journal, 50 (suppl. 7), 20.

Smith, D.H., Van Otto, B. and Smith, A.L. (1972), New England Journal of Medicine, 286, 583.

St. John, J.B. (1970), Analytical Biochemistry, 37, 409.

Strehler, B.L. and Totter, J.R. (1952), Archives of Biochemistry and Biophysics, 40, 28.

Ten Krooden, E. and Darrell, J.H. (1974), Journal of Clinical Pathology, 27, 452.

Van Dyke, K., Stitzel, R., McClellen, T. and Szustkiewicz, C. (1969), Clinical Chemistry, 15, 3.

THE PROBLEM OF ANTIBIOTIC MIXTURES IN SERUM SAMPLES

D.S. REEVES* AND H.A. HOLT

DEPARTMENT OF MEDICAL MICROBIOLOGY

SOUTHMEAD HOSPITAL, BRISTOL, BS10 5NB, ENGLAND

The treatment of bacterial infection by the giving of more than one antibiotic simultaneously is a common and frequently justifiable practice. Clinical microbiological laboratories are therefore often faced with the problem of assaying an antibiotic in a sample of body fluid in the presence of one or more other antibiotics. Even when the antibiotics are given sequentially as treatment the residual presence of an antibiotic which has ceased being administered can prove an unexpected hazard to accurate assay. Microbiological assays are the commonest method used in clinical laboratories and although convenient they are usually lacking in specificity. This review will explore methods of increasing the specificity of microbiological assays and also briefly examine other more specific assays suitable for serum samples.

A wide variety of methods are available for assaying the antibiotic components in mixtures (Table 1), many of them developed by the needs of industry for research and development purposes. Unfortunately not all of them are suitable for use with serum samples from patients. Proteins and other substances may interfere in the method of separation or estimation. Serum samples usually contain relatively low concentrations of antibiotic and a method designed to operate on production samples may lack sensitivity. Some methods of separation may employ strong acids or alkalis which could denature the relatively unstable antibiotics.

SPECIFIC ASSAYS

Highly specific assays are not available for all the antibiotics in common use without employing some sort of separation proce-

133

Specific assay – chemical or physico-chemical method
                  – radioimmuno assay
                  – radio-tagging assay

Remove activity of unwanted component – degradation
                                       – absorption
                                       – filtration
                                       – antagonism

Separate components before assay – electrophoresis
                                 – T.L.C.
                                 – filtration

Semi-specific microbiological assay

Table I: Methods Available for Assaying Components of Mixtures

dure first.   Chemical or physico-chemical procedures are often
needed and there is only space to give two examples here (Table 2).

The sulphonamide method is relatively crude by normal analytical standards but succeeds because of the high concentration of
drug present.   The trimethoprim method relies on double extraction
since it is a highly lipid soluble drug and stable at extremes of
pH, two properties not possessed by the commonly used penicillin
and cephalosporin antibiotics.   With non-microbiological assays
it is important to check the relevance of the values obtained in
the context of use since ultimately it is microbiological activity
that is required.   For example, some chemical assays will measure
microbiologically inactive metabolites.

Bacterial transferase enzymes have been exploited to attach
various radioactive labels to aminoglycoside antibiotics.   Assays
by this method are specific for aminoglycosides but there is cross
reactivity between various members of the group depending on which
transferase is employed (Haas and Davies, 1973; Broughall and
Reeves, 1975).   Radio-immunoassays are often highly specific.   For
example, the different isomers of gentamicin may be assayed individually, and different aminoglycosides can be assayed individually.
The aminoglycosides are particularly suitable for assay by this
method because under normal circumstances they are metabolised very
little.   This is important since in other fields it has been

Agent	Method
Sulphonamide	Bratton–Marshall (1939) procedure.
Trimethoprim	Extraction, oxidation, and spectrofluorimetry (Schwartz et al, 1969).

Table 2: Chemical Assays of Commonly Used Anti-Bacterial Agents

suggested that radioimmunoassay techniques may sometimes measure
inactivated drug. In spite of their advantages the complexity of
many specific assays presents difficulties to the average clinical
laboratory. It is for this reason that less specific techniques
for detection and quantitation are often prefered, perhaps preceded by one of the techniques described in the next two sections.

REMOVAL OF ACTIVITY OF COMPONENTS BEFORE ASSAY

(i) Degradation

Destruction of a component by enzyme is widely used for penicillin and cephalosporin antibiotics (Sabath et al, 1971; Stroy
and Preston, 1971).   Suitable broad spectrum B-lactamase preparations are available commercially (e.g. Whatman B-lactamase broad
spectrum mixtures; see Waterworth, 1973) which are capable of
removing the activity of all the B-lactam antibiotics at present in
clinical use. The introduction of the cephamycins may present a
problem. Selective degradation of particular types of penicillin
may be possible using different types of B-lactamases but the enzymes
are not commercially available and the procedure would need precise
control.   Thus although the use of B-lactamases will permit the
assay of other antibacterials from mixtures containing B-lactam
antibiotic they cannot help in the routine differential assay of
penicillins and cephalosporins at present.

Other enzymatic degradations represent the means of resistance
of many bacteria to antibiotics.   Although many enzymes have been
isolated and identified from a wide variety of bacteria against a
number of antibiotics they are unlikely to be used routinely unless
commercial preparations are available.   Particularly useful would
be a preparation for the destruction of aminoglycoside activity.

Less specific methods of destruction of activity can be tried.
For example, heating or changes in pH (e.g. erythromycin – Grove and
Randall, 1955) may inactivate the less stable antibiotics while
stable drugs like aminglycosides remain.   A number of well-designed
controls would be essential. Ultra-violet light has been used to
inactivate cephalothin (Sabath et al, 1968).

(ii) Absorption

Absorption onto activated charcoal is relatively non-specific
but ion-exchange resins can be selective to the extent that differential absorption of basic and acidic antibiotics occurs. Using
the acid Dowex resin 50-X8 we could absorb completely aminoglycoside antibiotics in both serum and buffer at concentrations found

Completely absorbed		Partially absorbed		Not absorbed
Compound	Max.conc. tested (mg/l)	Compound	Max.conc. tested (mg/l)	Compound
Kanamycin	10	Lincomycin	20	Benzyl penicillin
Gentamicin	20	Clindamycin	20	Ampicillin
Streptomycin	50			Cephaloridine
Tobramycin	20			Erythromycin
Neomycin	100			Doxycycline

Table 3:   Absorption of Antibiotics by Dowex 50-X8 Resin

during therapy (Table 3).   An interesting difference between the
absorption of the aminoglycoside and the lincomycin is that the
former seems to follow a first-order reaction while the latter
reaches a limit of absorption (Fig.1).   The level at which this
limit occurs depends on the proportion of resin to serum.   The
rate of absorption and, in the case of lincomycin, the final value
is dependent on pH (Fig.1).   The absorption is more efficient in
buffer medium than in serum but aminoglycoside antibiotics can still
be rapidly removed from the latter by Dowex 50-X8.   As the resin
is in large beads it settles out rapidly after agitation without
centrifugation.

To a lesser extent the absorption of acidic antibiotics onto
basic resin (Dowex 1X8-50) does occur but while the absorption of
cephalothin, cephacetrile, cephazolin, benzyl penicillin, ampicillin,
carbenicillin, cloxacillin, fusidic acid, novobiocin and doxycycline
occurred from buffer solutions it was much more inefficient from
serum, with the possible exception of cloxacillin.   The basic antibiotics (the 5 aminoglycosides in Table 3, plus clindamycin, lincomycin, erythromycin and rifampicin) are not absorbed.

(iii) Filtration

Differential molecular filtration through collodion membranes
has been described but the separation was thought to be insufficient
for clinical purposes (Barza et al, 1973).

(iv) Antagonism

Antagonism of activity at a microbiological level without destruction of the drug is well known (Table 4).   While again it must
be emphasized that these manoeuvres be controlled to ensure the
effectiveness of antagonism, we have found 50 mg/l of para-amino-
benzoic acid and 5 mg/l of thymidine sufficient to neutralise the
activity of co-trimoxazole in the sera of patients receiving this
combination.

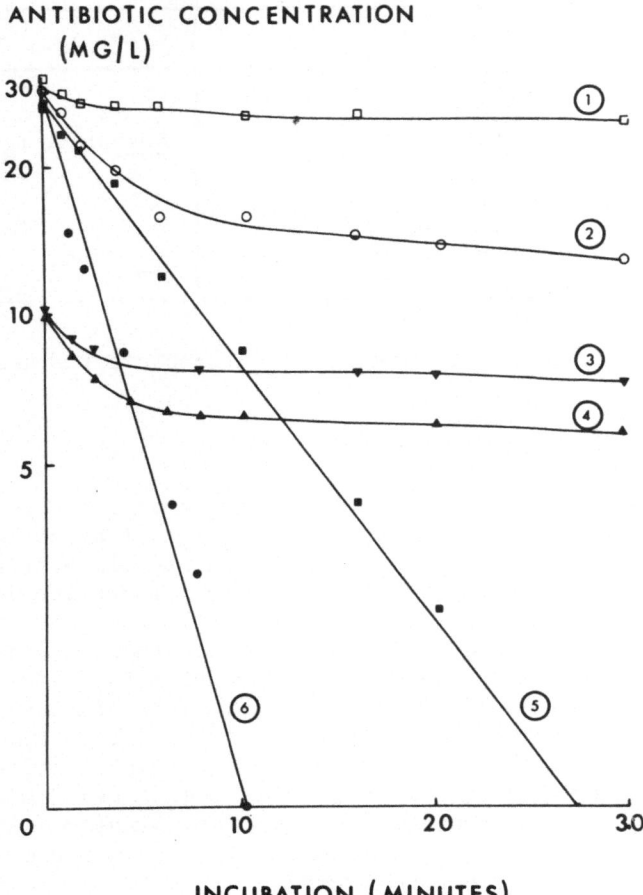

Fig.1: Use of the acidic ion-exchange resin Dowex 50–X8 to absorb
two basic antibiotics, lincomycin and gentamicin.
1. lincomycin (starting conc. 30 mg/l). Resin 0.07 g/ml pH 8.4
2. lincomycin (" " 10 mg/l). " " " pH 6.7
3. lincomycin (" " 10 mg/l). Resin 0.07 g/ml pH 7.6
4. lincomycin (" " 10 mg/l). Resin 0.2 g/ml pH 7.6
5. gentamicin (" " 30 mg/l). Resin 0.07 g/ml pH 8.4
6. gentamicin (" " 30 mg/l). " " " pH 6.7

SEPARATION BEFORE ASSAY

Separations of components of mixtures and their individual
assay by a non-specific method are widely practised for research
and control applications but little used in clinical microbiology.
This is a pity since such methods are capable of offering adequate
sensitivity with high specificity.

Drug	Antagonist	Typical Conc.*
Sulphonamide	para-amino benzoic acid	50 mg/l
Trimethoprim	thymidine	5 mg/l
Streptomycin	semicarbazide	<u>See</u> Grove and Randall 1955
Cycloserine	D-alanine	
Aminoglycosides	lauryl sulphate or divalent cations	20 g/l <u>See</u> Ervin and Bullock 1974

*   for use in a suitable culture medium

Table 4:   Antagonism of Antibacterial Drugs

(i) High Voltage Electrophoresis (HVE)

HVE offers a rapid means of separating mixtures. The use of
paper as a carrier medium has the disadvantage of allowing the
application of only small samples and it is therefore difficult to
obtain sufficient sensitivity.   Agar, with its greater depth and
the possibility of applying samples in a well, was first described
for the electrophoresis of antibiotics by Lightbown and de Rossi
(1965). By further development we have adapted the method so as to
render it suitable for separating the components of mixtures in
serum samples.   The method is described in detail elsewhere (Reeves
and Holt, 1975), but briefly samples are electrophoresed from wells
in a sheet of buffered agarose on a water-cooled bed for approximately one hour.   The position (and also sometimes concentration)
of antibiotics is developed and measured by bio-autography in an
applied seeded layer of nutrient agar.

(ii) Thin Layer Chromatography (TLC)

Reports on the use of TLC for separating antibiotics in serum
samples have been few, doubtless because of the problems of lack of
sensitive detection methods and interferance from protein. Since
these problems do not usually apply to urine samples many reports
illustrate the value of TLC in dealing with mixtures.   In spite
of the difficulties Konno and Fujii (1970) reported briefly on the
separation of penicillins in serum samples.   The ready and rapid
availability of protein-free ultrafiltrates of serum using membrane
cones should encourage further exploration.   We have recently
experimented with TLC as a means of separating antibiotics in
aqueous solutions.   Various methods of chemical detection were
tried but none gave as good sensitivity as bioautography on a thin
layer of nutrient agar seeded with <u>Bacillus</u> <u>subtilis</u>.   The results
in Table 5 are preliminary but suffice to show that useful separation can be achieved at the range of concentrations found in the

Antibiotic	R_m (relative to benzyl penicillin)	Minimum Conc. Detected (mg/l)
benzyl penicillin	100	< 1
ampicillin	60	1
carbenicillin	100	20
cloxacillin	129	20
flucloxacillin	128	20
pivampicillin	0	10
cephacetrile	87	15
cephalexin	60	100
cephaloridine	56	4
cephalothin	87	4
cephazolin	66	15
erythromycin	130	10
clindamycin	72	10
lincomycin	64	100
trimethoprim	76	10
novobiocin	126	200
rifampicin	124	10

Support: cellulose 100 u thick
Solvent: butanol/acetic acid/water (12/3/5)
Application: 5 ul

Table 5:   Thin Layer Chromatography of Antibiotics in Aqueous Solution

Antibiotic	Minimum Conc. Detected (mg/l)	R_m (benzyl penicillin 100)
ampicillin	100	163
cephaloridine	10	124
cephalothin	5	90
cephazolin	20	113
cephacetrile	20	160
clindamycin	100	166
cloxacillin	50	57
doxycycline	10	49
erythromycin	500	158
gentamicin	50	228
kanamycin	100	218
lincomycin	300	202
mecillinam	10	195
minocycline	100	51
rifampicin	10	34
streptomycin	200	260
tobramycin	100	270

Table 6: Results of TLC on Sephadex G15 followed by bio-autography

urine and, in some instances, in the blood. Doubtless the sensitivity could be increased further for some individual drugs by
appropriate adjustments to the bio-autographic method.

Thin layer gel filtration (TLGF). Sephadex has been advocated
in that an aqueous solvent can be used (Zuidweg et al, 1969).
Following and developing the technique described we were unable to
achieve sufficient sensitivity for assaying typical serum samples.
However, separations which may be of use for urine samples were
achieved (Table 6).

SEMI-SPECIFIC MICROBIOLOGICAL ASSAY

Use of an indicator organism sensitive to the drug to be
assayed but resistant to other antibiotics often provides a practical solution to the problem of mixtures. For therapeutic
reasons it is fortunate that combinations of antibiotics with
closely similar antimicrobial activities are not often given and
in practice laboratories are rarely asked, for example, to assay a
mixture of aminoglycosides or penicillinase-resistant penicillins.
This is just as well since finding and keeping a range of indicator
organisms appropriate to this purpose would be near impossible.
Furthermore, each organism would have its own characteristics in
the assay itself and it would therefore be difficult to maintain
a satisfactory degree of accuracy in the occasional assay. Other
problems are the instability of acquired resistance in indicator
strains and slowness of growth. Nevertheless, numerous examples
of this type of assay have been described (see review Reeves and
Bywater, 1976). Special condition as, for example, an alteration
in the medium pH may render an assay specific.

Sometimes large differences in the relative concentrations of
two antibiotics in typical serum samples may be put to use. For
example, a fully sensitive Pseudomonas aeruginosa can be used to
assay carbenicillin in patients also receiving gentamicin because
the dilution required to measure the high concentrations of the
former dilutes out the activity of the gentamicin. Finally, when
all other methods have failed the concentration of an antibiotic
can be deduced by subtracting the activity of the interfering substance or by preparing standards containing the exact amount of
interfering antibiotic as in the sample to be assayed. The very
tedium of such a method makes it unwelcome and it is likely the
result will not be of clinical relevance by the time it is obtained.

UNSUSPECTED MIXTURES

Although one often suspects an assay result of being inaccurate due to a contaminating antibiotic it is salutory to know that

nearly 20% of serum samples submitted for assay in our hospital contained undisclosed antibiotics (Reeves and Holt, 1975). Clearly this situation is alarming and apart from emphasising the need for improving communications with clinical colleagues and better education, specific assays of sufficient simplicity for routine use are urgently required.

REFERENCES

Bratton, A.C., and Marshall, E.K. (1939). Journal of Biological Chemistry, 128: 537-50.

Broughall, J.M. and Reeves, D.S. (1975b). Antimicrobial Agents and Chemotherapy. In press.

Ervin, F.R., and Bullock, W.E. (1974). Antimicrobial Agents and Chemotherapy, 6, 831-835.

Grove, D.C., and Randall, W.A. (1955). A Laboratory Manual. New York. Medical Encyclopaedia.

Haas, M.J., and Davies, J. (1973). Antimicrobial Agents and Chemotherapy, 4, 497-499.

Konno, M., and Fujii, R. (1970). Progress in Antimicrobial and Anticancer Chemotherapy, Vol. 1, Baltimore University Park Press, 1027-1032.

Lightbown, J.W., and de Rossi, P. (1965). Analyst, 90, 89-98.

Reeves, D.S., and Bywater, M.J. (1976). Balliere, Tindall and Cox, London. (In press).

Reeves, D.S., and Holt, H.A. (1975a). Journal of Clinical Pathology (in press).

Sabath, L.D., Casey, J.I., Ruch, P.A., Stumpf, L.L., and Finland, M. (1971). Journal of Laboratory of Clinical Medicine, 78, 457-463.

Sabath, L.D., Loder, P.B., Gerstein, D.A., and Finland, M. (1968). Applied Microbiology. 16: 877-880.

Schwartz, D.E., Koechlin, B.A., and Weinfeld, R.E. (1969). Chemotherapy, 14, 22-29.

Stroy, S.A., and Preston, D.A. (1971). Applied Microbiology, 21, 1002-1006.

Waterworth, P.M. (1973). Journal of Clinical Pathology. 26, 596-598.

Zuidweg, M.H.J., Oostendorp, J.G., and Bos, C.J.K. (1969). Journal of Chromatography, 42, 552-554.

SOME FACTORS INFLUENCING THE ASSAY OF GENTAMICIN

J.D. Jarvis and T.W.C. Leung

Department of Clinical Microbiology
The London Hospital
Whitechapel, London E1 1BB

When it was decided to change from the urease method to plate
assay method for the monitoring of gentamicin therapy, sufficient
variables in the methods of plate assay currently being practised
were noted, such that it seemed worthwhile re-examining some of
the more obvious factors which might influence results in clinical practice.

We therefore decided to review four culture media:

Difco Antibiotic Medium No. 5 (Grove and Randall formula)

Difco Antibiotic Medium No.11 (Grove and Randall formula)

Oxoid Sensitest

B.B.L. Mueller Hinton Medium (Baltimore Biologicals Ltd.)

and to attempt to establish performance criteria for these media
in the light of

a) the effect of buffering the standards

b) the effect of buffering the serum

c) the use of horse or human serum

d) the inactivation of serum

e) the effect of contaminating solution in samples collected
   via CVP lines

The assays were done in large square plates (235 mm)
using Klebsiella spp. (NCTC 10896) as a surface seeded inoculum

143

of 5×10^6 organisms/cm^3. Samples were randomized following a
latin square pattern.

Gentamicin in concentrations from 20μg/cm^3 falling to
1.25μg/cm^3 were prepared in horse serum (pH 8) and also in
phosphate buffer at pH 6, 7 and 8. (Standards were checked by the
adenylase method).

It was found that reductions in zone size are related to pH.
This is least noticeable with Sensitest and Mueller Hinton medium
whilst with Difco No. 5 a dramatic difference may be discerned.
Difco 11 was almost as severely affected by pH shift.

Table I summarises the results for Sensitest and Difco No.
11 for an arbitrary zone size yielding a result of 5μg/ml for
the standard.

One of the inherent difficulties with plate assay is the
quality and crispness of the zones of inhibition, and this may
be so especially with surface seeded plates. Nevertheless the
advantage of rapidity makes surface seeding worthwhile and it
seems that zones on Sensitest, Mueller Hinton and Difco 11 are all
clearly defined and therefore easy to measure, whilst Difco 5
gave rise to fuzzy indefinite zones.

Obviously the advantage lies with any medium that gives more
sensitivity in terms of larger zones and whilst all three are
good in this respect it must be noted that Sensitest and Mueller
Hinton tend to fall off more rapidly at the lower concentrations.

TABLE I

Medium	Zone Size (mm)	Values (μg/ml) obtained from standards of			
		Horse Serum	Buffer pH 6	Buffer pH 7	Buffer pH 8
Sensitest	19.2	5	8	6.2	5
Difco No.11	20.7	5	Off the graph	>20	6.4

Table II summarises our findings:

<u>TABLE II</u>

Gentamicin conc. (μg/ml)	Zone Diameter (mm)			
	Difco No.11	Difco No.5	Sensitest	Mueller Hinton
20	23.8	23.5	23.8	24
1.25	18	18	14.5	14

and it will be apparent that all the media tested were similarly sensitive at high concentrations of gentamicin. However, the Difco media gave consistently larger zones at concentrations at and below 1.25 μg/cm^3. The standard curves are consequently steeper and accuracy in measurement remains critical.

A comparison between standards made up in horse serum, human serum and cerebro-spinal fluid showed some slight degree of divergence but on Difco 11 particularly, this was minimum so that it was possible to adopt horse serum as a standard vehicle.

The pooled cerebro spinal fluid had a total protein of 100 mgm% which is outside the normal (10 - 40 mgm%) and it was difficult to obtain sufficient material to make sufficient numbers of observations.

The horse and human sera which were used were tested before and after inactivation at 56°C for 30 minutes no measureable differences were detected.

Variation in pH of batches of commercially available horse serum had then to be established or excluded. Over a period of some months the pH had ranged from 7.4 to 8.0 with the majority of batches at 7.8 or 8.0.

We were able to compare working standards of four other laboratories, three in serum and one in buffer, and the pH ranged between 8.0 to 8.5.

Gentamicin standards were therefore prepared in horse serum adjusted to pH 7.5, 8.0 and 8.5 after the addition of gentamicin.

Sensitest shows virtually no variation with sera at this range except for a slight reduction in zone size with pH 7.5 serum.

Mueller Hinton was very similar to Sensitest.

Difco 5 demonstrated reduced zone sizes at lower pH values.

With Difco 11 the differences were not discernible.

A study was undertaken to eliminate the possibility of contaminating intravenous solutions affecting the assay of serum samples. Vamine which contains Na 50 mg/ml, K 20 mg/ml, Mg 3 mg/ml, Ca 3 mg/ml and Aminosol and intra lipid were used as diluent for gentamicin standards in concentrations of 2% and 10% in serum. There was no significant effect upon the assays.

Conclusion

Table III summarises the results of conclusions drawn from our experiences with the four media tested.

At present with surface seeding Difco 11 medium seems on balance in our hands to give the most reliable results.

TABLE III

Media	Susceptibility to pH change in buffer	in serum	Crispness of zones	Sensitivity at 1.25 μg/ml	20 μg/ml	Shape of standard curve
Sensitest	+	±	good	poor	poor	flat
Mueller Hinton	+	±	good	poor	good	flat
Difco No.11	+++	±	good	good	good	steep
Difco No.5	+++	+	poor	good	good	steep

ASSAY OF GENTAMICIN AND TOBRAMYCIN BY A RELIABLE 2½ HOUR

KLEBSIELLA PLATE METHOD

D.C. Shanson, C. Hince and J.V. Daniels

Department of Medical Microbiology
The London Hospital Medical College
Turner Street, London E1 2AD

SUMMARY

A 2½ hour Klebsiella plate diffusion method for serum gentamicin and tobramycin assays is described which involves increasing the incubation temperature to $40^{\circ}C$ and the use of a heavy inoculum. The accuracy of the method compares favourably with that of the conventional 4 to 5 hours or overnight assays at $35^{\circ}C$. The advantage of the more rapid assay is that results can be given the same day on specimens which arrive in the late morning or early afternoon. Results would then be available before the next injection of aminoglycoside so that the dose can be adjusted accordingly.

INTRODUCTION

There is often a need to perform rapid serum gentamicin assays to ensure adequate dosage and to avoid toxic levels in patients with impaired renal function (Noone,P. et al, 1974). Tobramycin has similar properties to gentamicin (Waterworth, P.M. 1972) and a rapid assay of this drug is sometimes required. Most laboratories attempting rapid aminoglycoside assay use a plate diffusion method. Klebsiella used as the assay organism allows the assay to be shortened to about 5 hours (Reeves, D.S.,1972) but a 5 hour assay still does not allow serum assays to be read the same day if the specimens arrive later in the day (Noone,P., and Pattison, J.R., 1975). A 2½ hour Klebsiella assay can be performed if surface seeded plates are previously incubated for 2½ hours, with more accurate results at $40^{\circ}C$ than at $35^{\circ}C$ (Shanson, D.C., 1975). However, long pre-incubation of the assay plates presents practical difficulties in a routine laboratory.

An improved Klebsiella assay at 40°C has been developed which is
simple, not requiring long pre-incubation of seeded plates, and
which gives accurate results at $2\frac{1}{2}$ hours.

MATERIALS AND METHODS

Media and Methods of Assay

Oxoid Diagnostic Sensitivity Test Agar (DST), CM261, was
used for gentamicin and tobramycin assay at pH 7.3. 30 ml agar
was poured into 100 mm square plates and 120 ml agar into 235 mm
square plates and all these plastic plates were levelled. Plates
were stored from 1 to 4 days at room temperature before use. On
the day of use, small plates were pre-dried for 30 min. at the
temperature of assay and large plates for 20 to 30 minutes in a
35°C hot room.

Aliquots of an overnight peptone water culture of <u>Klebsiella
edwardsii var. atlantae</u> NCTC 10896 were stored at -70°C and a
fresh sample thawed each week. From this the Klebsiella was sub-
cultured onto blood agar and the next day several colonies were
emulsified into peptone water. A few drops of the peptone water
suspension were added to 100 ml nutrient broth and this was
incubated at 35°C overnight. Dilutions in nutrient broth of the
overnight culture were used to surface seed plates. For the 40°C
assay a 1 in 10 dilution was used and for the 35°C assays various
dilutions from 1 in 10 to 1 in 100 were used. After seeding the
plates were drained well. Each day a fresh subculture of the
organism was made onto blood agar and 100 ml nutrient broth
inoculated for overnight culture, as described above.

Plates for 4, 5 and 16 hour assays were left at room temperature after seeding with the lids on, for 15 min. Seeded plates
for $2\frac{1}{2}$ hour assay were dried with their lids off for exactly 30
min. at the temperature of assay. Immediately after drying 7 mm
wells were cut.

The results obtained with No.5 inactivated horse serum
(Wellcome Reagents Ltd.) used for diluting standard and test sera,
were the same as those with human serum (Shanson, D.C. and
Daniels, J.V., 1975). As preliminary experiments showed that this
also applied to tobramycin assays, the above horse serum was used
as a diluent for standards and tests for all the assays.

Immediately after the wells were cut they were quickly and
completely filled with sera. Standard and test sera were introduced in duplicate in small plates and all the wells of one plate
were filled before proceeding to the next. In 30 well large
plates sera were randomly introduced in triplicate. Assays at
35°C were incubated in a hot room (35 to 36°C) and assays at 40°C

in a 40 - 41°C incubator. The zone sizes were measured on a zone
reader (Leebrook Instrument Co. Ltd).

RESULTS

Increasing the temperature of assay

At 40°C, using a 1 in 10 dilution of an overnight culture,
the assay could be read easily after $2\frac{1}{2}$ hours. The growth of the
Klebsiella was much lighter than on a conventional 5 hour assay
but was still clearly visible. The zones had sharp edges and
were easy to read on the zone reader. In contrast at 35°C
identical assays could only be read with great difficulty after
$2\frac{1}{2}$ hours. The plates showed very little growth and the zones had
poorly defined edges which could only just be seen on the zone
reader. Zone sizes at 40°C were much larger than those at 35°.
The accuracy of assays was also much greater at 40°C than at 35°C
(see results below).

$2\frac{1}{2}$ hour gentamicin assay compared with 4 hour and overnight assay

The discrimination, as shown by the slopes of the standard
curves, was similar for the $2\frac{1}{2}$ hour at 40°C and 4 hour at 35°C
assays (Figure 1). However neither of the rapid assays showed as
good discrimination as the 16 hour assay. The most sensitive
method was the $2\frac{1}{2}$ hour assay at 40°C which gave the largest zone
with the 1.25 µg/ml gentamicin standard.

Accuracy of assay was indicated by 95% confidence limits
($\pm$ mean % error + twice the standard deviation % error). As
shown by Table I, the $2\frac{1}{2}$ hour method at 40°C was the most accurate of the 3 assays for estimating the concentration of a
3.0 g/ml gentamicin test serum. In Table II the % errors for
100 consecutive assays were used to calculate the 95% confidence
limits for each rapid assay. The $2\frac{1}{2}$ hour assay was more accurate
than the 4 hour assay, with respective 95% confidence limits of
$\pm$ 15.9% and $\pm$ 25.4%, and as accurate as the overnight assay which
gave 95% confidence limits of $\pm$ 17.5%.

$2\frac{1}{2}$ hour compared with 5 and 16 hour tobramycin assay

The discrimination for 5 and 16 hour assays was better than
for the $2\frac{1}{2}$ hour assay (Figure 2). $2\frac{1}{2}$ hour assay zone sizes were
larger at 40°C than at 35°C (Figure 2). The $2\frac{1}{2}$ hour, 40°C assay
was associated with the largest zone size produced by the
1.25 µg/ml tobramycin standard.

The accuracy of the $2\frac{1}{2}$ hour assay was much greater at 40° than
at 35°C as indicated by respective 95% confidence limits of $\pm$ 16.6%
and $\pm$ 41.3% (Table III).

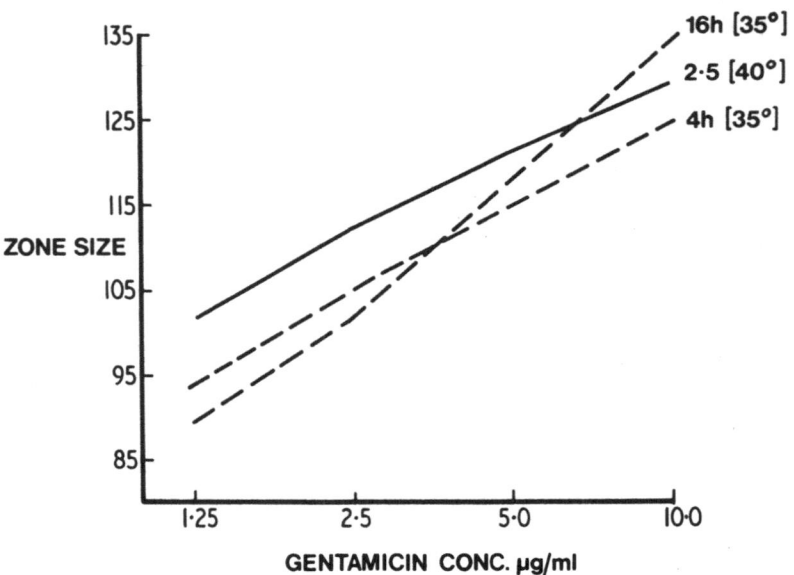

Fig. 1 Comparison of standard curves for small plate assays of
       gentamicin

- - - - = 1/20 dilution of overnight culture as inoculum
───────── = 1/10 dilution of overnight culture as inoculum
Zone size measured in mm on a zone reader. n = 12.

TABLE I

RESULTS OF ASSAY OF 3.0 μg/ml SERUM GENTAMICIN BY 3 METHODS

	Assay		
	$2\frac{1}{2}$ hr at 40°C	4 hr at 35°C	16 hr at 35°C
No. of assays	50	50	15
Mean result (μg/ml)	3.0	3.2	3.1
Mean % error	5.3	10.1	7.5
95% confidence limits	$\pm$ 14.0%	$\pm$ 33.0%	$\pm$ 20.3%

The assays at 35°C used a 1/20 dilution of overnight culture as
the inoculum. Assays were in small plates.

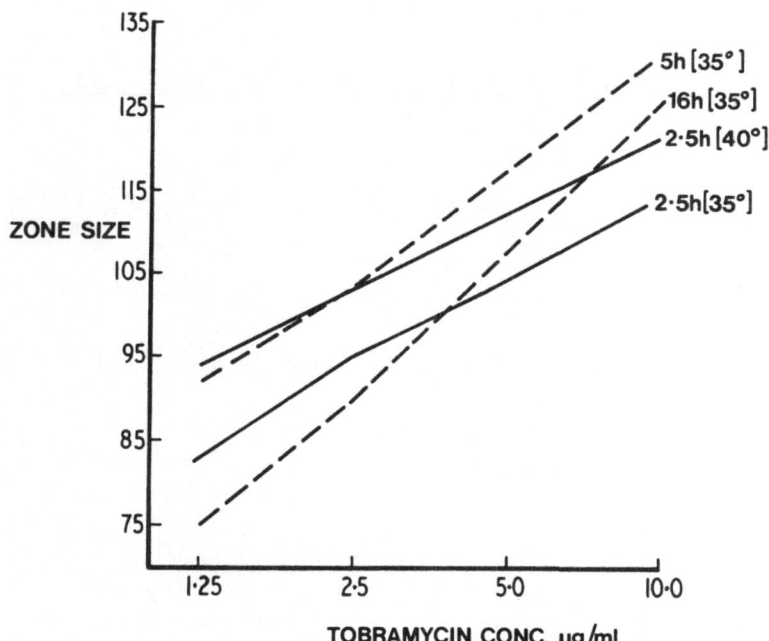

Fig. 2 Comparison of standard curves for large plate assays
        of tobramycin
- - - - = 1/50 dilution of overnight culture as inoculum
————— = 1/10 dilution of overnight culture as inoculum
Zone size measured in mm on a zone reader. n = 16

TABLE II

% ERRORS OF SERUM GENTAMICIN ASSAY

	Assay Method		
	$2\frac{1}{2}$ hr at 40°C	4 hr at 35°C	16 hr at 35°C
No.of assays	100	100	30
Mean % error	6.24	8.78	7.33
Standard deviation % error	4.84	8.29	5.10
95% confidence limits	$\pm$ 15.9%	$\pm$ 25.4%	$\pm$ 17.5%

All assays were in small plates, poured 1 to 4 days previously.
The % errors for assays of a 3.0 μg/ml test serum were combined
with the % errors for an equal number of assays of a 7.7 μg/ml
test serum

TABLE III

MEAN RESULTS (μg/ml) AND % ERRORS OF TOBRAMYCIN SERUM ASSAYS

ASSAY

	$2\frac{1}{2}$ hr at 40°C	$2\frac{1}{2}$ hr at 35°C	5 hr at 35°C	16 hr at 35°C
Mean result with 2.0 μg/ml test serum	2.0(0.17)	2.1(0.50)	2.0(0.12)	2.0(0.17)
Mean result with 7.7 μg/ml test serum	7.8(0.45)	8.3(1.19)	8.3(0.65)	8.1(0.78)
2.0 and 7.7 test sera combined (n = 32):				
Mean % error	5.0	18.8	6.9	7.1
95% confidence limits	$\pm$ 16.6%	$\pm$ 41.3%	$\pm$ 19.0%	$\pm$ 20.3%

Assays were in large plates. n = 16 for each test serum.
( ) = standard deviation. The 5 and 16 hr. assays used as
inoculum a 1/50 dilution of overnight culture. The $2\frac{1}{2}$ hr. assays
used as inoculum a 1/10 dilution of overnight culture.

DISCUSSION

More rapid growth of the assay Klebsiella occurred at 40°C than
at 35 or 37°C. As increasing the temperature of assay to 40°C also
resulted in greatly increased zone sizes and sharpness of zone
edges, it became possible to use a much heavier inoculum than at
35°C. This heavier inoculum further increased the speed of assay.
In the gentamicin Klebsiella assay at 40°C described previously
(Shanson, D.C.,1975), the inoculum was a 1 in 100 dilution of an
overnight peptone water culture. With this light inoculum it was
necessary to have prolonged pre-incubation of seeded plates in
order to read the assay after $2\frac{1}{2}$ hours. In the present method
which uses a heavy inoculum (a 1 in 10 dilution of an overnight
nutrient broth culture), long pre-incubation becomes unnecessary.
One further difference between the previous and present methods of
40°C assay is that the assay medium has now been changed from Sensitest agar to DST which gives slightly earlier growth of the
Klebsiella.

Well dried plates are essential for rapid Klebsiella assays.
Small plates were easier to dry than large plates. The pre-drying

of plates was often carried out some hours before they were used.
Although small plates were usually dried for 30 min. this time
could be varied between 20 and 40 min. After arrival of a specimen
in the laboratory, an assay plate could be seeded and then dried
for 30 min. exactly. During this time the blood sample can be
centrifuged and the serum separated.

Pre-diffusion errors are more likely to occur with large plates
than with small plates as large plates have many more wells. If
large plates are used a random order of filling the wells should be
adopted. For routine use, small plates can be recommended for
reliability, accuracy and convenience with the new $2\frac{1}{2}$ hour assay.

A 40°C is preferred to a 42°C incubator for the $2\frac{1}{2}$ hour assay
as growth of the Klebsiella becomes less rapid when the temperature
exceeds 42°C.

Discrimination of assays was reduced as the assay time was
decreased but this did not necessarily affect the accuracy of assay.
The $2\frac{1}{2}$ hour assay was more accurate than the 4 hour assay and as
accurate as 5 or 16 hour assay. Often the edges of 4 to 5 hour
assays at 35°C were more difficult to read than those of the $2\frac{1}{2}$
hour assay at 40°C.

REFERENCES

Noone, P., Pattison, J.R. and Garfield Davies, D. (1974) Post-
    graduate Medical Journal, 50 (Suppl.7, 9-16.

Noone, P. and Pattison, J.R. (1975) J. Clin.Path., 28, 83-84.

Reeves, D.S. (1972) Lancet, ii, 1369-1370.

Shanson, D.C. (1975) Journal of Antimicrobial Chemotherapy, 1,
    247-249.

Shanson, D.C. and Daniels, J.V. (1975) Journal of Antimicrobial
    Chemotherapy, 1, 219-227.

Waterworth, P.M. (1972) J. Clin. Path., 25, 979-983.

PUNCH HOLE METHOD. A SIMPLIFIED BIO-ASSAY TECHNIQUE

OF ANTIBIOTIC CONCENTRATIONS

Shigeru Kondo

Osaka Medical College

Takatsuki, Osaka, Japan

Introduction

In the bio-assay of antibiotic concentrations in body fluids such as bile, blood, urine, etc., the diffusion of antibiotics into an agar medium is commonly utilized, and the techniques of these bio-assay are usually that of horizontal diffusion and that of vertical diffusion. In the former, the cup method, the paper cisc method, and the band culture method (okubo and Fujimoto, 1970) are the most commonly used, while in the latter, the super-position method (Torii, 1959) is the most common.

Each of these bio-assay methods has its merits and demerits when compared with the others so that the method of choice depends on the purpose, conditions, and materials of the research.

Recently, the speaker has conceived a new bio-assay method for antibiotic concentrations and has named it "Punch Hole Method".

Technique of the Punch Hole Method

1) Bacillus subtilis PCI 219 is most convenient test organism as the bacillus is harmless and it has a wide application range. Bacillus sibtilis PCI 219 can be cultivated on an oblique agar medium (A) for seven days (at least more than four days) to form spore.

2) Five platinum loops of the above cultivated bacillus are suspended in 10 ml of distilled water or physilogical saline. The suspension is warmed to 60°c for thirty minutes to make a pure suspension of the spore.

After this procedure, the suspension includes 10^9 to 10^{10} spores per ml, thus prepared suspension can be used for about two weeks when it is kept in a refrigerator.

3) A 1.5 per cent agar culture medium (B) is used as the test media, which is liquified in a water bath and then the temperature is brought down to 60-50°C. 1 ml of the spore suspension is
added to 100 ml of the liquified test media and mixed throughly;
at this temperature range, the media does not become solid and
he spores are not killed.

4) Petri dishes, the diameter of which is 90 mm are prepared
and 6.4 ml of the liquified agar media is pored into each Petri
dish and extended horizontally. The agar media becomes solid very
soon and the thickness of the plate medium is approximately 1 mm,
when it is solified: this thickness is the same as the agar medium
of Okubo's band culture method.

5) A metal tube, whose diameter is 4.0 mm is connected with
a water-jet aspirater. The speaker prefers to use an ophthalmolo-
gical tube drill for this purpose. The solodified plate media is
punched out with the tube drill to make a hole; this is easily
done by inserting the tube into the medium layer to remove the
agar by water-jet aspiration.

6) Samples of unknown antibiotic concentrations and a series
of standard antibiotic solutions at known concentrations are filled into the pinched holes; the speaker prefers to use capillary
pipetts in this technique to prevent over-flow of the samples or
the standard solutions.

7) The plate medium to which the samples and the standard
antibiotic solutions have been added is kept in a closed box, the
bottom of which is covered by water containing gauze or filter
paper to protect the agar from drying. After that the box is
placed in an incubator at 37°C.

8) During the incubation period, the antibiotics both in the
samples and in the standard solutions diffuse into the surrounding
afar medium by the passage of time while the spored of the bacillus subtilis PCI 219 in the agar plate awake, grow, and multipli-
cate to make colonies. Certain hours after incubation, an inhibi-
tationzone ring is formed around the punch hole; within the ring
the colonies of bacillus subtilis do not develop, because of the
diffused antibiotic so that the surface of the agar medium remains
clear.

9) The diameter of the each inhibition ring is measured to
o.o5 mm.

10) By plotting the diameter of the inhibition ring (mm) in
ordinary scale while the known concentrations of standard solutions in logarithmic scale of semi-logarithmic section paper, a standard curve can be drawn.

11) From the X-interception on the thus obtained standard
curve, the unknown concentrations of the samples can be obtained.
Over a wide experimental range, a linear relationship between the
diameter inhibition ring and the logarithm of the antibiotic
concentrations can be demonstrated.

12) In ampicillin, cephaloridine, cephalothin, cefazoln, oxytetracycline, chloramphenicol, streptomycin, kanamycin, aminode-
oxykanamycin, and ribostmycin, this relationship can be recognized
and in these antibiotics the punch hole method is an excellent one
to assay their concentrations.

Discussion

Although there are few experimental results, the speaker's
punch hole method, when compared with other bio-assay methods,
seems to have the following metits and demerits:

In the cup, paper disc, abnd culture, and punch hole methods,
cultivation time is short, while in the super-position method the
time required is long; the reason may be that in the former four
methods the groeth conditions are aerobic whereas in the super-
position method, they are rather anaerobic.

Accordingly, in the former four methods, the growth of the
test organism is good and the border of the inhibition zone is
sharp and easy to read, while in the super-position method the
growth is often so poor that the border is sometimes too vague to
read.

As to the most important condition of freedom from error due
to disturbance, in the cup and surposition methods, antibiotic
diffusion is often disturbed by precipitate to promote error.
But in the band culture and punch hole methods the diffusion is
not disturbed by precipitate.

As for the sample amount required for each assay technique,
in the cup method it is large, in the super position method it is
small, in the band culture method it is smaller (16 mm^3), and in
the punch hole method it is minimum (12 mm^3); this is an important
condition when assaying antibiotic concentration in the bone marrow. If a large quantity of bone marrow sample is aspirated, the
circulating blood necessarily enters the sample to produce error
in assaying concentration.

As for handing, in the cup, paper disc, band culture, and
punch hole methods, the washing of the implements after assay is
simple and easy, but in the super-position method the washing is
difficult and troublesome.

As for equipment, for the cup, paper disc, superposition, and
punch hole methods, both Petri dishes and small test tubes are
easily obtainable, to say nothing of cups, paper discs, and an
ophthamological tube drill. On the other hand, the band culture
method, requires a special assay plate and a special boring pipet
and the external edges of the boring pipet should be of the same
width as the grooves of the assay plate.

From these reasons, the speaker believes that the punch hole
method may prove to be an excellent technique for assaying antibiotic concentrations in body fluids and tissues, especially in
the bone marrow, since the sample required is minimal.

Summary
1)   The details of the punch hole method for assaying the antibiotic concentrations in body fluids is introduced.
2)   The merits and demerits of the punch hole method are discussed, and compared with other bio-assay methods such as the cup,
paper disc, super-position, and band culture methods.
3)   From these standpoints, the speaker is convinced that the
punch hole method may prove to be an excellent technique for assaying antibiotic concentratuions in the body fluids and tissues,
especially in bone marrow since the sample required is very small.
4)   Moreover, the punch hole method seems to be the most reliable and simple technique, when the sample amount is very small.
Although an ophthlmogical tube drill of 4 mm diameter was used in
this description when comparison was made with Okubo's band culture method, the sample requirement can be still further decreased,
when a tube of smaller diameter is used.

Reference
Okubo, H. and Fujimoto, Y. (1970), Progress in Antimicrobial and
Anticancer Chemotherapy,1, 495.

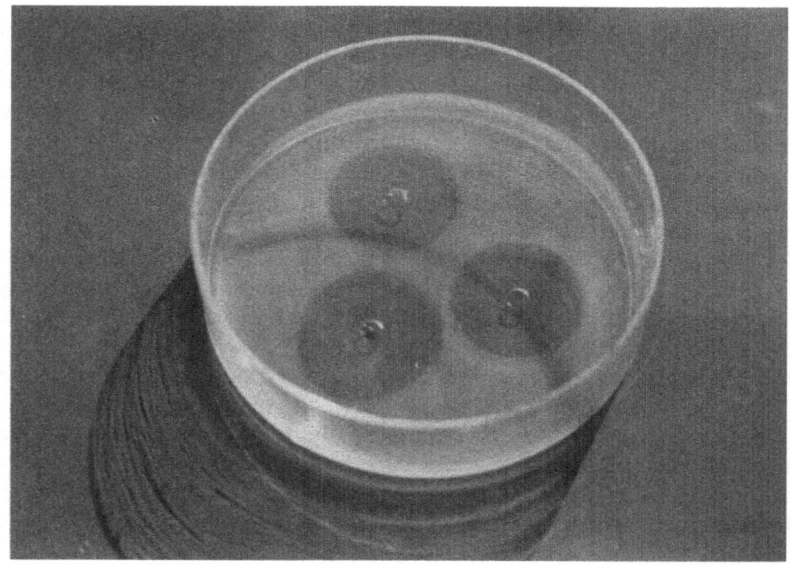

Figure 1

THE ASSAY OF SERUM AMINOGLYCOSIDE CONCENTRATIONS BY THE (^{14}C)-ACETYL TRANSFERASE TECHNIQUE

J.M. BROUGHALL* and D.S. REEVES

SOUTHMEAD GENERAL HOSPITAL

DEPT. OF MEDICAL MICROBIOLOGY, BRISTOL, ENGLAND

The recently introduced technique of labelled group transfer (1-3) for the assay of serum gentamicin concentrations enables hospital laboratories with suitable radioisotope measuring equipment, i.e., a liquid scintillation counter for β radiation, to offer a quicker and more accurate service than that possible with traditional agar plate diffusion methods, especially when the acetyl transferase technique is used (3).

The technique involves the transfer of a group (either adenyl or acetyl) labelled with ^{14}C to the gentamicin. The transfer reaction is catalysed by specific transferase enzymes isolated from E. coli strains resistant to various aminoglycoside antibiotics (4). Once labelled the gentamicin can be separated from the unreacted donor molecule by absorption to phosphocellulose paper, (P-81 paper), which enables any unreacted (^{14}C) – adenosine triphosphate or (^{14}C) – acetyl coenzyme A to be removed by washing. When the washed papers are dried the radioactivity, expressed as counts per minute (cpm) is a direct measure of the gentamicin originally present in the serum sample. This relationship for the (^{14}C) acetyl transferase method is illustrated in Fig. 1. It can be seen that a variety of other aminoglycoside antibiotics can be assayed with this technique, including the two other commonly encountered types of aminoglycoside, kanamycin and tobramycin.

The absolute number of counts obtained for each assay is dependant on both the quantity of serum containing gentamicin added to each assay tube and also the specific activity of the (^{14}C) acetyl coenzyme A. For the standard curves shown in Fig. 1 the respective values were 20 μl and 30 μCi/μmole acetyl coenzyme A. The cost of each assay tube is approximately 6p at current prices.

159

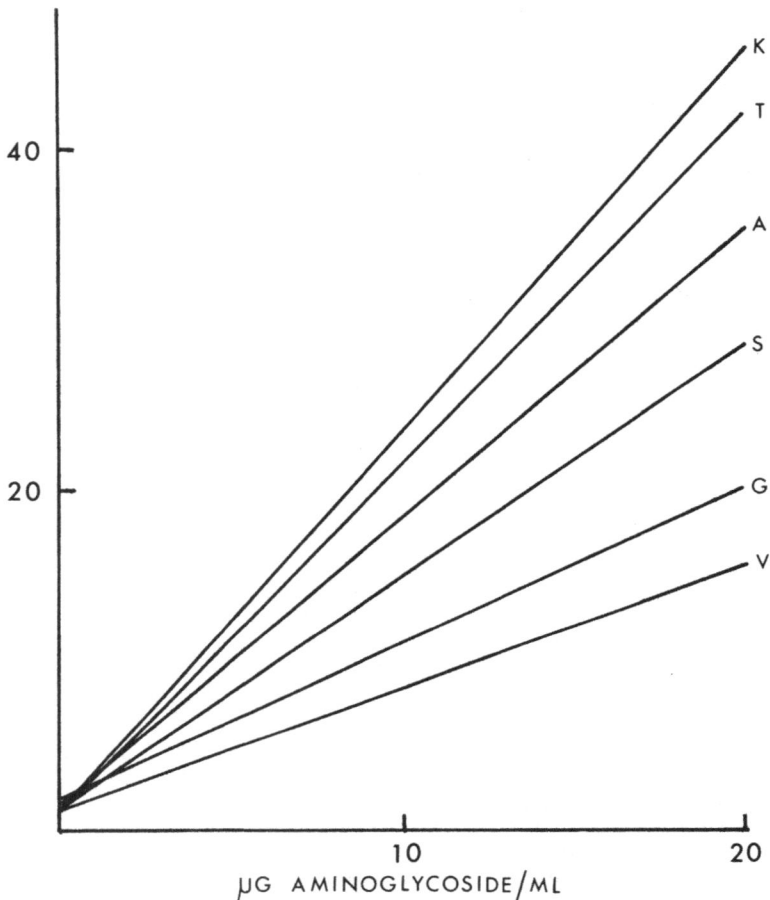

CPM X 10^{-3}

μG AMINOGLYCOSIDE/ML

Fig.1   Standard graphs for aminoglycoside antibiotics.
        K : kanamycin, T : tobramycin, A : amikacin,
        S : sisomycin, G : gentamicin, V : verdamycin.

The assay result is obtained within 1 hour of the receipt of
a clotted blood specimen at the laboratory bench.   This speed and
also the good accuracy of the acetyl transferase method (2,3) compared to other assay methods dependant on microbiological growth
are significant advantages.   The high specificity for aminoglycoside antibiotics is illustrated in Table 1.   Here a second antibiotic was introduced into a serum sample containing a known
concentration of gentamicin and then the serum was assayed for the

gentamicin concentration.   The % error was calculated for the
known $_\mathrm{V}$ found concentrations.

2nd antibiotic	Concentration of 2nd antibiotic (µg/ml)	% error in gentamicin concentration
Tobramycin	10.0	+ 425
Neomycin	37.5	+ 160
Kanamycin	10.0	+ 480
Amikacin	5.0	+ 306
Sisomycin	5.0	+ 240
Verdamycin	5.0	+ 215
Streptomycin	37.5	< 2.0
Penicillin	7.5	< 2.0
Ampicillin	7.5	< 2.0
Clindamycin	22.5	< 2.0
Erythromycin	7.5	< 2.0
Lincomycin	22.5	+ 7.7
Rifamycin	7.5	< 2.0
Fucidin	5.0	− 4.5
Novobiocin	75.0	− 5.0
Trimethoprim	6.0	< 2.0
Nalidixic acid	10.0	+10.0
Cloxacillin	10.0	< 2.0
Cephacetrile	3.75	< 2.0
Cephalothin	3.75	< 2.0
Cephazolin	15.0	+ 6.0

Table 1 :   Effect of Secondary Antibiotics

The results demonstrate that other commonly encountered non-
aminoglycoside antibiotics do not significantly affect the accuracy
of this method.   This is important since up to 20% of serum samples
presented for gentamicin assay have been found to contain other undisclosed antibiotics, (5) which may seriously affect a microbiological assay of gentamicin.

The enzyme used in the assay was isolated from E. coli W677/R5
which is resistant to tobramycin but not to gentamicin.   The
acetyl transferase enzyme system which confers resistance to the
organism will acetylate gentamicin isomers C_{1A} and C_2 but not the
C_1 isomer (isomers kindly supplied by Nicholas Laboratories Ltd.).

By using affinity chromatography it has been possible to
isolate the acetyl transferase enzyme and stablize it in a lyophilized state.   The affinity chromatography column was prepared
by conjugation of gentamicin sulphate to cyanogen bromide activated

Sepharose 4B (Pharmacia Ltd.).   The technique used was that described in the literature from Pharmacia Ltd.   Following conjugation the gentamicin – Sepharose 4B column was equilibrated with
0.025 M NaCl.   The enzyme applied to the column was the 14,000 g
supernatant from a sonicate of an E. coli W677/R5 washed cell
suspension in 10 mM Tris–Cl pH 7.5.   Following application of the
enzyme the non linear gradient of 0.025M to 2.0 M NaCl was passed

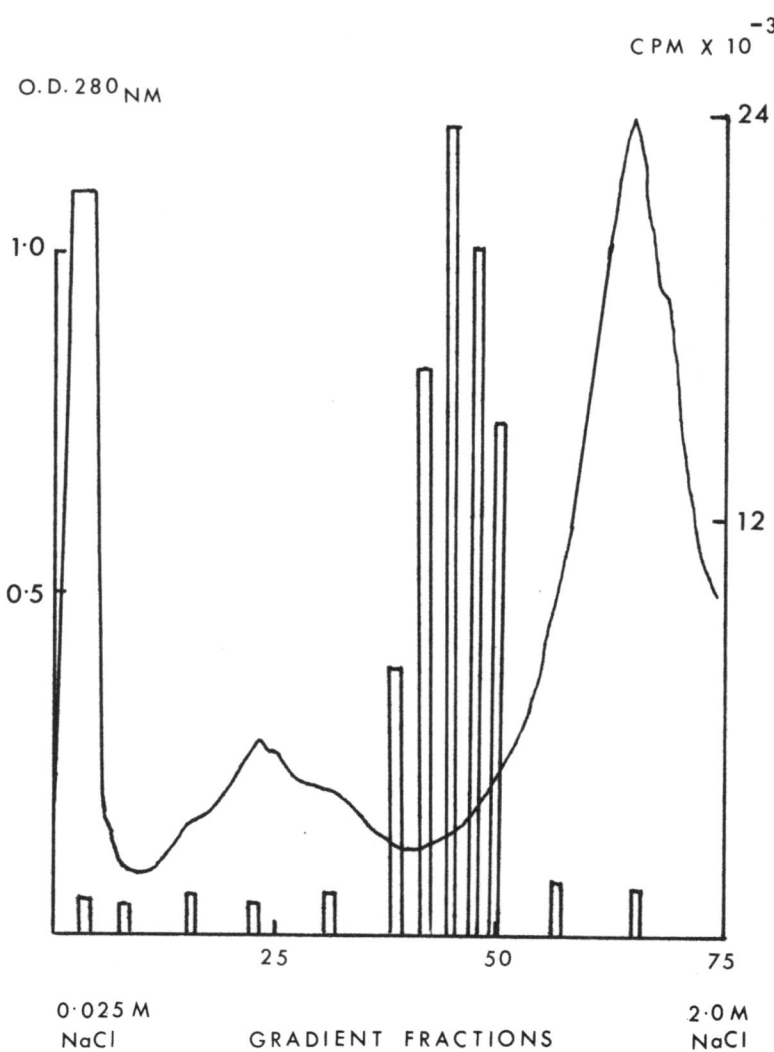

Fig.2   Elution profile of acetyl transferase enzyme from gentamicin
        – Sepharose 4B column.

down the column.   The acetyl transferase enzyme activity eluted
approximately mid-way through the gradient as is illustrated in
Fig. 2.

   The large final peak of material absorbing in the UV region was
probably nucleic acid as judged by the maximal absorption at 256 nm.
The enzymatically active fractions were determined, pooled and then
dialysed against distilled water at $4^{\circ}C$ for 12 hours.   The distilled water dialysis solution was changed twice over this period.
Following dialysis the enzyme solution was dispensed into 2.0 ml
volumes and lyophilized, then stored at $-20^{\circ}C$.   For reconstitution
of the enzyme 250 µl of 10 mM Tris Cl pH 7.5 was added to each vial.

   The reconstituted enzyme solution is as active as the crude
E. coli sonicate as is shown in Fig. 3.   When lyophilized the
enzyme may be kept up to 72 hours at room temperature without too
great a loss of activity.   Due to this stability it is possible
to send the enzyme in the post and we are prepared to supply
limited quantities of this preparation to other laboratories who
may wish to set up this assay technique.

   At present there is only one contra-indication for this assay
technique and this is when the patient has recently been on intravenous lipid therapy so that the serum sample has a very high lipid
content.   In this case the serum will be seen to be opaque.   The
excess lipid coats the P-81 phosphocellulose paper and prevents
effective washing to remove residual (^{14}C)-acetyl coenzyme A,
thus giving an apparent result which is far greater than the true gentamicin concentration.

   The technique also demands that the standards be made up in
the same media as the samples.   It is necessary to have pooled
human serum for preparing the standards, standards made up in
bovine serum will give slightly different results.   Similarly for
assaying gentamicin in other body fluids a suitable medium must be
found for the standards – for urine phosphate buffer at pH 7.3 is
adequate, the samples being diluted in the same buffer.   Although
standards in a non-protein medium may not give a straight standard
graph it is quite possible to obtain accurate results from a curved
graph.   For routine assays of gentamicin sera samples standards
at 1.25, 2.5, 5.0, 10.0 and 20.0 µg/ml are assayed singly and each
sample in duplicate.

   This assay technique is now in routine use in this laboratory
and appears to offer several advantages over conventional microbiological plate diffusion methods with the only one disadvantage
being that of non specific interference from lipids.

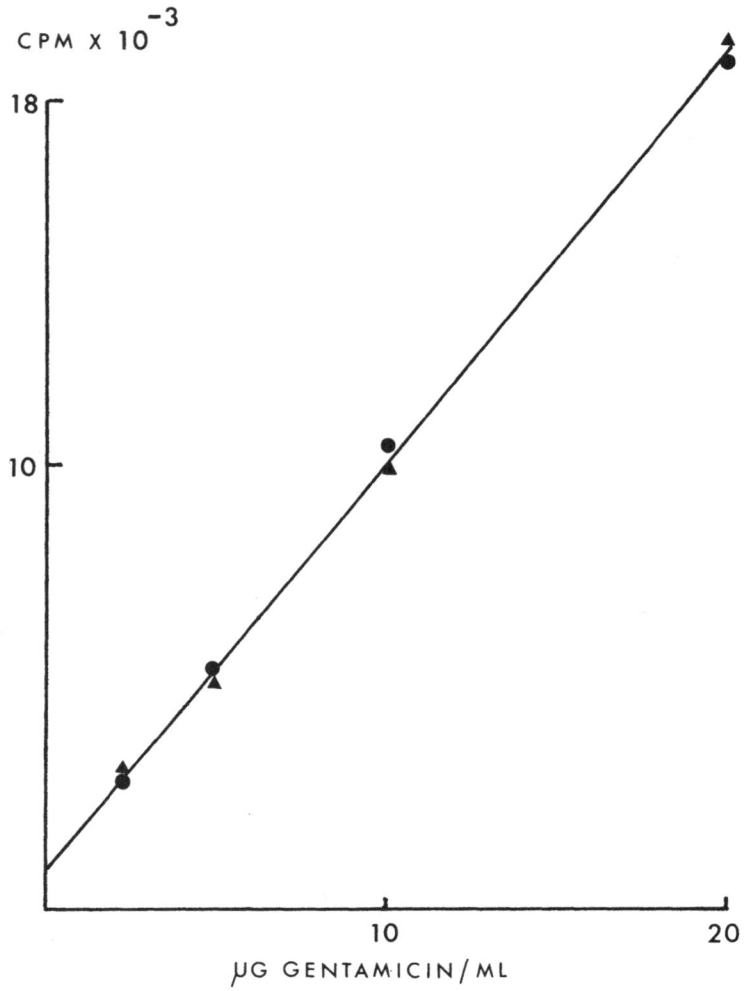

Fig.3   Comparative Activity of Reconstituted Lyophilized Enzyme
        and the Crude Sonicate.

        ▲ : reconstituted freeze-dried enzyme.   ● : crude sonicate.

REFERENCES

1. Ten Krooden, E., and J.H. Darrel, (1974). J.Clin.Path. 27,
    452–456.
2. Phillips, I., C. Warren and S.E. Smith, (1974). J.Clin.Path.
    27, 447–451.
3. Broughall, J., and D.S. Reeves, (1975). J.Clin.Path. 28, 140–145.
4. Davies, J., M. Brzezinska and R. Benveniste, (1971). Annals New
    York Acad. Sci., 128, 226–233.
5. Reeves, D.S., and H.A. Holt, (1975). J.Clin.Path. 28, 435–442.

IMMUNOCHEMICAL STUDY OF THE STRUCTURAL SPECIFICITY OF AN ANTI-GENTAMYCIN ANTISERUM, USEFUL ALSO FOR RADIOIMMUNOASSAY OF SISOMYCIN

S. Jonsson

Department of Medical Microbiology, University of
Lund, Sölvegatan 23, S-223 62 Lund, Sweden

At this Department a piece of collaborative work has resulted in a new method for the radioimmunoassay of gentamycin
levels in biological fluids (Jonsson et al., 1974 and 1975).
It differs in two important respects from the techniques applied by the first two groups in the field (Lewis et al., 1972,
Mahon et al., 1973). The most important difference lies in the
choice of the radioactive tracer. Since there is no commercial
source supplying a reproducible preparation of tritiated gentamycin, and since it is technically much simpler to measure
gamma radiation than beta radiation, a large effort was put
into establishing a method for the reproducible preparation of
a conjugate of gentamycin and human serum albumin (HSA). This
product is easily labelled with radioactive iodine, ^{125}I, in
a reproducible fashion without loss of the antigenic activity
of the coupled gentamycin. The second difference lies in the
choice of technique for the separation of antibody-bound and
free antigen. We have applied a solid phase separation reagent
of killed protein A-containing Staphylococcus aureus (Jonsson
and Kronvall, 1974) with a high capacity for binding more than
90 per cent of the serum IgG of some mammals such as man and
rabbit.
    In running the summarized radioimmunoassay for gentamycin
we have confirmed the results of earlier workers that a number
of other antibiotics in clinical use - including streptomycin,
kanamycin and also tobramycin - do not interfere in the reaction between radiolabelled gentamycin and anti-gentamycin antiserum raised in rabbits that had been immunized with a conjugate of gentamycin and ovalbumin prepared with a water-soluble
carbodiimide according to the directions of Lewis et al. (1972).

165

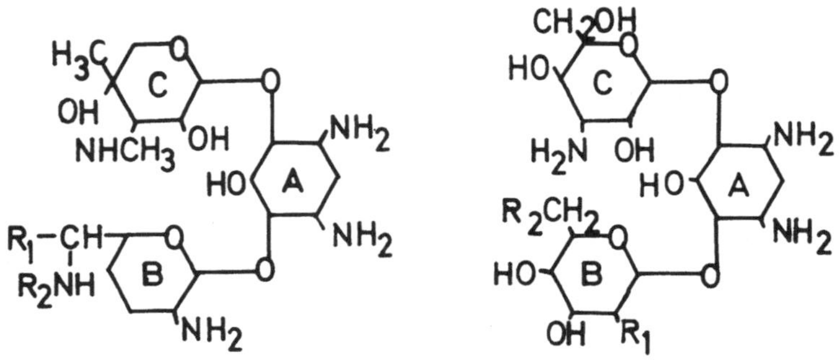

Gentamycin

Kanamycin

C_1	$R_1 = CH_3$	$R_2 = CH_3$		A	$R_1 = OH$	$R_2 = NH_2$
C_2	$R_1 = CH_3$	$R_2 = H$		B	$R_1 = NH_2$	$R_2 = NH_2$
C_{1a}	$R_1 = H$	$R_2 = H$		C	$R_1 = NH_2$	$R_2 = OH$

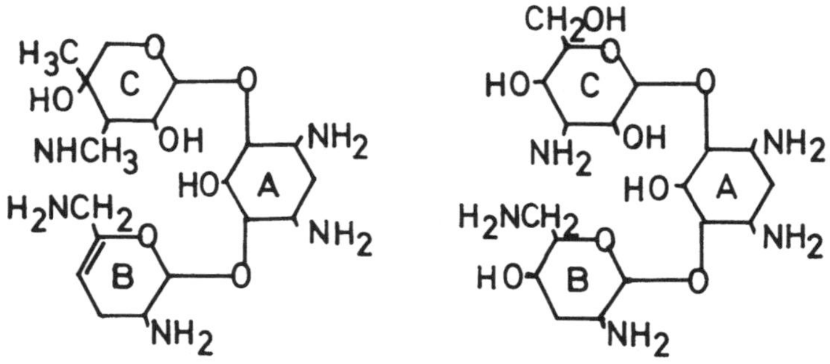

Sisomycin

Tobramycin

Fig. 1. Structural formulas of four closely related aminoglycoside antibiotics: gentamycin, kanamycin, sisomycin, and tobramycin. Of the latter three only sisomycin cross-reacts immunologically with gentamycin in its reaction with an anti-gentamycin antiserum.

However, we have found that a new aminoglycoside antibiotic, sisomycin, significantly cross-reacts in our radioimmunoassay for gentamycin. Sisomycin is about 50 per cent as effective as gentamycin in the assay, irrespective of the use of genta-mycin-HSA-^{125}I or sisomycin-HSA-^{125}I as the radioactive tracer. After submission of the abstract of this communication I have become aware of a recent paper by Minshew et al. (1975), who have registered the same results in a radioimmunoassay with tritiated gentamycin as the tracer.

These findings raise the question of the structural specificity of the antisera obtained from rabbits subjected to the
mentioned immunization procedure. Fig. 1 demonstrate structural
formulas of four closely related aminoglycoside antibiotics:
gentamycin, kanamycin, sisomycin and tobramycin. For simplicity,
the three ring structures of each have been designated A, B, and
C, resp. It is readily apparent that the A rings of all four
aminoglycosides are identical. The B rings of the four antibiotics have many substituents in common. The B ring of sisomycin
with its double bond stands out, however. The C rings are identical between gentamycin and sisomycin on the one hand and between kanamycin and tobramycin on the other. In comparing the
C rings between the two groups, four or five distinct differences are found.

The lack of cross reactions of kanamycin and tobramycin,
resp., with gentamycin in the various radioimmunoassay methods
could be explained by the fact that the A ring carries two
primary amino groups, which might be destroyed by action of the
water-soluble carbodiimide, used in excess for the preparation
of the macromolecular immunogen. The other primary amino sub-
stituent groups of gentamycin, present in its B ring, should
also be expected to be subjected to the same changes as the
A ring. Then, antibodies to gentamycin's A and B rings, structurally changed, would not recognize structures identical or
similar to those of native gentamycin. The finding that our two
antigentamycin antisera are practically incapable of binding
kanamycin-HSA-^{125}I supports the proposed interpretation. The
C ring common to gentamycin and sisomycin is unique in that it
carries no primary amino group at all. The presented data
point to this C ring as being the most important antigenic
determinant of gentamycin when one uses the type of antiserum
described. The findings also indicate that coupling procedures,
alternative to the carbodiimide technique applied sofar, might
be necessary for the production of immunogenic conjugates of
aminoglycosides which carry primary amino substituents on all
ring structures.

REFERENCES.

S. Jonsson, G. Kahlmeter, T. Hallberg, and G. Kronvall, Communication to the VIth Int. Congr. of Inf. and Parasitic Diseases,
Warszawa, Poland, Sept. 1974, Abstracts volume p. 323.

S. Jonsson, G. Kahlmeter, T. Hallberg, and G. Kronvall (1975),
Manuscript submitted for publication.

S. Jonsson and G. Kronvall (1974), Europ. J. Immunol. 4: 29

J.E. Lewis, J.C. Nelson, and H.A. Elder (1972), Nature New

Biology <u>239</u>: 214.

W.A. Mahon, J. Ezer, and T.W. Wilson (1973), Antimicrob. Agents
Chemother. <u>3</u>: 585

B.H. Minshew, R.K. Holmes, and C.R. Baxter (1975), Antimicrob.
Agents Chemother. <u>7</u>: 107.

Another paper on a related subject is published also
in the proceedings

SERUM ACTIVITY DETERMINATION AS CONNECTING LINK

BETWEEN EXPERIMENT AND CLINIC

Enno Freerksen and Magdalena Rosenfeld

Forschungsinstitut Borstel

2061 Borstel / West Germany

Today, the evaluation of chemotherapeutic agents usually is carried out separately within the two fields

| Experiment | | Clinic |

generally looked upon as two independent areas. As the results are not just interchangeable, we directed investigations towards methods and procedures to fill the gap between experiment and clinic (2,3,6).

A kind of connecting link was found in the determination of serum activity in man (healthy volunteers). The measured values reflect the attainable and therapeutically utilizable activity in the organism and allow to compare the effectivity of different substances and combinations. The problems and implications are well known, but cannot be discussed here. Only a few typical results can be demonstrated.

Our methods, including in vitro-tests, animal experiments and preliminary clinical use, show the potentiating effect of certain substances on others, so far scarcely profited of in the therapy of tuberculosis.

Thus it is possible to apply Prothionamide (PTH) in the well tolerated, by itself nearly ineffective dose of 5 mg./kgm. Potentiating properties has also Diaminodiphenylsulfone (DDS) in a dose of 1-2 mg./kgm. Besides its own therapeutic action, Ethambutol (EMB) enhances the action of other substances and can be potentiated by others (Fig. 1).

FIGURE 1

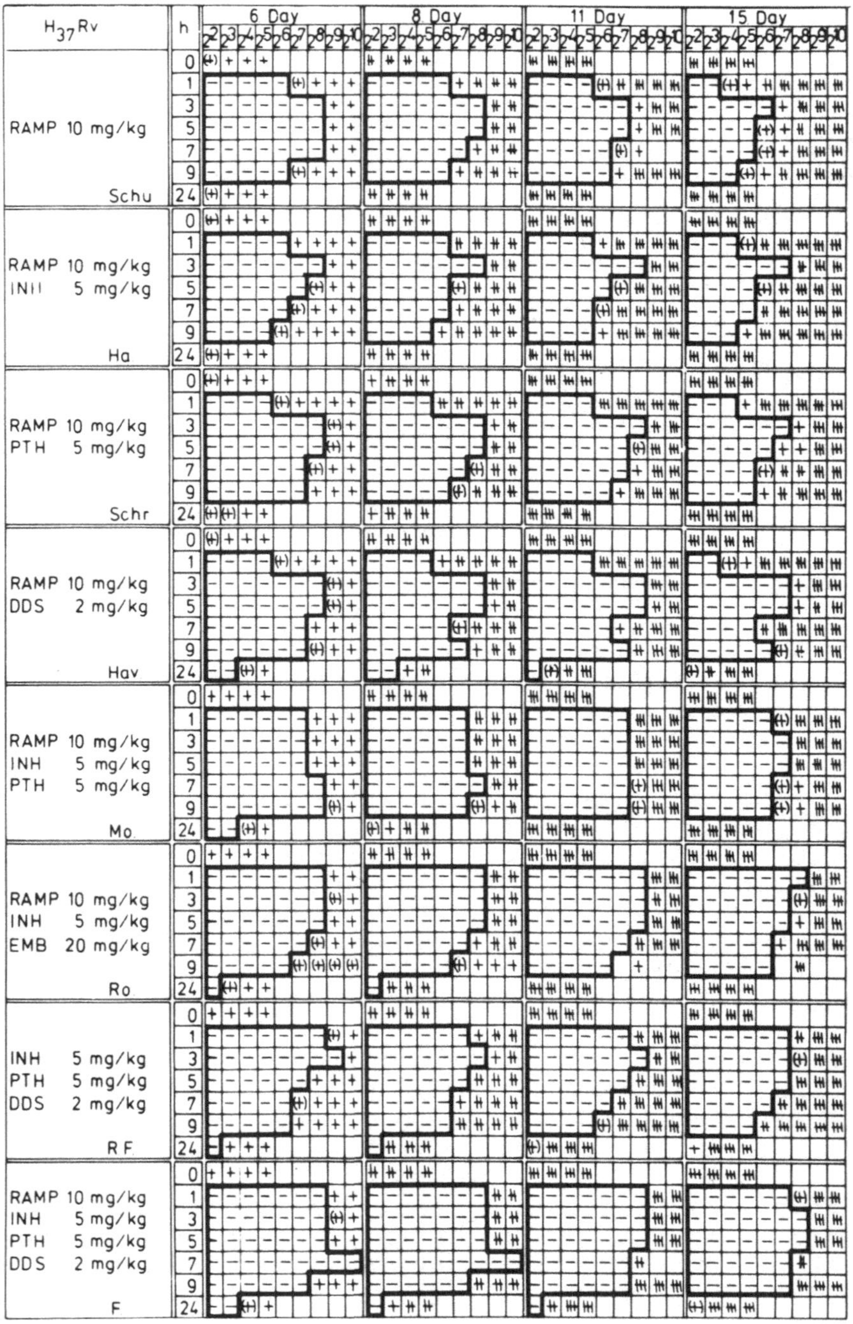
$H_{37}Rv$
h
6 Day
8 Day
11 Day
15 Day
RAMP 10 mg/kg
Schu
RAMP 10 mg/kg
INH 5 mg/kg
Ha
RAMP 10 mg/kg
PTH 5 mg/kg
Schr
RAMP 10 mg/kg
DDS 2 mg/kg
Hav
RAMP 10 mg/kg
INH 5 mg/kg
PTH 5 mg/kg
Mo
RAMP 10 mg/kg
INH 5 mg/kg
EMB 20 mg/kg
Ro
INH 5 mg/kg
PTH 5 mg/kg
DDS 2 mg/kg
R.F.
RAMP 10 mg/kg
INH 5 mg/kg
PTH 5 mg/kg
DDS 2 mg/kg
F

As a consequence, a series of combinations was developed for the treatment of tuberculosis. As twin combination

RMP + INH

is nowadays commonly used. Serum activity determinations indicate that at least an equivalent effect can be expected of

RMP + PTH
RMP + DDS
RMP + Sm
RMP + EMB

Besides the generally used triple combination

RMP + INH + EMB

already recommended on the basis of serum activity determinations, new alternatives are available:

RMP + PTH + INH   as purely oral medications
RMP + DDS + INH
RMP + PTH + EMB

RMP + INH + SM   as partially parenteral
RMP + PTH + SM   medications

Of special interest is the combination

INH + PTH + DDS,

the first one (definitely not the last one) being worked out in full consideration of the potentiating phenomenon. As dosis-proportions play an important role to obtain optimal effectivity and to simplify administration, a fixed combination (ISOPRODIAN) has been prepared.

Such medications allow ambulatory, highly effective treatment, are applicable even under difficult circumstances and, in addition, are inexpensive. The therapeutic effect is similar to that of RMP+INH+EMB and that of the "classical" triple combination INH+SM+PAS.

Using this principle, leprosy treatment was entirely changed. Up till now, leprosy bacilli cannot be satisfactorily cultivated in vitro. Therefore we take atypical mycobacteria, mainly M.marinum, as substitutes (3).

Carrier S. oranienburg since 22 years
Pre-treatment: Chloramphenicolum   Cholecystectomy
               Streptomycine
               Ampicilline
               Autovaccine
Determination of serum activity: healthy test-persons
Strain: S. oranienburg

h	Ampicilline 2 g							Trimethoprime-Sulfamethoxazole 960 mg							Rifampicine 600 mg							Trimethoprime-Sulfamethoxazole 960 mg Rifampicine 600 mg						
	Serumdilution																											
	2^{-2}	2^{-3}	2^{-4}	2^{-5}	2^{-6}	2^{-7}	2^{-8}	2^{-2}	2^{-3}	2^{-4}	2^{-5}	2^{-6}	2^{-7}	2^{-8}	2^{-2}	2^{-3}	2^{-4}	2^{-5}	2^{-6}	2^{-7}	2^{-8}	2^{-2}	2^{-3}	2^{-4}	2^{-5}	2^{-6}	2^{-7}	2^{-8}
0	+++	+++	+++	+++	+++	+++	+++	+++	+++	+++	+++	+++	+++	+++	+++	+++	+++	+++	+++	+++	+++	+++	+++	+++	+++	+++	+++	+++
1	+	+	++	+++	+++	+++	+++					+++	+++	+++	+++	+++	+++	+++	+++	+++	+++					+++	+++	+++
3		++	+++	+++	+++	+++	+++					+++	+++	+++	+++	+++	+++	+++	+++	+++	+++					+++	+++	+++
5	+	+++	+++	+++	+++	+++	+++					+++	+++	+++	+++	+++	+++	+++	+++	+++	+++						+++	+++
7	+++	+++	+++	+++	+++	+++	+++					+++	+++	+++	+++	+++	+++	+++	+++	+++	+++						+++	+++
9	+++	+++	+++	+++	+++	+++	+++					+++	+++	+++	++	+++	+++	+++	+++	+++	+++				+	+++	+++	+++
24	+++	+++	+++	+++	+++	+++	+++	+++	+++	+++	+++	+++	+++	+++	+++	+++	+++	+++	+++	+++	+++			(+)	+++	+++	+++	+++

Determination of serum activity: patient M.K.
Strain: S. oranienburg
Treatment: Trimethoprime-Sulfamethoxazole 480 mg
           Rifampicine 300 mg

h	Serumdilution						
	2^{-2}	2^{-3}	2^{-4}	2^{-5}	2^{-6}	2^{-7}	2^{-8}
3					+++	++	+++
7					+++	+++	+++

Therapy: twice daily
Duration of treatment: 30 days
Negative culture results since first week after onset of therapy
Follow-up period: 2 years

FIGURE 2

The "Marinum-model" revealed that RMP is superior
to DDS. Today, the following combinations are to be considered the most potent ones:

```
(INH + PTH + DDS) + RMP
(INH + PTH + DDS) + EMB
 RMP + PTH + EMB
 RMP + PTH + INH
 RMP + PTH + DDS
 RMP + PTH
 RMP + EMB
 RMP + DDS
 RMP + LSA
```

Their efficacy in leprosy treatment has been testified
meanwhile at different places (1,4,5).

This combination principle made possible another
step ahead in the treatment of mycobacterioses. Now we
dispose of therapeutical possibilities no longer to
classify as "therapy of tuberculosis" or "therapy of
leprosy", but as a general kind of treating mycobacterioses. In cases suffering simultaneously from more
than one mycobacterial disease, now only one basic
treatment is required.

Suitable combinations for this purpose are:

```
RMP + (PTH + INH + DDS)
EMB + (PTH + INH + DDS)
RMP + (PTH + EMB)
```

Concerning treatment of salmonellosis, only
carriers will be briefly mentioned today. Testing serum
activity, we determine an optimal and individual therapy.
Good results were obtained also in unsuccessfully pre-
treated cases, including cholecystectomy. A typical
case is demonstrated in Fig. 2. Urine- and stool-
specimens, bacteriologically negative after the first
days of treatment, are followed up daily during the
first phase, then in weekly, later in monthly intervals.
Bile is tested just before stopping treatment which,
depending on individual requirements, takes 4 to 8 weeks.

As example for other infections, urological or pulmonary, we will demonstrate only the results obtained
with a Klebsiella-Aerob. strain (Fig. 3).

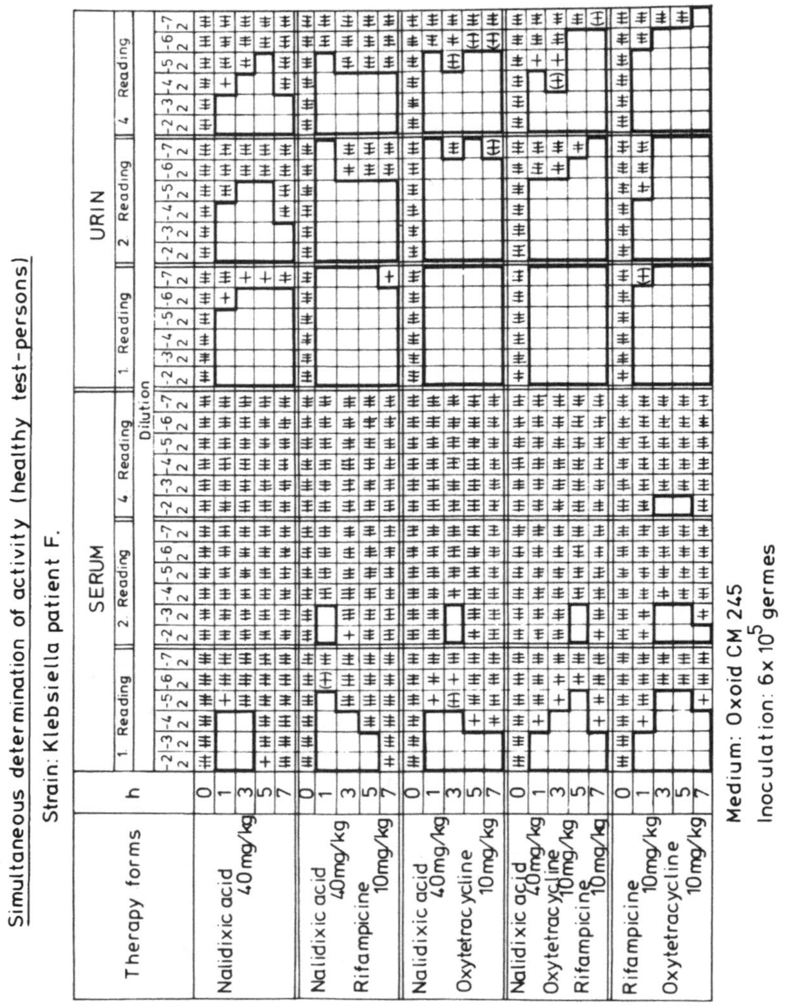
Simultaneous determination of activity (healthy test-persons)
Strain: Klebsiella patient F.
Therapy forms
h
SERUM
URIN
1. Reading
2. Reading
4. Reading
Dilution
Nalidixic acid 40 mg/kg
Nalidixic acid 40mg/kg
Rifampicine 10mg/kg
Nalidixic acid 40mg/kg
Oxytetracycline 10mg/kg
Nalidixic acid 40mg/kg
Oxytetracycline 10mg/kg
Rifampicine 10mg/kg
Rifampicine 10mg/kg
Oxytetracycline 10mg/kg
Medium: Oxoid CM 245
Inoculation: 6x10^5 germes

Fig. 3

Despite lack of time, we hope to have been able to indicate the possibility to determine the value of new substances and medications by means of testing activity in human serum - the only human material relatively safely and nearly unlimited to obtain. With this method the therapeutic value can be predicted. In consequence, clinical evaluation is getting a new aspect.

References:

1. Bonnici, E., G. Depasquale:
   The Leprosy Eradication Programme of Malta. 2nd International Leprosy Colloquium, October 1974, Borstel (in the press)

2. Freerksen, E., R. Bönicke, M. Rosenfeld, W. Reif:
   Antibakterielle Wirkstoffe und Substanzen im Makroorganismu. Jahresbericht 1952/53, Borstel.

3. Freerksen, E.:
   The Technique of Evaluation of Antileprosy Medication at the Forschungsinstitut Borstel. 2nd International Leprosy Colloquium, October 1974, Borstel (in the press)

4. Krenzien, H.N.:
   Preliminary Experience with Rifampicin and Isoprodian in Combination in Leprosy Treatment. 2nd International Leprosy Colloquium, October 1974, Borstel (in the press)

5. Rohde, R.:
   Report of Combined Therapy in Leprosy with Rifampicin and Isoprodian Conducted at the Bisidimo-Center, Ethiopia. 2nd International Leprosy Colloquium, October 1974, Borstel (in the press).

6. Rosenfeld, M.:
   Rifampicin, Myambutol, Isoxyl, and Capreomycin as Combination Partners in Animal Experiments. Antibiotica et Chemotherapia. Vol. 16, 501-515. Karger, Basel/München/New York 1970.

ANIMAL MODELS IN THE ASSESSMENT OF ANTIMICROBIAL AGENTS:

WHAT SHOULD WE EXPECT OF THEM?

FRANCIS O'GRADY

UNIVERSITY OF NOTTINGHAM
DEPARTMENT OF MICROBIOLOGY
CITY HOSPITAL, NOTTINGHAM NG5 1PH

The properties required of an effective therapeutic antibiotic are few in number but demanding in character. The agent must be absorbed from the site of administration and survive the processes of metabolic destruction and excretion to the extent that it reaches the site of infection in sufficient concentration to inhibit the growth of bacteria or better still to kill them.

Since it is too much to hope that agents will ordinarily seek out the site of infection in the sense that they will be preferentially concentrated there, access of the agent to the lesion must inevitably be accompanied by its widespread distribution throughout the body. It follows that its antibacterial benefit must not be obtained at the cost of deleterious effects on remote tissues uninvolved in the infectious process.

PREDICTIONS FROM PRELIMINARY STUDIES

On the basis of these few identifiable properties, it might seem that the potential therapeutic value of a new antibiotic ought to be predictable from a thorough preliminary examination of three things: its in vitro antibacterial activity; its detailed pharmaco- kinetics and the nature and magnitude of its toxicity. Any agent that reached potential infection sites in concentrations sufficient to exert a potent antibacterial effect on doses far below those likely to produce untoward manifestations must surely be identifiable as a therapeutic winner. Unfortunately, in practice the situation is not quite so straightforward and at least some of the reasons why predictions made on this kind of basis generally lack confidence can be readily identified.

In the first place, the conditions in which the activity of antibiotics and bacteria interact in the infected lesion are very different. In in vitro sensitivity tests, the number of bacteria exposed to the antibiotic is small and the conditions are arranged so that the bacteria will grow since it is interference with growth that is the essence of antibacterial effect. In the lesion, on the other hand, the number of bacteria is large and in established infection, except where active extension is proceeding, the bacterial population is close to its climax state and its rate of turnover is low.

In laboratory tests, the nutritional conditions and antibiotic concentrations are intended to be stable. In the lesion they are constantly changing, often so that the antibiotic concentration to which the organisms are exposed rises and falls over a range far exceeding that studied in the laboratory not once but several times over the period of a conventional in vitro test. Moreover, in order to secure the necessary bacterial growth, cultural conditions are favourably adapted to whatever degree the organism demands. In the lesion, on the other hand, if there is to be any hope of successful resolution of infection, the conditions are as hostile to bacterial survival as the body can make them. In a word there is no major respect in which laboratory tests and real life therapeutic situations resemble one another.

When we come to look at the pharmacokinetic studies, extensive though they often are, the quantity and quality of data is often found to increase in proportion to its distance from the lesion. A good deal is usually known, for example, about the absorption of the compound and the shape of its plasma profile: the height and time of its peak and the shape and rate of its decay. Much is often known of its excretion, but if its metabolism is at all complex the fate of a greater or lesser proportion of the drug is frequently obscure; and as we approach the pharmacokinetic heart of the matter - the concentration of the agent in potentially infected tissues - our knowledge of the situation in many important sites, for example the lung or the CSF, is frequently seriously defective. Moreover, even where the agent can be shown to reach the infected site in concentrations that would be expected from in vitro studies to exert a useful antibacterial effect we have generally no way of knowing whether those effects will occur in the peculiar and complex humoral and cellular environment of the infected lesion.

POTENTIAL RÔLE OF ANIMAL MODELS

In the face of all these difficulties, the possibility that the therapeutic place of antibiotics might be predictable from the results of treating experimental animal infections appears very attractive. In such infections the bacteria must be living in conditions characteristic of lesions - whatever they may be - and an agent that exerts a favourable effect on the course of the experimental disease must by definition be reaching the lesion in sufficient concentration to exert a useful antibacterial effect within the environment of the lesion. In fact at first glance, the information provided by such experiments appears so comprehensive and therapeutically relevant as to raise the question whether they make preliminary in vitro sensitivity tests and pharmacokinetic studies entirely superfluous. Before the question can be answered it is necessary to explore three other questions of increasing difficulty.

TYPES OF ANIMAL INFECTION

The first question is 'To what extent do experimental infections resemble anything that occurs spontaneously in nature?' The second, more difficult, question, is "To what extent do these infections resemble anything that occurs spontaneously in man?' - bearing in mind that the predictions of therapeutic value must relate to man and not to the rodents to which we devote so much of our time and energies. The third question, which is so difficult that almost all of it will be left to Professor Mawer (p. 000) to answer, is 'To what extent do differences in the ways in which antibiotics are handled by experimental animals and man, modify or even negate any conclusions that might otherwise be drawn about the human therapeutic usefulness of the agent?' In attempting to answer these questions it is useful to distinguish three types of experimental infection.

TYPE I 'INFECTION'

These are typified by the lesion produced by local injections, or by challenge to death by the intravenous or intraperitoneal routes. They are better described as 'bacterial challenges' rather than 'infection'. Almost invariably treatment, if it is successful, must begin at the time of, or very shortly after, injection. The outcome cannot usually be influenced by later treatment and Type I procedures are not infections in the ordinary sense of the term. They nevertheless provide valuable information in that a protective effect indicates that the antibiotic reaches the site of infection and operates in the environment of the lesion. Dose-ranging studies utilising such challenges might fairly be described as 'titrations in vivo'. To be useful Type I 'infections' must exhibit two features. Their effect must be readily measured (for example the time to death) and the measurement must be reproducible within fairly narrow limits. It may reasonably be argued that almost any device however 'unnatural' (for example the use of mucin in the

bacterial inoculum, or treatment of the animals with immunosuppressive agents) is acceptable in Type 1 tests providing the
measurement and its reproducibility are facilitated.

TYPE II INFECTIONS

These are quite different. They attempt to mimic as precisely
as possible particular human infections and their value depends
directly on the extent to which they succeed in that objective.
Examples are pyelonephritis in the rat, meningitis in the dog or
endocarditis in the rabbit. In some such infections, rabbit
endocarditis for example, the mimicry of the corresponding human
infection in pathogenesis, course and outcome is reasonably
convincing. In other experimental infections, the correspondence
with man is a good deal less faithful. Histopathological
correspondence may be close but that in itself may not provide
very strong evidence of identity because the range of reactions
that an organ (for example, kidney) can mount to a whole variety
of insults may be distinctly limited.

The most important test of competence of Type II models in
therapeutic predictions is, not surprisingly, the therapeutic one:
the infection must respond to appropriate treatment after the
lesion has been established and its natural course already begun
to unfold. A lesion that responds only to treatment instituted
shortly after initiation should be regarded, notwithstanding close
histological similarity to the corresponding human disease, as a
Type I challenge.

TYPE III INFECTIONS

These utilise a natural pathogen for the animal species
employed. Some such infections have clear human equivalents: for
example, Salmonella typhimurum infections in the mouse and
systemic salmonellosis in man. Some, like Streptobacillus
moniliformis infection in the mouse, have no such obvious
corresponding human disease. Diseases artificially induced, but
utilising natural pathogens, may have a special part to play in
predictive therapeutic assessments. In appropriate experimental
circumstances, they may be transmitted by the natural route
(permitting not only therapeutic but prophylactic assessments); but
even where this is not employed, the interaction between the host
and its natural pathogen - even in those cases where the animal
disease possesses no obvious direct human equivalent - may well
represent more faithfully fundamental pathological features of
human infections than do challenges by unlikely routes with
specifically human pathogens.

CHOICE OF ANIMAL

The essential issues of 'naturalness' of experimental infections and the degree of human correspondence plainly involve not only the choice of organism and the route of its administration but the choice of animal. It must appear that experimental airborne tuberculosis in the primate provides better guidance to the treatment of human tuberculosis than streptococcal infection in the mouse foot-pad provides for the treatment of human sore throat.

If a near-perfect model of a human infection can be devised, then it might well render laboratory tests of antibacterial activity and pharmacokinetic studies superfluous. At the moment, however, the deficiencies of the great majority of animal models are all too obvious; but so too are the deficiencies of current in vitro sensitivity tests and general pharmacokinetics. As long as the nature of these deficiencies is recognised and the particular contribution made by all three kinds of study is identified, then each can make a valuable contribution towards constructing a sufficiently comprehensive view of the behaviour of the agent to enable a reasonably secure prediction of its likely therapeutic place to be made.

LOCAL LESIONS

G. N. Rolinson

Beecham Pharmaceuticals Research Division

Brockham Park, Betchworth, Surrey, England

The term local lesion is used here to mean infections of skin
or soft tissue which result in a lesion which is localized with
only limited systemic spread of the infecting organism.   A number
of experimental models of this type have been described, involving
intramuscular, subcutaneous or intracutaneous infection and also
infections of abraded or burnt skin.   In general the number of
organisms required to cause infection in these models is high and
various procedures or agents have been used to enhance infection
including shock (Miles and Niven, 1950) and the administration of
adrenaline (Evans et al., 1948), malonate (Berry and Mitchell,
1953) or ferric iron (Weinberg, 1966).   The presence of a foreign
body such as a suture (Elek and Conen, 1957; James and MacLeod,
1961) or cotton dust (Noble, 1965) has also been used to enhance
infection.

In this contribution to the Symposium some results will be
presented which have been obtained using an intramuscular
infection in the mouse, first described by Selbie and Simon (1952).
In this model, 0.2 ml of a bacterial suspension is inoculated into
the back of the thigh section of the hind leg of the mouse and the
injection is made so that as far as possible the bacteria are
inoculated between, rather than into, the muscle fascicles.
Following the inoculation a lesion develops resulting in a marked
swelling of the leg.   This enlargement can be measured and an
example of the results obtained are shown in Fig. 1.   In this
experiment mice were inoculated with a strain of Escherichia coli
and the number of colony-forming units (CFU) injected per thigh
are shown on the graph.   The enlargement of the thigh reaches a
maximum 24-48 hours after inoculation and then remains relatively
constant for several days.

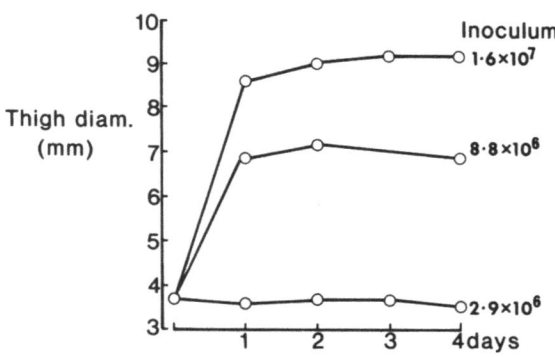

FIG. 1. Thigh enlargement in mice infected with <u>E. coli</u>.
(Data from Hunter, Rolinson and Witting, 1973)

     Prevention of thigh enlargement is used as an index of
therapeutic effect following antibiotic dosage and results are
shown in Fig. 2.   In this experiment mice were again inoculated
with a strain of <u>E. coli</u> and ampicillin was injected subcutaneously
at the time of inoculation.   It can be seen that increase in
antibiotic dosage resulted in a correspondingly greater prevention
of thigh enlargement and in this experiment a dose of 100 mg/kg
prevented the formation of a lesion completely.   From results of
this type a value for percentage protection can be calculated

$$\left(\% \text{ Protection} = \frac{\substack{\text{enlargement of the} \\ \text{infected controls}} - \substack{\text{enlargement of} \\ \text{test group}}}{\text{enlargement of infected controls}} \times 100 \right)$$

and plotted against dose from which an ED_{50} value can be obtained.

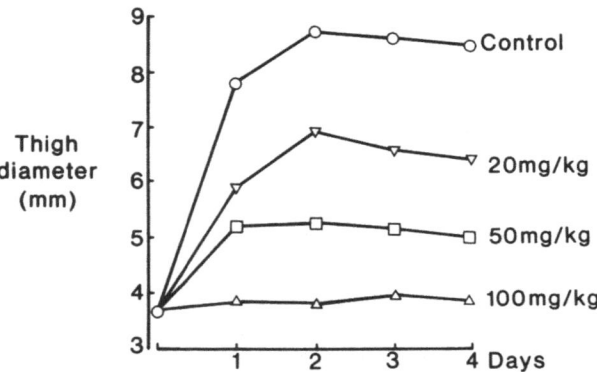

FIG. 2. Effect of ampicillin subcutaneously in the thigh
lesion test using <u>E. coli</u>.
(Data from Hunter, Rolinson and Witting, 1973)

An example of the dose-response plots so obtained is given in
Fig. 3.   In this experiment ampicillin or amoxycillin was administered orally to groups of ten mice and E. coli was again used as
the infecting organism.   The points on the graph represent the
mean values for the groups of mice and indicate the variation which
occurs between one experiment and another.   This variation is due
in part to the fact that the severity of the lesion and hence the
percentage protection is dependent on the virulence and the number
of organisms injected.

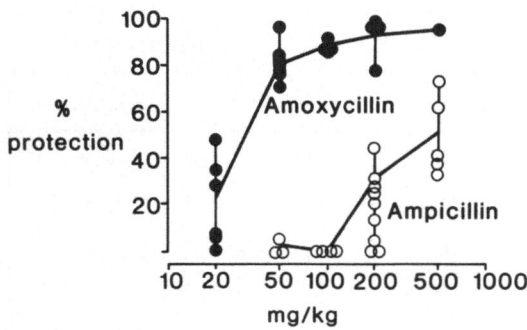

FIG. 3.   Effect of oral dosage of ampicillin or amoxycillin
          in the thigh lesion test using E. coli.
     (Data from Hunter, Rolinson and Witting, 1973)

In order to obtain a lesion the size of the infective
inoculum is critical and this can be expressed in terms of the
number of viable bacteria injected.   Below a certain number the
bacteria are cleared by body defences and no lesion develops.
Above a critical number, clearance by body defences is unable to
keep pace with bacterial multiplication, an increase in the
numbers of viable cells occurs, and a lesion is produced.   Certain
organisms are highly virulent in this model and even with an
inoculum as small as a few cells, rapid bacterial multiplication
occurs with the formation of a lesion.   On the other hand, with
many organisms the critical infective number is relatively high
and is in the order of 10^6-10^7 CFU injected per thigh.   After
inoculation bacterial multiplication or clearance by defence
mechanisms can be followed by homogenizing the entire infected
thigh section and performing viable counts in the usual way.
In Fig. 4 the critical infective number is shown for Pseudomonas
aeruginosa, E. coli and Staphylococcus aureus.   The number of
viable bacteria per thigh (CFU) shown at time 0 is the number
recovered in the homogenate and is slightly lower than the true
number injected.   Recovery of viable cells in the homogenate,
however, is good and is in the order of 50-70% of the number
injected (Table 1).   It will be seen from Fig. 4 that in the

case of <u>Ps</u>. <u>aeruginosa</u>, using an inoculum of 10^6 CFU or more, bacterial multiplication is rapid, cell numbers reaching a maximum at approximately 24 hours after inoculation and remaining relatively constant for several days. This pattern of bacterial growth is always accompanied by the formation of a lesion.

TABLE 1. Recovery of viable organisms after intramuscular inoculation in mice.
(Hunter, Witting and Rolinson, unpublished data)

E. coli			Pseudomonas		
Injected	Recovered	%	Injected	Recovered	%
1.1×10^7	7.5×10^6	68	4.8×10^6	3.4×10^6	71
8.4×10^6	6.5×10^6	77	4.2×10^6	2.8×10^6	67
5.6×10^6	4.3×10^6	77	5.3×10^6	3.2×10^6	60
3.8×10^6	3.5×10^6	92	6.3×10^6	3.1×10^6	49
2.4×10^6	1.6×10^6	67	5.0×10^6	2.9×10^6	58
2.1×10^6	1.4×10^6	67	5.5×10^6	2.8×10^6	51
4.2×10^5	2.3×10^5	55	8.9×10^6	3.4×10^6	38
	Mean	72		Mean	56

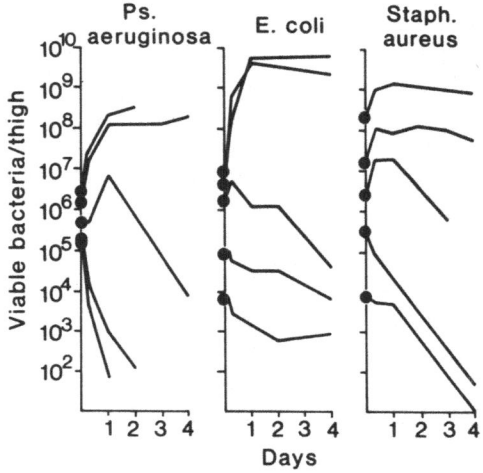

FIG. 4. Counts of viable organisms in the thigh of mice following intramuscular infection.
(Hunter, Witting and Rolinson, unpublished data)

With an inoculum of 5×10^5-10^6 CFU some bacterial multiplication
may occur over the first 24 hours but thereafter the bacteria may
be cleared by defence mechanisms and in such cases the lesion is
small.   With an inoculum of 5×10^5 CFU or less the bacteria are
cleared rapidly and no lesion is produced.   A similar picture is
seen with E. coli except that the critical infective number is
slightly higher than it is with Pseudomonas and below the critical
inoculum bacterial clearance is very much slower.   As with
Pseudomonas there is a direct correlation between bacterial multiplication or clearance and the formation or absence of a lesion.
With Staph. aureus the critical infective number is higher again
and only with an inoculum of 10^7 CFU or more is there multiplication and approximately 10^8 CFU are required for the formation
of a consistent lesion which is maintained for several days.   The
clearance rate with Staph. aureus is intermediate between that of
E. coli and Pseudomonas.

The determination of the number of viable bacteria present
in the infected thigh allows the effect of antibiotic dosage to
be studied not only in terms of prevention of the formation of a
lesion, but also in terms of the inhibition of growth or rate of
killing of the infecting organism in vivo.   Results are shown in
Fig. 5 for the viable counts obtained in mice infected with
E. coli following dosage with ampicillin subcutaneously at the
time of infection.   Using a dose of 50 mg/kg a slight bactericidal effect occurred over the first hour after infection but
thereafter bacterial multiplication took place at a rate parallel
with that seen in the untreated controls and lesion formation was
only partially prevented.   With 100 mg/kg a more pronounced antibacterial effect was seen but bacterial multiplication again
occurred after approximately 2 hours with only partial prevention
of lesion formation.   With 200 mg/kg inhibition of bacterial
growth was maintained for at least 7 hours after infection and
thigh enlargement was almost completely prevented although at
24 hours bacterial numbers had increased to give a count only
slightly below that in the controls.   At 400 mg/kg bacterial
numbers remained relatively low even at 24 hours and no lesion
developed.   These results show that a clear dose response can be
obtained with this model in both bacteriological and therapeutic
terms.

The model can also be used to study the effect of dosage
schedules and some results are shown in Fig. 6.   In this experiment mice were infected with Ps. aeruginosa and carbenicillin
administered subcutaneously at the dosage indicated.   Using a
dosage regimen of 500 mg/kg at 0, 2 and 4 hours after infection a
marked bactericidal effect occurred and bacterial numbers continued
to fall steadily over a period of 24 hours.   In these animals no
lesion developed.   On the other hand, with a dose of 500 mg/kg at
the time of infection only, a brief bactericidal effect could be

seen over the first 2 hours after infection but thereafter
bacterial multiplication occurred and this was accompanied by the
formation of a lesion.

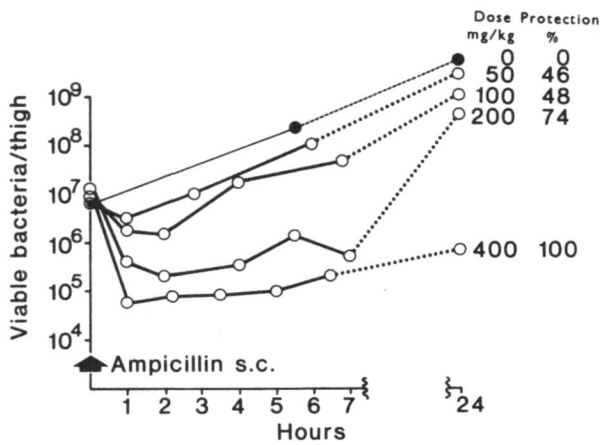

FIG. 5. Effect of ampicillin in the thigh lesion test
using E. coli
(Data from Hunter, Rolinson and Witting, 1973)

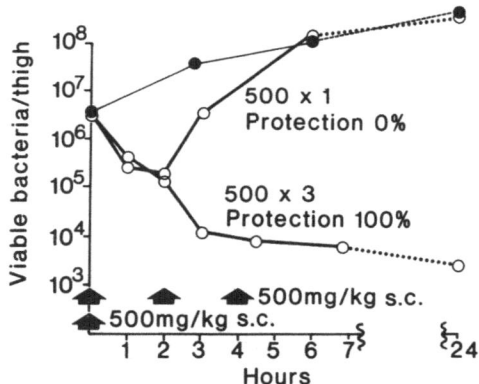

FIG. 6. Effect of carbenicillin in the thigh lesion test
using Ps. aeruginosa
(Hunter, Witting and Rolinson, unpublished data)

     In addition to determinations of the number of viable bacteria
present in the infected tissue and the formation or absence of a
lesion the levels of antibiotic in blood and tissue homogenate can
also be measured.   In this way it is possible to correlate antibiotic dosage, antibiotic levels, antibacterial effect and therapeutic effect in the one model.

It is important to bear in mind that the pharmacokinetic aspects of antibiotic distribution and elimination in this model are those which apply to the mouse and they may be different from those in man.   Moreover, the infection itself does not necessarily parallel a clinical infection in man and the model does not purport to do this anyway.   The model does provide a system, however, in which bacterial growth occurs in vivo, and in which the antibiotic also exerts its effect in vivo, and as a consequence of this antibacterial action a therapeutic effect is achieved which can be measured in terms of prevention of a definable lesion.

[Data in figs. 1, 2, 3 and 5 are reproduced by courtesy of the American Society for Microbiology, Bethesda, Md.]

REFERENCES

Berry, L. J. and Mitchell, R. B.   1953.   J.Infec.Dis., 93, 75.

Elek, S. D. and Conen, P. E.   1957.   Brit.J.Exp.Path., 38, 573.

Evans, D. G., Miles, A. A. and Niven, J. S. F.   1948.
    Brit.J.Exp.Path., 39, 20.

Hunter, P. A., Rolinson, G. N. and Witting, D. A.   1973.
    Antimicrob.Ag.Chemother., 4, 285.

James, R. C. and MacLeod, C. J.   1961.   Brit.J.Exp.Path., 42, 266.

Miles, A. A. and Niven, J. S. F.   1950.   Brit.J.Exp.Path., 31, 73.

Noble, W. C.   1965.   Brit.J.Exp.Path., 46, 254.

Selbie, F. R. and Simon, R. D.   1952.   Brit.J.Exp.Path., 33, 315.

Weinberg, E. D.   1966.   Bact.Rev., 30, 136.

INTRAPERITONEAL CHALLENGE

K. R. Comber, C. D. Osborne, R. Sutherland

Beecham Pharmaceuticals Research Division

Brockham Park, Betchworth, Surrey, England

Experimental intraperitoneal mouse infections are used universally in the assessment of the therapeutic potential of novel antibacterial agents and in the majority of cases the virulence of the infecting organism is enhanced by the concomitant administration of hog gastric mucin to the animal. Much effort has been devoted to studies of the preparation, biological mode of action, and active constituents of hog gastric mucin and there is a considerable body of knowledge concerning these aspects, as can be seen from the excellent reviews of Olitski (1948, 1957). Surprisingly, there appears to have been much less study of the effects of therapy on the development of the intraperitoneal infection in the animal host, despite the extensive use of these routine tests in the evaluation of compounds.

The influence of hog gastric mucin on the development of infection in mice after intraperitoneal injection of a strain of <u>Escherichia coli</u> is illustrated in Fig. 1, where it can be seen that when an inoculum of 10^5 cells of an overnight culture of the organism was administered in saline, the bacterial count in the peritoneal cavity fell rapidly to a count of about 10^3 cells/ml and remained at about this level for the next 7 hours. There was a rapid appearance of bacteria in the blood following intraperitoneal injection, reaching a count of about 50 bacteria/ml., but thereafter the count barely increased over the next 7 hours. In contrast, when the inoculum was injected as a suspension in 3% hog gastric mucin, the bacterial count in the peritoneal cavity increased rapidly to in excess of 10^9 cells/ml of washings within 8 hours. Similarly, the blood bacterial count rose rapidly to a count of 7×10^8 cells/ml at 8 hours. In the presence of mucin, therefore, the culture was able to proliferate rapidly in the peritoneal cavity after intraperitoneal injection, resulting in the rapid appearance of bacteria in blood and the production of progressive bacteraemia.

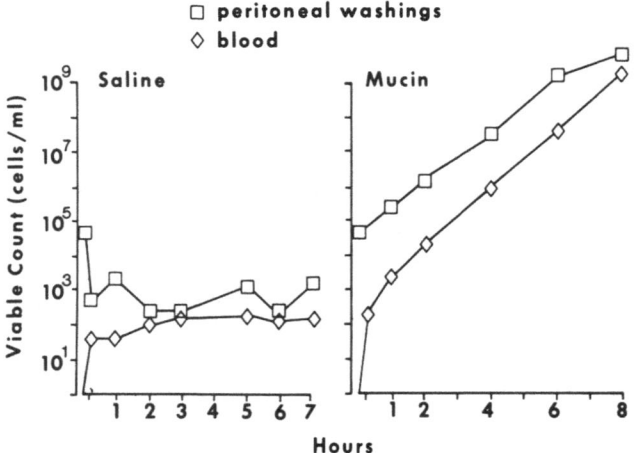

FIG. 1. Effect of mucin on the proliferation of E. coli (8) in mice after intraperitoneal injection

      The development of bacterial growth in the animal after intraperitoneal injection of mucin suspensions of different bacteria varies according to the organism. For example, the multiplication of the Smith strain of Staphylococcus aureus in the peritoneal cavity and the blood of mice was very similar indeed to that of Escherichia coli (strain 8), but with Pseudomonas aeruginosa (strain 11), a rather different pattern was observed (Fig.2). Thus, bacterial growth was very much slower, so that 4 hours after injection the peritoneal bacterial count had barely increased by one order of magnitude and by 8 hours the count was less than 10^8 cells/ml, in contrast to the counts of $>10^9$ cells/ml observed with E. coli and Staph. aureus. Likewise, in blood the bacterial numbers increased at a slow rate, and after 8 hours the pseudomonas count had reached a level of only 10^4 cells/ml. With Salmonella typhimurium (strain 10) growth of the organism was relatively slow in the peritoneal cavity, (Fig. 2) reaching a count of only 10^7 cells/ml by 8 hours, but the blood bacterial count rose rapidly to the levels observed in the peritoneum. It is apparent, therefore, that there are distinct differences in the growth of bacteria in the animal after intraperitoneal injection of bacterial suspensions in mucin and it would be expected that these differences would result in varying responses to therapy.

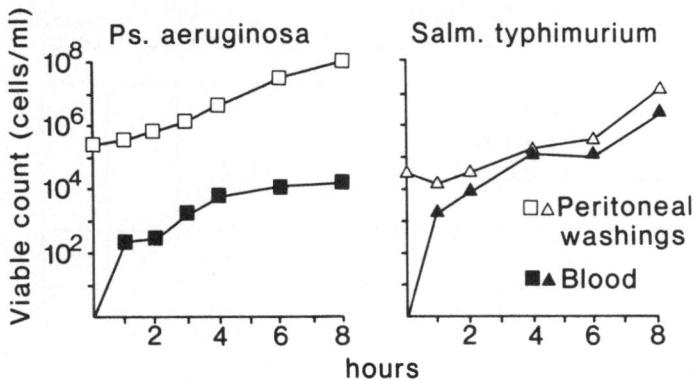

FIG. 2. Bacterial counts in mice after intraperitoneal injection
of mucin suspensions of Ps. aeruginosa (11) and
Salm. typhimurium (10).

As might be expected, the virulence of an organism may be
influenced significantly by the concentration of mucin in which
the inoculum is administered. Thus, with Escherichia coli
(strain 8) an inoculum of 10^5 cells in 1% mucin was considerably
less virulent than the same inoculum in 3% mucin - producing
only 40% mortality compared with 100% deaths caused by the latter.
With the same inoculum in 5% mucin, no increase in mortality
could be expected beyond the 100% deaths obtained with 3% mucin,
but response to penicillin therapy was much less pronounced
showing that the virulence was increasing in proportion to the
quantity of mucin injected into the peritoneal cavity. This is
probably due to the prolongation of the length of time the mucin
remains in the cavity and consequent persistence of its virulence-
enhancing properties in the host. For example, with an inoculum
of E. coli (8) in 3% mucin the infection-promoting effects of the
mucin disappear within 4 hours after injection. This was
demonstrated by administering sterile mucin intraperitoneally to
non-infected mice, and subsequently injecting, at intervals,
broth suspensions of E. coli 8 by the same route (Table 1).
When administration of the bacteria was delayed for 4 hours
after injection of the mucin there was a significant reduction in
mortality compared with results obtained between 0 and 2 hours,
and by 7 hours, the virulence-promoting effects of the mucin were
minimal. The rate of disappearance of mucin from the peritoneal
cavity has therefore, a marked influence on the virulence of the
infection and its response to therapy.

TABLE 1. Effect of intraperitoneal injection of E. coli 8
in mice pre-dosed intraperitoneally with sterile mucin

Time of infection after dosing with sterile mucin (hours)	0	1	2	4	6	7
% survivors	0	10	10	70	70	90

The effects of a single subcutaneous dose of amoxycillin on
the multiplication of bacteria in the peritoneal cavity after
intraperitoneal injection of E. coli (8) in 3% mucin are shown in
Fig. 3. In untreated mice the peritoneal counts rose rapidly to
greater than 10^9 cells/ml by 6 hours. Effective doses of
amoxycillin (200, 50 and 12.5mg/kg) produced rapid bactericidal
effects and caused 99% reduction in viable counts within 1 to 2
hours after infection. Between 2 and 6 hours, following elimination
of the antibiotic from the animal, there was a gradual increase
in the bacterial count and 6 to 12 hours after infection the count
rose sharply to levels of between 5×10^6 and 10^8 cells/ml.
Between 12 and 16 hours the count remained stationary and persisted
at a level of about 10^6 cells/ml up to 40 hours after injection
after which the count decreased to 10^2 cells/ml at 72 hours.

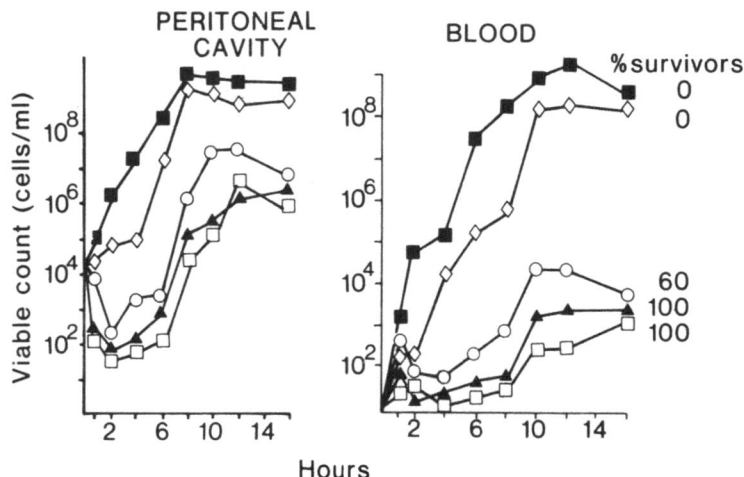

FIG. 3. Effects of a single subcutaneous dose of amoxycillin on
the bacterial counts in the peritoneal cavity and blood of mice
infected intraperitoneally with E. coli (8)
■, control; □, 200mg/kg; ▲, 50mg/kg; ○, 12.5mg/kg; ◇, 3.1mg/kg

   The cessation of growth at 12 hours following the phase of
rapid increase in count between 6 and 12 hours was unexpected
in view of the high numbers of bacteria reached in the peritoneal
cavity during this period and one possibility considered for the
apparent lack of virulence of these organisms was that bacteria
surviving exposure to the penicillins were in some way deficient.
In order to investigate this possibility, healthy mice were
infected with **E. coli** (strain 8) (Table 2) and dosed immediately
after infection with a single subcutaneous 200mg/kg or 100mg/kg
dose of amoxycillin, doses normally resulting in 90-100%
protection of the infected animals. A dose (0.5ml) of sterile
mucin was injected intraperitoneally into these mice 6, 8 or
10 hours after infection, and it can be seen that administration
of the mucin between 6 and 10 hours to the amoxycillin-treated
animals resulted in a significant reduction in survivors,
suggesting that the bacteria exposed to amoxycillin in the
peritoneal cavity had not been damaged and were capable of showing
normal virulence. It would appear then that the decline in the
peritoneal growth of treated animals from 12 hours onwards was
a direct result of cellular response within the animal.

TABLE 2. Effect of administering a second dose of sterile mucin
          to mice infected with **E. coli** 8 and treated with
                  subcutaneous amoxycillin

Time of addition of 2nd dose of mucin (hr. after infection)	% survivors	
	100 mg/kg	200 mg/kg
0*	90-95	100
6	15	35
8	30	10
10	10	10

                  * No 2nd dose

   Examination of bacterial growth in the blood of the infected
mice (Fig. 3) showed a similar pattern of bactericidal activity
and a similar dose response, reflecting events in the peritoneal
cavity. Thus, after injection of amoxycillin, the blood counts
in animals treated at the higher dose levels remained between
10^2 cells/ml from 1 to 4 hours after infection, followed by
gradual growth between 4 and 8 hours and a phase of more rapid
growth from 8 hours to 10 hours. From 10 hours onwards the rate
of growth declined and counts remained stationary at about

10^3 cells/ml for up to 24 hours, after which there was a gradual fall until no bacteria were detected in the blood 72 hours after infection.

These findings show that after intraperitoneal injection of bacteria the blood bacterial counts are related to the rate of proliferation in the peritoneal cavity and demonstrate that the inhibitory effects of penicillins on blood bacterial counts depend not only upon the antibiotic concentrations present in blood, but also upon the bactericidal effects of the compounds in reducing the numbers of bacteria in the peritoneal cavity in the early stages of infection. In turn, reduction of the blood bacterial count resulted in greater ability of the immune mechanism of the infected animal to eliminate the high bacterial counts appearing in the peritoneal cavity after excretion of the antibiotic from the animal.

In conclusion, the results reported illustrate some of the factors that influence the development of experimental intra-peritoneal mouse infections and demonstrate the value of chemo-therapeutic tests in the evaluation of antibacterial agents by measurement of therapeutic effects that could not be predicted from knowledge of in vitro antibiotic sensitivity of the organism or of antibiotic blood concentrations alone. The intraperitoneal mouse infection is often criticised as being a highly artificial model with little relevance to the clinical situation but proper understanding of the model and of the effects of treatment of the infection may contribute significantly to the assessment of the therapeutic potential of a novel agent.

REFERENCES

Olitski, L., 1948. Bacteriological Reviews, 12, 149.
Olitski, L., 1957. Bulletin of the Research Council of Israel,
    6E, 193.

ENDOCARDITIS

Lawrence R. Freedman and Georges Demierre

Department of Internal Medicine
Centre Hospitalier Universitaire Vaudois
University of Lausanne

Infective endocarditis has undergone a spectacular transformation since the development of antibiotics. As Lou Weinstein put it recently, "now young physicians are often disturbed by failure of defervescence within 24 - 48 hr. after initiation of treatment, and older ones are upset by a fatal outcome when, not too many years ago, they were amazed by a spontaenous recovery" (1).

It soon became apparent, however, that the available antibiotics or the way we were using them, left a series of important questions unresolved. The diagnosis was being made with increasing frequency in older patients without known underlying heart disease. The major cause of death became congestive heart failure due to acute perforation of the aortic valve - despite "effective" antibiotic treatment of "subacute" bacterial endocarditis, that is, infection with relatively "non-virulent" bacteria.

Subsequently, the temporary placement of foreign bodies in the heart, cardiac surgery, chronic renal dialysis, and finally drug addiction, have produced a new population of patients often infected with unusual and antibiotic resistant microorganisms (2).

Clinical evaluation of antibiotic treatment and prophylaxis of infective endocarditis are severely limited by the length of treatment, the potentially fatal outcome of inadequate treatment and the low frequency of risk of establishment of or certain complications of infection. Thus, modern antibiotic usage is empiric.

---

*Supported by the Swiss National Fund for Scientific Research grant 831.272.74 and F. Hoffmann-La Roche & Co., Limited.

It is no wonder that there have been many efforts to establish a useful laboratory model of infective endocarditis. Such a
model would have application not only in the assessment of antimicrobial agents but also to study the unique biology of endocardial
infection. We are thinking here particularly of the lack of participation of polymorphonuclear leucocytes as an important host
defense mechanism and the presence of extraordinarily high antibacterial antibody titres simultaneous with the circulation in the
blood of the responsible antigen, extracellular bacteria.

Until recently, animal models of this disease have had the
disadvantage of being inconsistant, technically difficult to accom-
plish, or have involved the need for cardiac surgery resulting in
the placement of intravascular suture material in contact with circulating bacteria (3).

What we sould like to do today is describe a simple model for
the production of infective endocarditis in small animals and review some of the studies which have been conducted with this model,
including those to evaluate the action of antimicrobial agents.

Some years ago we were impressed with the role of indwelling
intravenous polyethelene catheters in provoking bacteremia in
man (4). We reasoned that the insertion of open catheters filled
with bacteria into the vena cava of rabbits might simulate the conditions of endocarditis in man. When we carried out these experiments in rabbits, we were surprised to find that nothing happened.
Filling these catheters with staphylococcus aureus did not produce
positive blood cultures or metastatic abcesses.

Recalling that one of our original patients had developed
infective endocarditis following placement of a central venous catheter in the right auricle, we modified the animal experiment by
advancing the bacteria filled catheter to the entrance to or within the right heart. The result was convincing. Virtually all
of the animals developed infective endocarditis (3).

Insertion of sterile catheters resulted in the formation of
lesions of non-bacterial thrombotic endocarditis which were then
easily infected by injecting microorganisms intravenously (5). The
same sequence of events could be reproduced by inserting a catheter into a carotid artery and passing it into the left side of the
heart (6, 7).

As far as we are aware, all vegetative forms of bacteria
which have been tested have shown themselves capable of initiating
infection. In addition, infections have been established with Candida albicans and aspergillus (8, 9).

We have noticed a difference in the number of microorganisms
required to initiate infection after intravenous inoculation among
different bacteria. It was easier to induce infection with staphylococcus aureus than with streptococcus viridans and both of these were infective at lower inocula than Echerichia coli (10).

To date, efforts to produce infection with viruses, or stable cell-wall deficient bacteria have been unsuccessful, althouth Linneman et al. have recovered staphylococci from the blood stream after penicillin treatment in hypertonic but not ordinary media (11, 12).

The clinical picture of endocarditis in rabbits is similar in many respects to that seen in man. Infection is accompanied by bacteremia fever, anemia, and embolic phenomena.

In the few years the model has been investigated, it is already possible to point to a wide variety of biological phenomena which have been or will be susceptible to experimental study.

Infection can be initiated by either filling the catheter with microorganisms thus encouraging local heart valve infection or by intravenous inoculation of microorganisms, as soon as a few moments after introducing the catheter.

The initial events after inoculation of bacteria have been studied by Durack who has demonstrated the rapid deposition of bacteria on the surface of the vegetation followed by the progressive encircling of groups of multiplying bacteria by layers of fibrin and platelets (13).

The inability of host phagocytes to participate in the elimination of bacteria enmeshed in these vegetations poses a therapeutic problem similar to that of patients with agranulocytosis.

Hook and Sande and Valone have studied the effect of anticoagulation with warfarin on these early events (10, 14). Despite prevention of the development of a macroscopic vegetation, susceptibility to infection was unchanged, but the course of infection was catastrophic. Levels of bacteremia were higher and survival shorter in anticoagulated animals. Interestingly, Hook and Sande found it considerably easier to sterilize such vegetations with penicillin as compared with animals which were not anticoagulated.

For the moment, it is thought that the dense packing of bacteria in a confined space facilitates the establishment of maximal bacterial populations which Durack and Beeson showed were metabolically less active, thus making conditions less favorable for any antibiotic depending for its effectiveness on the speed of metabolic processes (15).

The pattern of evolution of infection depends on the infecting microorganisms and the location of the infection, i.e., right or left side of the heart (16). We were early impressed by the benign nature of right sided as compared to left sided infection. Right sided infection due to the streptococcus we use heals spontaneously, even with the catheter in place. On the left side of the heart, however, the infection is lethal, even when the catheter is removed. Consistant with this difference in evolution of infection is the finding that microbial populations are 200 - 300 times greater on the left side of the heart than on the right.

I think this phenomenon is important in determining the natural
history of infection. It is not known why bacterial densities are
different on the two sides of the heart.

We looked very hard for evidence of glomerulonephritis in
these animals but found none. Macro and micro embolic lesions were evident but not diffuse glomerulonephritis. Reasoning that bacteremic animals with left sided streptococcal infection might not
live long enough to develop glomerulonephritis, animals were pre-
immunized before inducing streptococcal endocarditis. In this way,
it was possible to induce the changes of proliferative glomerulonephritis (16, 17).

Lesions of pulmonary arteritis have been noted in right sided
staphylococcal endocarditis, but have as yet not been further investigated (3).

Splenomegaly is a regular finding and has been shown by Joyce
and Sande to increase with duration of left sided infection and to
correlate well with increasing anemia and reticulocytosis. These
authors have presented convincing data to show that the anemia in
this model infection is a result of red cell sequestration and ex-
tra-vascular hemolysis due to changes taking place in the enlarged
spleen (18).

We have recently succeeded in establishing the technique for
this model infection in mice. Sterile vegetations are easily produced by placement of a thin wire in the left side of the heart via
the carotid artery. Infection of such lesions is accomplished by
intravenous inoculation of bacteria. The advantage of the mouse
model is that it permits experiments to be conducted in genetically
pure strains of animal thus permitting the possibility of various
immunological investigations. In addition, the entire heart can be
used for bacteriological studies, thereby eliminating the risk of
neglecting to sample areas of infection that are not easily visible
to the naked eye (19).

Another interesting area of study is the mechanism by which
mouth bacteria enter the blood stream following dental manipulation.
Mcgowan and Hardie and Bahn et al. have succeeded in infecting non-
bacterial thrombotic endocarditis by introducing appropriate bacteria into the region of dental manipulation (20, 21).

Placement of cardiac pacemaker electrodes in rabbits instead
of a polyethylene catheter has also been effective in producing
lesions (22) and the model system has been used to study the effectiveness of blood culture systems (23).

The effect of antibiotics on experimental endocarditis has
proven to be a most fruitful area of investigation and has already
had an important impact on patient management. Durack and Petersdorf, testing right sided infection in rabbits with a strain of
streptococcus sanguis, demonstrated the failure of even massive doses (the equivalent by weight of 20,000,000 units) of penicillin

given 30 minutes before inoculation of bacteria. Streptomycin a-
lone had some effect, but the combination was clearly effective.
Vancomycin was a highly effective agent for prophylaxis and penicillin alone was effective when preparations were given which gave
a combination of high peak and prolonged serum levels. Bacteriostatic antimicrobials were without effect (24, 25).

Thus it is evident that if the experience in rabbits were
applicable to man, current recommendations for antibiotic prophylaxis are inadequate. There are clinical observations to support
this concern (26).

It is likely, however, that the situation will prove to be
more complex. We find differences in the protection afforded on
the right and left sides of the heart and even see an effect of
penicillin in preventing right sided infections when bacteria are
inoculated 2 hours after administration of antibiotics - a time
when bacteria are inoculated 2 hours after administration of antibiotics - a time when serum concentrations have fallen to very low
levels (27).

It is evident that serum antibiotic concentrations at the
time of bacteremia are not well correlated with the efficacy of
antibiotic prophylaxis in this model infection. The role of tissue
antibiotic levels has not as yet been examined.

In contrast to the difficulty in preventing alpha-strepto-
coccal infections, a single injection of 5 fluorocytosine 40 min.
before inoculating candida albicans in rabbits with non-bacterial
thrombotic endocarditis has proven very effective in preventing
infection of these vegetations (28).

Studies of penicillin and penicillin-streptomycin treatment
of established endocarditis in rabbits have demonstrated a decreasing effectiveness the longer the interval following establishment
of infection (29). In addition, the in-vivo effectiveness of peni-
cillin-aminoglycoside combinations has been clearly established
for infections with streptococcus sanguis, enterococci and staphylococcus aureus (30, 31, 32, 33, 34).

To date, there has been a good correlation between in-vivo
and in-vitro synergism, but in a study by Hook, Roberts and Sande
a synergistic effect of adding streptomycin to penicillin was seen
with an enterococcus resistant to more than 2000 µgm/ml of streptomycin (35). This model infection has also been used to demonstrate antibiotic antagonism between penicillin and chloramphenicol
in an infection due to S. viridans (36).

In conclusion, we have described a simple model for producing infective endocarditis in small animals developed from observations in man of the infections complicating use of indwelling
intravascular plastic catheters. The model has proved useful in
investigating the role of blood clotting in vegetation formation
as well as the anemia and glomerulonephritis seen in endocarditis.

Studies of antibiotic activity have raised serious questions about current practices in antibiotic prophylaxis and have been important in altering treatment programs in man. Because of the unique biology of this infection, its importance in clinical practice, and the difficulty of conducting studies in man, this simple model provides a useful investigative tool.

- B I B L I O G R A P H Y -

1 - WEINSTEIN, L. and SCHLESINGER, J. Treatment of Infective Endocarditis. Progress in Cardiovasc. Dis. 16, 275, (1973).
2 - MANDELL, G.L. and SANDE, M.A. Some newer aspects of infective endocarditis. Geriatrics, 30, 97 (1975).
3 - GARRISON, P.K. & L.R. FREEDMAN. Experimental endocarditis. I. Staphylococcal endocarditis in rabbits resulting from placement of a polyethylene catheter in the right side of the heart. Yale J. Biol. Med. 42 : 394 (1970).
4 - SMITS, H. & L.R. FREEDMAN. Prolonged venous catheterization as a cause of sepsis. New Engl.J.Med. 276 : 1229 (1967).
5 - DURACK, D.T. & P.B. BEESON. Experimental bacterial endocarditis. I. Colonization of a sterile vegetation. Brit. J. Exp. Pathol. 53 : 44 (1972).
6 - PERLMAN, B.B. & L.R. FREEDMAN. Experimental endocarditis. III. Staphylococcal infection of the aortic valve following placement of a polyethylene catheter in the left side of the heart. Yale J. Biol. Med. 44 : 206 (1971).
7 - PERLMAN, B.B. & L.R. FREEDMAN. Experimental endocarditis. III. Natural history of catheter induced staphylococcal endocarditis following catheter removal. Yale J. Biol. Med. 44 : 214 (1971).
8 - FREEDMAN, L.R. & M.L. JOHNSON. Experimental endocarditis. IV. Tricuspid and aortic valve infection with Candida albicans in rabbits. Yale J. Biol. Med. 45 : 163 (1972).
9 - J. CARRIZOSA, C. KOHM and M.E. LEVINSON. Experimental Aspergillus Endocarditis in Rabbits. Clinical Research 22, 438 A (1974).
10 - VALONE, J. and L.R. FREEDMAN. In preparation (1974).
11 - DURACK, D.T., P.B. BEESON & R.G. PETERSDORF. Experimental bacterial endocarditis. III. Production and progress of the disease in rabbits. Brit. J. Exp. Pathol. 54 : 142 (1973).
12 - LINNEMAN, C.C., Jr., C. WATANAKUNAKORN & C. BAKIE. Studies on the pathogenicity of stable L-phase variants of Staphylococcus aureus. Failure to colonize experimental endocarditis in rabbits. Infec. Immunity 7 : 725 (1973).
13 - DURACK, D.T. Experimental bacterial endocarditis. IV. Structure and evolution of very early lesions. J. Path. 115, 81 (1975).

14 - HOOK, E.W. III and Sande, M.A. Role of the vegetation in experimental Streptococcus viridans endocarditis. Infection and Immunity 10, 1433 (1974).

15 - DURACK, D.T. & P.B. BEESON. Experimental bacterial endocarditis. II. Survival of bacteria in endocardial vegetations. Brit. J. Exp. Pathol. 53 : 50 (1972).

16 - FREEDMAN, L.R., ARNOLD, S., VALONE, J. Experimental endocarditis. Annals N.Y. Acad. Sci. 236, 456 (1974).

17 - ARNOLD, S.B., VALONE, J.A., ASKENASE, P.W., KASHGARIAN, M. and FREEDMAN, L.R. Diffuse Glomerulonephritis in Rabbits with Streptococcal Viridans Endocarditis. Lab. Invest. 1975 in press.

18 - R.A. JOYCE and M.A. SANDE. Mechanism of Anemia in Experimental Bacterial Endocarditis. Clinical Research 22, 396 A (1974).

19 - DEMIERRE, G., VALONE, J. and FREEDMAN, L.R. In preparation.

20 - McGOWAN, D.A. and HARDIE, J.M. Brit. Dent.J. 137, 129 (1975).

21 - BAHN, S.L., BITTERMAN, P., ROSS, D. and BAHN, A.N. J. Dent. Res. 54, L 101 (1975).

22 - D. TANPHAICHITRA, K., RIES, M.E. LEVISON. Clinical Research, 22, 455 A (1974).

23 - J.W. EAKINS. Rabbit Endocarditis Model to test the Effectiveness of Five Blood Culture Systems. Clinical Research 23, 27 A (1975).

24 - DURACK, D.T. & R.G. PETERSDORF. Chemotherapy of experimental streptococcal endocarditis. I. Comparison of commonly recommended prophylactic regimens. J. Clin. Invest. 52 : 592 (1973).

25 - SOUTHWICK, F.S. and DURACK, D.T. Chemotherapy of experimental streptococcal endocarditis. III. Failure of a bacteriostatic agent (tetracycline) in prophylaxis. J. Clin. Path. 27, 261 (1974).

26 - DURACK, D.T. and LITTLER, W.A. Failure of "adequate" penicillin therapy to prevent bacterial endocarditis after tooth extraction. Lancet 2, 846 (1974).

27 - ARNOLD, S., DEMIERRE, G. and FREEDMAN, L.R. In preparation.

28 - DEMIERRE, G. and FREEDMAN, L.R. In preparation.

29 - L.L. PELLETIER, K. NIELSON, R.G. PETERSDORF. Dynamics of Infection and Response to treatment of streptococcus Sanguis Experimental Endocarditis. Clin. Research 23, 416 A (1975).

30 - SANDE, M.A. & R.G. IRVIN. Penicillin aminoglycoside therapy in experimental endocarditis. J. Inf. Dis. 129 : 572 (1974).

31 - SANDE, M.A. & M.L. JOHNSON. Antibiotic therapy of
experimental endocarditis caused by staphylococcus aureus.
J. Inf. Dis. 131 : 367 (1975).
32 - DURACK, D.T., PELLETIER, L.L., PETERSDORF, R.G.
Chemotherapy of experimental streptococcal endocarditis. II.
Synergism between penicillin and streptomycin against
penicillin-sensitive streptococci.
J. Clin. Invest. 53, 829 (1974).
33 - J. CARRIZOSA, D. KAYE. Choice of aminoglycoside
in Enterococcal Endocarditis. Clin. Res. 23 , 415 A (1975).
34 - J. CARRIZOSA and M.E. LEVISON. Minimal Concentrations
of Ammoglycoside for Synergy Against Enterococci.
Clinical Research 23, 301 A (1975).
35 - E.W. HOOK III, R.B. ROBERTS, M.A. SANDE. Antimicrobial
Therapy of Experimental Enterococcal Endocarditis.
Clinical Research 23, 305 A (1975).
36 - CARRIZOSA, J., KOBASA, W.D. and KAYE, D. Antagonism
Between Chloramphenicol and Penicillin in Streptococcal
Endocarditis in Rabbits. J. Lab. Clin. Med. 85 : 307 (1975).

THE USEFULNESS OF EXPERIMENTAL MODELS OF URINARY TRACT
INFECTIONS IN THE ASSESSMENT OF CHEMOTHERAPEUTIC COMPOUNDS

D.M. Ryan

Glaxo Research Limited

Greenford, Middlesex, England

The literature relating to experimental chemotherapy is reviewed and the factors influencing the chemotherapeutic response discussed. It is concluded that experimental models of urinary tract infection are useful in assessing chemotherapeutic compounds.

The effectiveness of an antibacterial agent for use in specific infections in man cannot always be deduced by its activity in vitro (Hunter et al 1963), Prat et al 1968a, Greenwood and O'Grady 1970), nor from its ability to cure experimental septicaemia in the mouse (English et al 1966, Gorrill 1968). For this reason it is desirable to have an experimental model closely imitating the condition seen in man, in order to evaluate agents intended for treating infections of the urinary tract (Fisher et al 1960, Hunter et al 1963 Sunshine 1964, English et al 1966, Lipman et al 1966, Prat et al 1968a, Miraglia 1970).

A variety of systems exists for investigating experimental urinary tract infections and two reviews are available (Jackson 1965 and Gorrill 1968). Infections of the human urinary tract range from the chronic condition of pyelonephritis without attendant bacteriuria at one extreme, to single uncomplicated bacteriuria at the other. There are specific animal models imitating most situations, the exception being chronic pyelonephritis. This is still an obscure disease, both in its pathology and resistance to treatment (Gorrill 1968). The experimental urinary tract models commonly used in the assessment of antibacterial substances are summarised in Table 1. Basically they can be described as either haematogenous or ascending, depending on the primary route by which bacteria reach the kidney.

Table 1

Models commonly used in the assessment of
antibacterial substances

Haematogenous
infections

direct intrarenal injection
direct intravenous injection (IV)
(IV) plus temporary ureteral ligation
(IV) plus kidney massage

Ascending
infections

transurethral
intravesicular inoculation
intravesicular + foreign body

Experimental chemotherapy

Experimental urinary tract infections have been used to
evaluate many antibacterial agents, including tetracyclines,
sulphonamides, penicillins, cephalosporins, aminoglycosides,
macrolides, polypeptides, nitrofurantoin and nalidixic acid. Most
of the experiments involved the use of Gram-negative organisms.

(a) Tetracyclines

Several groups of workers tested the tetracyclines in rats
and rabbits, using haematogenous Escherichia coli infections
involving renal massage or temporary ureteral ligation. The
results were variable, some workers reporting tetracyclines to be
therapeutically effective (Weyrauch et al 1957, Amar 1961, English
1971, Lipman et al 1971), whilst others found them to be only
marginally active (Dutz 1962, Lipman et al 1966). In the treatment
of ascending infections in rats, the tetracyclines were effective
(Miller et al 1956, English et al 1971), and they also eradicated
sphaeroplasts of Proteus vulgaris from rabbit kidneys (Gnarpe
1973).

(b) Sulphonamides

Several sulphonamides, when tested against a wide range of
infecting organisms, did not show much in vivo activity.
Sulfisoxazole was ineffective against haematogenous E. coli and
Proteus mirabilis infections induced by renal massage (Hunter
et al 1963), and only marginally effective when the infections
were induced by direct renal puncture (Burrous and Cawein 1969).
Sulphamethoxazole was also ineffective or marginally active,
against E. coli and P. mirabilis renal infections (Burrous & Cawein

1969), but was later reported to be effective against ascending
infections with E. coli, P. mirabilis and Aerobacter aerogenes
(Vischer 1971). Konickova and Prat (1969) found that another
sulphonamide, sulphamethiazole was ineffective against E. coli
ascending infections. In earlier work Dutz (1962) showed that
sulphisomidine had low activity against haematogenous infections
in rabbits, but later found it active against haematogenous
infections in rats (Dutz 1965). Overall, the sulphonamides have
little activity in experimental urinary tract infections.

(c) Penicillins

Penicillin G has been used to induce and investigate the
viability and chemotherapy of protoplast and sphaeroplast forms of
Streptococcus faecalis and Proteus vulgaris in the kidneys of
experimental animals (Guze and Kalmanson 1964, Eastridge and Farrer
1968, Montgomerie et al 1966, Gnarpe 1970, 1973). Lipman et al
(1966) showed a significant decrease in the incidence of E. coli
in rats treated with penicillin G, but the kidneys of the animals
remained infected.

The results obtained with ampicillin have been conflicting.
It did not eradicate E. coli and P. mirabilis infections induced
by renal massage (Hunter et al 1963, Lipman et al 1966), and has
been reported as both effective and ineffective against E. coli
infections induced by direct renal puncture (Levison et al 1972,
Burrous and Cawein 1969). Variable results were obtained by other
workers against haematogenous and ascending infections with E. coli
and P. mirabilis; in some instances the results were poor
(Miraglia et al 1968, Burrous and Cawein 1969, Kalmanson et al 1969,
Jones and Shapiro 1970, Thiele 1974), while in other cases
ampicillin was effective (Fritsche 1969, Miraglia 1970 and Ryan
1970).

Carbenicillin was reported by English et al (1972) to be
active against a haematogenous E. coli infection, and against
ascending infections with P. vulgaris and Pseudomonas aeruginosa
in rats. In contrast Thiele (1974) found carbenicillin relatively
ineffective against ascending P. aeruginosa infections in rats.

(d) Cephalosporins

Compared with the penicillins less work has been done with the
cephalosporins. Parenterally administered cephaloridine,
cephalexin and cephaloglycin and oral cephalexin were all effective
against haematogenous E. coli and P. mirabilis infections in rats
(English et al 1972). Cephalothin was not active in the more
severe model using renal massage (Hunter et al 1963), but

cephaloridine, cephalothin and cephalexin were all effective
against ascending infections with E. coli and P. mirabilis (Prat
et al 1969, 1970, Kradolfer et al 1970, Ryan 1970).

(e) Gentamicin

Gentamicin controlled E. coli and P. mirabilis ascending
infections in rats (Konickova and Prat 1969, Prat et al 1969,
Hatala et al 1971, Vischer 1972), but was less effective against
P. mirabilis haematogenous infections in mice (Miraglia et al 1968).
Burrous and Cawein (1969) used a technique of direct renal puncture
and observed that gentamicin given orally, cured P. mirabilis
infections, but was relatively ineffective against similar E. coli
infections. Parenteral kasugamycin was effective in rats infected
with Pseudomonas by direct kidney puncture (Misiek 1969) while oral
kasugamycin was only marginally effective against P. mirabilis
renal infections (Burrous and Cawein 1969). The positive results
with oral gentamicin and kasugamycin are surprising as there is no
other evidence that either of these aminoglycosides is orally
absorbed. Kanamycin was very effective in eradicating P. mirabilis
from rat kidneys rendered susceptible to infection by massage
(Hunter et al 1963) but did not control P. mirabilis ascending
infections in rats (Cotran 1963).

(f) Rifampicin

Rifampicin was reported as effective in ascending infections
with E. coli (Zak and Kradolfer 1971, Prat et al 1970), but only
marginally effective against P. mirabilis (Zak and Kradolfer 1971).
Contrary to this Konopka (1968) had previously reported that
rifampicin was effective against ascending P. mirabilis infections.

(g) Macrolides

Little work has been published about the activity of macrolides
in experimental urinary tract infections, although it is known that
erythromycin can eradicate L form infections with P. mirabilis even
though it is itself inactive against the parent bacillus in vitro
(Montgomerie et al 1966).

(h) Polypeptide antibiotics

These have not featured strongly in experimental chemotherapy.
Colistin was tested in an acute E. coli model and was relatively
ineffective (Prat et al 1969), but in conflict with these findings
Kaye and Rocha (1970) and also Levison et al (1973) reported good

therapeutic effects in a system where E. coli was injected
directly into the kidney parenchyma. Furtado and Gorrill (1968)
used an acute test where Ps. aeruginosa was injected intravenously
into mice, and found that a single dose of colistin given 4 hours
after infection was capable of completely eliminating the organism
from the kidney.

(i) Nitrofurantoin

     Nitrofurantoin has been tested in a variety of models against
E. coli and Proteus species. In haematogenous infections and those
induced by direct injection into the kidney with E. coli or
P. mirabilis, nitrofurantoin was variously reported as effective
(Rocha et al 1969, English 1971), marginally effective (Amar 1961),
and ineffective (Burrous and Cawein 1969, Hunter et al 1963). In
models of ascending infection against these organisms, nitrofurantoin was effective (Rocha et al 1969, Miller et al 1956,
Vischer 1972, Fritsche 1969, Kradolfer et al 1970 and English
1971), or of marginal effectiveness (Miraglia 1970). Hossak (1962)
found it to be marginally effective against ascending P. vulgaris
infections in rats.

(j) Nalidixic acid

     Nalidixic acid, like nitrofurantoin, is regarded as a urinary
antiseptic. It was less effective than nitrofurantoin against
haematogenous infections with E. coli and P. mirabilis (Burrous
and Cawein 1969, English 1971, Prat et al 1968a) but against
ascending infections nalidixic acid always provided effective
therapy (Konickova et al 1968, Prat et al 1968, Vischer 1972,
Ryan 1970, English 1971, Miraglia 1970).

     It is evident from all these conflicting chemotherapy results
that the effectiveness of an antibacterial agent in an experimental
situation depends very much upon the model system in which it is
tested. The systems used represent infections ranging from those
mainly in the renal parenchyma to those where the primary infection
is in the urine. The organisms used have varied in their invasive-
ness, their ability to induce pathological changes in the tissue
of the urinary tract, and their sensitivity to the antimicrobial
agents used. There are also other variables concerning the amounts
of antibacterial agent given, the routes of administration, and
the treatment regimens. The variability of results seen for
established therapeutic agents, will throw doubt on results
obtained with a novel compound prior to clinical trial. This is
becoming increasingly recognised and several workers have attempted
to isolate and investigate the factors which have the most

influence on therapeutic effectiveness and their results will be
briefly reviewed.

Factors influencing experimental chemotherapy

There are several components to a model system (Figure 1)
and each must constitute a factor which can influence the outcome
of experimental chemotherapy.

(a) Route of infection

A summary of the published results of the experimental
chemotherapy of haematogenous and ascending infections is given
in Table 2. Only those antibacterial compounds or classes of
compounds with at least seven published reports on in vivo activity
are included. For each published result the response to chemotherapy is scored as 0 (ineffective), 1 (marginally effective) or
2 (effective). The overall activity of the test substance, as
determined by several authors, is expressed as the sum of the
individual scores divided by the number of observations. Thus an
effective drug can score a maximum of 2. All the agents tested
showed better activity against the ascending infections, and
overall, renal infections were less responsive to chemotherapy.
In this respect the outcome of treatment of experimental infections
is similar to that seen in man (Reeves and Brumfitt 1968, Ronald
and Boutrous 1970). Although there are only a few observations,
there is evidence that infections enhanced with renal massage are
more difficult to eradicate than renal infections enhanced by
temporary ureteral ligation or by direct renal puncture. Thus the
effectiveness of experimental chemotherapy is significantly
influenced by the route of infection and the methods used to
enhance infections.

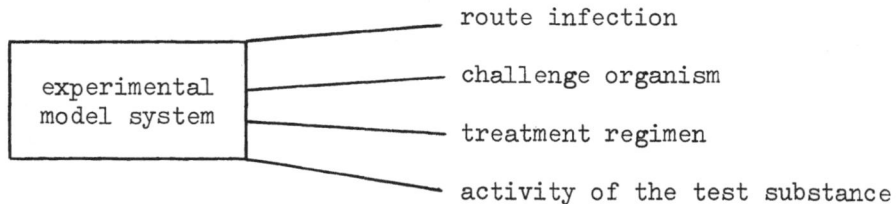

Figure 1

The compartments and factors in a model system
that can influence the outcome of experimental chemotherapy

Table 2

The effect of the primary route of infection* on the outcome of chemotherapy

Results from individual compounds or classes of compound

Compound	Route	No. published results	(Number of results with effectiveness scores of)			Average activity score (MAX = 2)
			0	1	2	
tetracyclines	haematogenous	6	0	2	4	1.7
	ascending	3	0	0	3	2.0
sulphonamides	haematogenous	7	4	3	0	0.43
	ascending	4	1	0	3	1.5
ampicillin	haematogenous	8	3	3	2	0.88
	ascending	4	0	1	3	1.75
gentamicin	haematogenous	3	0	2	1	1.3
	ascending	4	0	0	4	2.0
nitrofurantoin	haematogenous	6	3	1	2	0.83
	ascending	10	1	0	9	1.8
nalidixic acid	haematogenous	4	2	2	0	0.5
	ascending	7	0	0	7	2.0
cephalosporins	haematogenous	4	1	0	3	1.5
	ascending	6	0	0	6	2.0

* confined to E. coli and Proteus spp.

(b)   Challenge organism

     A number of different bacteria have been used to induce
experimental urinary tract infections. They show differences in
their abilities to colonise the renal tract and in the type of
infection they produce. Experimental infections with Staph. aureus
produce coagulative necrosis; Klebsiella and Proteus produce
chronic infections with attendant obstructive uropathy, S. faecalis
produces chronic disease with little or no scarring of the kidney
and E. coli usually produces a mild self limiting disease. The
outcome of therapy with the various species of bacteria will
obviously depend on the extent of renal damage and the persistence
of the bacteria in the urinary tract.

(c)   Treatment regimens

     Some workers have attempted to determine the effects of
different treatment regimens in a single system, in which
variables such as the route of infection and the species of
infecting organisms have been standardised. The time at which the
first treatment dose was given, or the frequency and duration of
the treatment period have been investigated. Better therapeutic
results were obtained in animals treated immediately or soon after
infection (Furtado and Gorrill 1968, Pitsch et al 1961, Konickova
et al 1969) but the validity of the better results obtained from
early treatments before the infection had become established was
questioned by Vermeulen and Goetz (1954). Beneficial effects of
prolonging treatment in a given model have been reported (Miller
et al 1956, Jones and Shapiro 1970, Pitsch et al 1961, Burrous and
Cawein 1969).

     From the results obtained in animals it is concluded that
variations in treatment regimens have a direct effect on the
outcome of therapy, and might account in part for the contradictory
reports on the in vivo activity of several antibacterial agents.

(d)   Activity of the therapeutic compound

     (i)   Antibacterial activity. It is assumed that the majority
of workers conduct therapy tests with bacteria sensitive to the
test compounds, even though the degree of in vitro sensitivity is
not always stated. This tacit acknowledgement of the importance
of drug sensitivity has been confirmed in the few cases where
moderately sensitive or resistant strains of bacteria have been
used, in that therapeutic effectiveness is directly related to
in vitro sensitivity.

     (ii) Pharmacokinetic activity. Antibiotic levels in serum

urine and renal homogenates have been measured in animals and the
results used to explain or interpret therapeutic activity (Lipman
et al 1966, 1971; Burrous et al 1971, Ryan 1970, English 1971,
Miraglia et al 1968, Pitsch et al 1961). While these factors are
important it should be remembered that normal and diseased kidneys
may handle chemotherapeutic substances in different ways
(Ritzerfeld et al 1969, Grafnetterova et al 1969, Kawamura 1969,
and Whelton et al 1972), and that the pharmacokinetics of some drugs
in man differ from those found in the usual laboratory rodents.

Conclusions

    It is concluded that the factors which influence the
chemotherapy of urinary tract infections in man, i.e. site of
infection, treatment regimens, and the antibacterial and pharmacokinetic activity of the test compounds, all operate in the
experimental animal. It is only when the conditions in the test
system are similar to or identical with the conditions likely to
be found in man can experimental models be of value in the
assessment of antibacterial compounds, and of predicting the
activity of novel compounds in the treatment of human urinary
tract infections.

References

AMAR, A.D., (1961), Journal of Urology, 85, 89.

BURROUS, S.E., and CAWEIN, J.B., (1969), Applied Microbiology, 18, 448.

BURROUS, S.E., FREEDMAN, R., CHAMBERLAIN, R.E., and BASSON, R.P., (1970), Applied Microbiology, 20, 598.

COTRAN, R., THRUPP, L.D., HAJJ, S.N., ZANGWILL, D.P., VIVALDI, E., and KASS, E.H. (1963), Journal of Laboratory and Clinical Medicine, 61, 987.

DUTZ, H., (1962), Chemotherapia, 5, 214.

DUTZ, H., (1965), Acta Biologica et Medica Germanico, 15, 480.

EASTRIDGE, R.R., and FARRAN, W.E., (1968), Proceedings of the Society of Experimental Biology and Medicine, 128, 1193.

ENGLISH, A.R., McBRIDE, T.J., CONOVER, L.H., and GORDON, P.N., (1966), In Antimicrobial Agents and Chemotherapy, ed. Hobby, Gladys; p 434, Philadelphia.

ENGLISH, A.R., (1971), Proceedings of the Society for Experimental Biology and Medicine, 136, 1094.

ENGLISH, A.R., RETSEMA, J.A., RAY, V.A., and LYNCH, J.E., (1972), Antimicrobial Agents and Chemotherapy, 1, 185.

FISHER, M.W., ERLANDSON, A.L., McALPINE, R.J., GAGLIARDI, L.A., and ROLL, D.E., (1960), In Biology of Pyelonephritis, ed. Quinn, E.L., and Kass, E.H., p 647, Boston.

FRITSCHE, D., (1969), Zentralblatt fur Bakteriologie, Parasitenkunde, Infektionskrakheiten und Hygeine; Erste Abteilung: originale (Stuttgart), 210, 181.

FURTADO, D., and GORRILL, R.H., (1968), Journal of Pathology and Bacteriology, 96, 65.

GORRILL, R.H., (1968), In urinary tract infections, ed. O'Grady, F., and Brumfitt, W., p 24, London.

GNARPE, H., (1970), in Acta Pathologica et Microbiologica Scandinavica, B., 78, 196.

GNARPE, H., (1973), Journal of Medical Microbiology, 6, 53.

GRAFNETTEROVA, J., HATALA, M., and PRAT, V., (1969), Časopis Lékařů Ceských, 108, 117.

GREENWOOD, D., and O'GRADY, F., (1970), Journal of Infectious Diseases, 122, 465.

GUZE, L.B., HUBERT, E.G., and KALMANSON, G.M., (1963), Journal of Laboratory and Clinical Medicine, 62, 90.

GUZE, L.B., and KALMANSON, G.M., (1964), Science, 143, 1340.

HATALA et al (1971), Zentralblatt fur Bakteriologie, Parasitenkunde, Infektionskrankheiter und Hygeine, 218, 49.

HOSSACK, D.J.N., (1962), British Journal of Pharmacology, 19, 306.

HUNTER, B.W., SOUDA, L.L. and SANFORD, J.P., (1963), Antimicrobial Agents and Chemotherapy, ed. Sylvester, J.C., p 608, Washington DC.

JACKSON, G.G., (1965), In Progress in Pyelonephritis, ed. Kass, E.H., p 191, Philadelphia.

JONES, and SHAPIRO, A.P., (1970), Investigative Urology, 7, 528.

KALMANSON, G.M., HUBERT, E.G., and GUZE, L.B., (1969), Anti-microbial Agents and Chemotherapy, ed. Sylvester J.C., p 458, New York.

KAYE, D. and ROCHA, H., (1970), Journal of Clinical Investigation, 49, 1427.

KAWAMURA, T., (1969), Japanese Journal of Urology, 60, 555.

KONICKOVA, L., PRAT, V., HATALA, M., and URBANOVA, D., (1968), Acta Biologica et Medica Germanica, 20, 195.

KONICKOVA, L., and PRAT, V., (1969), Arzneimittal - Forschung, 19, 1717.

KONICKOVA, L., PRAT, V., RITZERFELD, W., and LOSSE, H., (1969), Časopis Lékařů Ceských, 108, 117.

KONOPKA, A., (1968), Antimicrobial Agents and Chemotherapy, ed. Hobby, Gladys., p 519, New York.

KRALDOLFER, F., SACKMANN, W., ZAK, O., BRUNNER, H., HESS, R., KONOPKA, A., and GELZER, J., (1970) and Antimicrobial Agents and Chemotherapy, ed. Hobby, Gladys., p 150. Chicago.

LEVISON, Sandra P., PERLSTEIN, Deborah, & Kaye E., (1973), Journal of Infectious Disease, <u>128</u>, 251.

LIPMAN, R.L., TRYRELL, E., SMALL, J., and SHAPIRO, A.S. (1966), Journal of Laboratory and Clinical Medicine, 67, 546.

LIPMAN, R.L., McDONALD, R.H., CONNAMACHER, R.H., and SHAPIRO, A.P., (1971), Chemotherapy, 16, 300.

MILLER, G.H., CHAPMAN, W.H., SEIBUTIS and VERMEULEN, C.W. (1956), Journal of Urology, 76, 42.

MIRAGLIA, G.J., SCHERNER, N.I. and GADEBUSCH, H.H., (1968), Bacteriological Proceedings, Abstract from 68th Annual Meeting, p 99.

MIRAGLIA, G.J., (1970), Transactions of the New York Academy of Sciences, 32, 337.

MISIEK, M., CHISHOLM, D.L., LEITNER, F., and PRICE K.E., (1969), In Antimicrobial Agents and Chemotherapy, ed. Hobby, Gladys., p 225, Washington DC.

MONTGOMERIE, J.Z., KALMANSON, G.M., and GUZE, L.B. (1966), Journal of Laboratory and Clinical Medicine, 68, 543.

PITSCH, B., HERBERT, T. and CAREY, W.F., (1961), Antimicrobial Agents and Chemotherapy, ed. Finland, M., and Savage, G.M., p 54, New York.

PRAT, V., KONICKOVA, L., HATALA, M. and URBANOVA, D., (1968a), British Journal of Experimental Pathology, 49, 60.

PRAT, V., KONICKOVA, L., RITZERFELD., W. and LOSSE, H., (1968b), Arzneimittal-Forschung, 18, 1123.

PRAT, V., KNOICKOVA, L., RITZERFELD, W., and LOSSE, H., (1969), Časopis Lékařů Ceských, 108. p 470.

PRAT, V., KONICKOVA, L., HATALA, M., (1970), Arzneimittal-Forschung, 20, 554.

REEVES, D.S., and BRUMFITT, W., (1968), In Urinary Tract Infections, ed. O'Grady F., and Brumfitt, W., p 53, London

RITZERFELD, W., PRAT, V., KONICKOVA, L. and LOSSE, H., (1969), Internationale Zeitschrift fur Klinische Pharmakologic Therapic and Toxikologie, 2, 114.

ROCHA, H., da SILVA TELES, E., and BARROS, M., (1969), Applied Microbiology, 18, 547.

RONALD, A.R., and BOUTROUS, (1970), Journal of the American Medical Association, 219, 18.

RYAN, D.M., (1970), Postgraduate Medical Journal Supplement, 46, 19.

SUNSHINE, H., (1964), Journal of Urology, 92, 35.

THIELE, Elizabeth H., (1974), Journal of Antibiotics, 27, 31.

VERMEULEN, C.W., and GOETZ, R., (1954), Journal of Urology, 72, 93.

VISCHER, W.A., (1972), Chemotherapy, 17, 293.

WEYRAUCH, H.M., ROSENBERG, M.L., AMAR, A.D. and REDOR, M., (1957), Journal of Urology, 78, 532.

WHELTON, A., SAPIR, D., CARTER, G., GARTH, Mary A., WALKER, G.W., (1972), Journal of Infectious Diseases, 125, 466.

ZAK, O., and KRADOLFER, F., (1971), Seen in an abstract of the XI Interscience Conference on Antimicrobiological Agents and Chemotherapy.

AN ANIMAL MODEL FOR INTESTINAL INFECTIONS

E. Boehni

F. Hoffmann-La Roche & Co., Ltd.

CH-4002 Basle, Grenzacherstr. 124

SUMMARY

A model for intestinal infections with enteropathogenic bacteria in mice was established. The appropriate conditions for oral infections were achieved by alternate fasting with carbohydrate diet and sterilisation of the alimentary tract by antibiotics.

After treatment of the infected mice, the therapeutic action of various antibiotics, chemotherapeutics and various quinolines can be measured by colony counts per g bowel in comparison to that of untreated controls.

The usefulness of the model is supported by dose-dependent antibacterial effects, by structure-activity relationship of a new class of aminonaphtoquinones and further by the successful treatment of human dysentery with the most active derivative.

INTRODUCTION

Among the large number of chemical compounds that have to be screened in our laboratories for potential antibacterial properties, we encounter some compounds showing a more or less pronounced degree of antibacterial activity in vitro against gramnegative bacilli but are inactive against septicemia in mice when given orally, even in high dosages. This lack of effect may be explained either by metabolization into inactive compounds, or by poor gastrointestinal absorption; in the latter case they remain in the gastrointestinal tract without developing any activity. It is therefore

possible that in this group of substances potential agents against
bacillary dysentery may be discovered. For this reason we established
an oral infection in mice with enteropathogenic bacteria, which is
limited to the intestinal tract, i.e. an infection model ressembling
shigellosis in man. As pathogens we chose fresh clinical isolates
of Shigella sonnei (2220), Shigella flexneri (L 3947 2a) and a
dyspepsia-coli (086) from a seriously ill child.

According to McGuire and Floyd 1958[1], oral infections with
shigellae in normal, conventional mice are difficult to induce, or,
if a recognizable infection can be produced, the infective agent
persists in the intestine only for a few days. Many observations
have shown that susceptibility to intestinal infections can be markedly enhanced by feeding a carbohydrate-rich diet (Dubos and
Schaedler 1960), or by physical stress such as fasting (McGuire
and Floyd 1958[2]). In our own breed of conventional Swiss mice such
manipulations prove, however, unsuccessful.

In 1961, Formal et al. were able to prevent death in orally
Shigella-infected germ-free guinea pigs if a single oral administration of E. coli was given one or two weeks before the challenge;
Shigella-infected controls without E. coli died. Further investigations by the same authors (Sprinz et al., 1961) revealed that the
protective effect was caused by an immunological response of the
host to the coli-inoculation. The mucosa of the small and large
intestine in coli-challenged germ-free animals was larger and characterized by numerous plasma cells, macrophages, lymphocytes, neu-
trophils and eosinophils. The lymphatic tissue contained reactive
centers, compact lymphocytes and showed highly active cytophago-
cytosis.

We therefore decided to suppress the possible protective effect of normal enteric flora of our conventional mice (according to
Freter 1955) by antibiotic treatment prior to challenge and also
during the whole experiment in order to protect the mice from any
other possibility of recontamination.

EXPERIMENTAL SCHEDULE

The mice in groups of 5 are kept in sterile cages, protected
by a tent with ultraviolet radiation (Figure 1), during the whole
experiment (usually 10 groups). Corn grains (in the form of sterile
pop-corn) are fed from the beginning (Figure 2). The drinking-water·
contains 0.5 % piperazine as a nematocide during the first 4 days.
After this time the conditions for more or less sterile maintenance
of the animals are intensified by changing the cages every second
day. On the 5th day the animals are starved and their intestinal

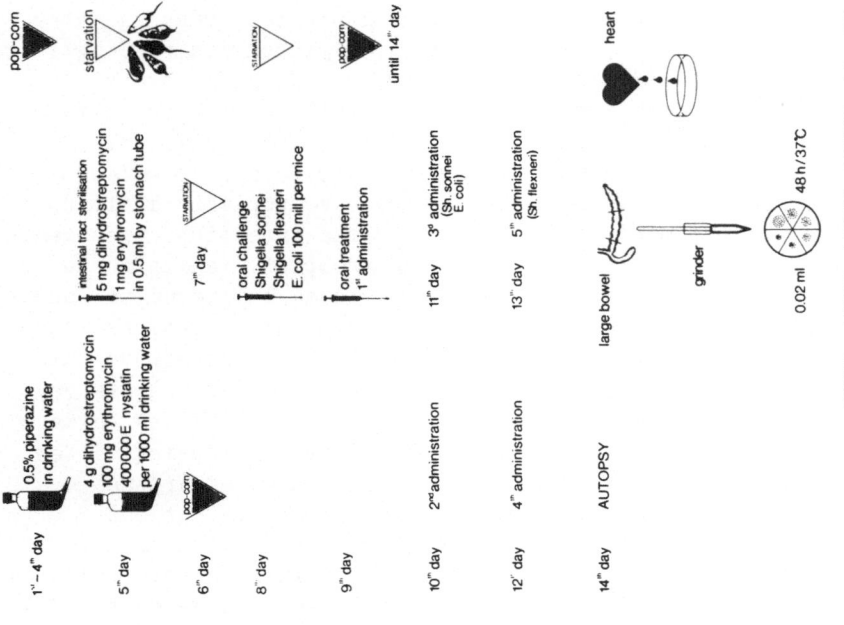

FIGURE 2: Experimental schedule for intestinal infections.

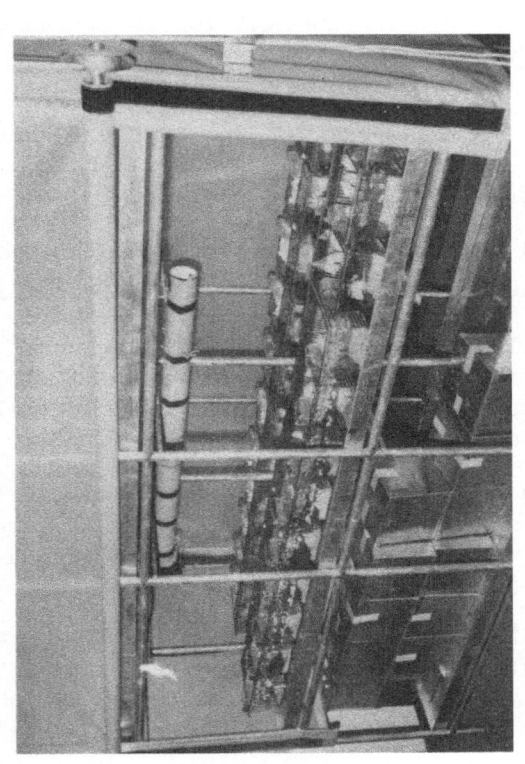

FIGURE 1: Ultraviolet radiated tent with 10 groups of Shigella-infected mice in sterile cages.

tract is sterilized by a single massive dose of dihydrostreptomycin
(5 mg/animal) and erythromycin (1 mg/animal), given by stomach tube.
Concomitantly, until the end of the experiment, the drinking-water
also contains dihydrostreptomycin (4 g/l), erythromycin (100 mg/l)
and nystatin (400'000 E/l). Then follows a feeding-day and again a
fasting-day. On the 8th day the mice are orally challenged either
by about 100 million Shigella sonnei or flexneri or by E. coli,
which are all highly resistant to dihydrostreptomycin (> 40'000
µg/ml). From the next day onwards they receive pop-corn daily until
the end of the experiment. 24 hours after the infection, treatments
are started with 9 groups. The remaining group of 5 animals are untreated controls. One dose of one compound is administered to one
group of 5 animals with Shigella sonnei or E. coli infections once
every 24 hours for 3 days. With Shigella flexneri infections this
treatment must be continued for 5 days in order to demonstrate any
activity of a known intestinal antiseptic. On the 14th day (6 days
after the infection), all animals are sacrificed, autopsied, a few
drops from the heart-blood are plated on Brain-Heart-Agar, and a
piece of the large bowel with 3 or 4 fecal pellets is cut out,
weighed and homogenized in phosphate-buffer of pH 7 with the aid of
a grinder. From this homogenized material 6 dilutions are made and
aliquots of 0.02 ml are dropped onto agar-plates (Brain-Heart-Infu-
sion Agar with 1000 µg dihydrostreptomycin per ml). After 48 hours
incubation at 37°C, the colonies are enumerated and counts per g
large bowel with feces are determined.

RESULTS

UNTREATED CONTROLS

One gram of large bowel usually contains about 500 million viable shigellae (average from 5 mice) (Table 1). In infections with
E. coli 086, the mean counts can exceed this number. In respect to
the challenge dose of 100 million per animal, i.e. about per 10 g
mouse intestine, apparently at least a 50-fold multiplication of
the infective germ in the intestine has developed representing a
true infection.

The infection develops first of all in the large bowel, then
spreads slowly into the cecum and small intestine. The duodenum is
never invaded. The infection persists with undiminished colony
counts for more than 20 days.

Routine blood checks are performed (as shown in the schedule)
to detect a possible transitory bacteremia. However, up to now the
occurrence of a blood phase has never been observed. Fatal septicemia only occurs if conventional mice are starved during the whole

Table 1: Intestinal infection with <u>Shigella flexneri</u> Colony counts in untreated mice and mice treated with Ro 8-5395 and % reduction of viable bacteria

	CONTROLS (untreated)	50 mg/kg Ro 8-5395 p.os	% Reduction
1.	557×10^6	$<2 \times 10^6$	99.9
2.	494×10^6	$<2 \times 10^6$	99.9
3.	388×10^6	16×10^6	96.0
4.	179×10^6	$<2 \times 10^6$	99.9
5.	614×10^6	$<2 \times 10^6$	99.9
mean	447×10^6 per g	$<5 \times 10^6$ per g	99.0
SD	$\pm 171 \times 10^6$	$\pm 6 \times 10^6$	
		$p = 0.01$	

Table 2: Dose-dependent activity of Ro 8-5395 and iodochlorhydroxyquin against 3 intestinal infections in mice

		Shigella sonnei	Shigella flexneri	E. coli 086
		% activity	% activity	% activity
Ro 8-5395	50	68	99	69
	25	75	64	58
	12.5	86	68	89
	6.25	39	32	63
	3.12	38	22	41
Jodochlor-hydroxyquin	50		74 ± 14.8	
	25	47 ± 14.7^0	52	71
	12.5	37 ± 14.5		18

^{0} Standard Deviation

experiment or with germ-free mice possessing an immature defense system. On the other hand, the infection is aborted in a short time if the animals drink water without an antibiotic supplement for a few days; latent contaminants such as Klebsiellae and other enteropathogens suddenly develop in the intestine and antagonize the shigellae.

Thus, host and parasite are maintained by antibiotic treatment and by alternate fasting in a susceptible labile equilibrium, which can be displaced to the advantage or disadvantage of the host by minimal deviation from the experimental procedure.

The infection is almost asymptomatic; the mice have no diarrhea or ulcerations. They occasionally show increased mucus production and very rarely hemorrhagic areas scattered throughout the mesentery and along the wall of the large intestine.

The aspect of the infection is therefore similar to the carrier-stage of shigellosis in man. The only criterium for evidence of a possible chemotherapeutic influence is therefore the recovery of the pathogen, i.e. a bacterial count.

Separate enumeration in the intestinal wall and in the feces reveal 10 to 50 times fewer bacteria in the wall than in its content. Because the antibacterial effect of a substance increases with reduced colony counts, we always observe better activity in the wall than in the feces. We therefore determine the viable counts in a homogenized aliquot of both wall and content.

TREATED ANIMALS

On the basis of the different average colony count means of 5 untreated and of 5 treated animals, we are able to calculate the percentual activity. Among hundreds of compounds examined we have found one derivative (Ro 8-5395) from a new class of aminonaphtoquinones that is able at a dosage of 50 mg/kg to reduce the viable Shigella flexneri by 99 % in comparison to the counts in untreated mice. In most treated animals, no shigellae are recovered in the first dilution step of 1 : 10'000. This means, calculated on 1 g intestine, less than 2 million. Taking into account the high colony counts in controls, we are therefore able to recognize germ reductions of more than 99 %.

With smaller dosages, a dose-dependent reduction of colony counts, i.e. a dose-dependent activity is observed in infections with all 3 pathogens (Table 2). However, after administration of higher dosages, 50 and 25 mg/kg, lower activity, which lies clearly outside the standard deviation, is often recorded. A possible explanation for this finding is that the antibiotically irritated

Table 3: CD_{50} (mg/kg) of Ro 8-5395 in comparison with intestinal antiseptics

	Shigella sonnei	Shigella flexneri	E. coli 086
Ro 8-5395	7	8	4
Jodochlorhydroxyquin	25	25	19
Broxyquinoline + Broxaldine	6	2.5	19
Sulfadimethoxine	12.5	50	50
Neomycin	25	1.5	3
Ampicillin	15	17	9
Chloramphenicol	—	11	18

Table 4:   Structure-dependent activity (CD_{50}) of aminoquinones

	Shigella sonnei	Shigella flexneri	E. coli 086
rac. exo- Ro 8-5395	7	8	4
rac. endo	>25	>12.5	>12.5
(−) endo	<50	>50	>50
(+) exo	>50	50	>50

intestinal wall causes a higher multiplication rate of the shigellae
and in consequence lower activity. For this reason, 50 mg/kg is in
all compounds about the highest possible dosage to be examined in our
model.

Based on the percentage of activities, the CD_{50} can be estimated
by means of the probit method (Table 3). The activity of Ro 8-5395
against infections with Shigella sonnei is comparable to that of the
usual intestinal antiseptics such as the combination broxyquinoline
+ broxaldine or drugs usually administered to combat dysentery such
as ampicillin and sulfadimethoxine. Ro 8-5395 has a stronger effect
than iodochlorhydroxyquin and neomycin. Against Shigella flexneri
we have observed with Ro 8-5395 an activity equivalent to that of
chloramphenicol and ampicillin, and a greater effect than with iodochlorhydroxyquin or sulfadimethoxine. Ro 8-5395 is not superior to
broxyquinoline + broxaldine or to neomycin. A good effect, comparable to that of neomycin and of ampicillin, is also observed against
infections with E. coli 086, whereas iodochlorhydroxyquin, broxyquinoline + broxaldine, sulfadimethoxine and chloramphenicol are
less active.

The usefulness of the test model is further supported by the
existence of a structure-dependent activity. In our model a comparison of the bornylamino-derivative Ro 8-5395 with closely related
aminonaphtoquinones revealed a remarkable structure-activity relationship, i.e. the configuration of the bornylamino-substituent is
essential: both antipodes and of course the racemate of the endo-
compound are practically inactive (Table 4).

The most impressive value of an animal model is proved by the
coincidence of the activity in animals and in humans. This could be
demonstrated in our case with Ro 8-5395, which exhibits a distinct
effect in human shigellosis and will be examined further in clinical double-blind trials in order to develop a useful intestinal antiseptic.

The correlation between experimental and clinical activity of
Ro 8-5395 has encouraged us to continue to maintain our experimental shigellosis model in spite of the considerable expenditure of
personnel, material and money involved.

REFERENCES

Dubos, R.J. and Schaedler, W.R. (1960), J. Exp. Med. 111, 407.

Formal, S.B., Dammin, G.J., Sprinz, H., Kundel, D., Schneider, H., Horowitz, R.E. and Forbes, M., (1961), J. Bacteriol. 82, 284.

Freter, R. (1955), J. Infect. Dis. 97. 57.

McGuire, D. and Floyd, T.M., (1958), J. Exp. Med. 108, 269 (1).

McGuire, D. and Floyd, T.M., (1958), J. Exp. Med. 108, 277 (2).

Sprinz, H., Kundel, D.W., Dammin, G.J., Horowitz, R.E., Schneider, H. and Formal, S.B., (1961), Am. J. Pathol. 39, 681.

ANIMAL MODELS IN THE ASSESSMENT OF ANTIMICROBIAL AGENTS:

SALMONELLOSIS

Edward W. Hook

University of Virginia School of Medicine

Charlottesville, Virginia   22901   USA

Two major clinical syndromes are observed in human beings infected with bacteria of the genus Salmonella: gastroenteritis and enteric fever.

Salmonella gastroenteritis is an actual infection of the intestinal mucosa which is characterized in man by fever, abdominal cramps and diarrhea. Although there is remarkable variability in the severity and duration of manifestations from a few cramps to severe fulminant diarrheal disease, the majority of patients who come under the care of physicians have an illness lasting 3 to 5 days. The disease is common and is the cause of appreciable morbidity, mortality and economic loss in the world each year (Hook 1975).

Availability of an acceptably nontoxic antimicrobial that would promptly kill the causative organisms in the gut might reduce the duration of disease and shorten convalescence, and certainly would aid in the management of the convalescent fecal carrier or the asymptomatic person found to harbor salmonella in the stool.

Evaluation of the efficacy of antimicrobial agents in salmonella gastroenteritis in man is difficult because of the brief and variable clinical course of the disease, the length of time required to establish a definitive diagnosis, and the spontaneous yet spotty elimination of the infecting organisms from the intestines by the normal defense mechanisms of the host. Controls receiving no antimicrobial therapy, or preferably receiving a placebo, and microbiologic observations into convalescence are essential to determine if therapy has decreased the duration of illness or the

period of excretion of organisms in feces after recovery. For
these reasons, there are relatively few adequately controlled
studies of the efficacy of antimicrobial agents in human salmonella
gastroenteritis. In fact, because of these problems, a number of
antimicrobials with excellent in vitro activity have not been
adequately tested in asymptomatic or symptomatic salmonella intestinal
infections.

The evidence that is available at the present time supports
the view that antimicrobial therapy does not exert a beneficial
effect on the course of salmonella gastroenteritis in man, either
by reducing the period of clinical illness or the period of excretion
of organisms in stools, despite marked susceptibility of the causative organisms to the antimicrobial agent administered. In fact,
contrary to evidence of benefit are increasing data that indicate
that antimicrobial therapy actually exerts a deleterious effect on
the course of intestinal infections with salmonellae by prolonging
the intestinal carrier state. In addition, by affecting the normal
flora of the gut, antimicrobial therapy also appears to enhance
susceptibility of animals and man to intestinal infection with
salmonella, as well as to convert the asymptomatic intestinal
carrier state to symptomatic gastroenteritis (Hook 1975, Hornick
1973).

The reasons for failure of antimicrobials in salmonella gastroenteritis are not well defined (Mandell and Hook 1971). The availability of suitable animal models of gastroenteritis would perhaps
permit an analysis of factors influencing antimicrobial action. It
is, of course, not possible to directly apply the results of such
observations to man; nevertheless, parallels exist between human
and animal salmonellosis, and at the least, the observations in
animals might aid in the selection of problems for study in man, or
in predicting the relative effectiveness of antibacterial agents in
treating gastroenteritis in man.

There are also many unanswered questions regarding antimicrobial
therapy of enteric fever (Hook 1970, 1974; Hornick 1973). One of
the most interesting and troublesome problems for those concerned
with evaluating new antibacterial agents is the potential for
discrepancy between in vitro susceptibility of a microbe to a
specific agent and response of infection by the same microbe to
therapy with the same antimicrobial agent. In searching for new
antimicrobial agents effective in salmonella infections, it seems
clear that we cannot rely on in vitro susceptibility tests as a
guide to the selection of effective drugs. Although in vitro
susceptibility tests provide the best method for the selection of
antimicrobial agents for treatment of many infections, typhoid
fever is one of the best examples of a microbial disease in which
in vitro susceptibility of the causative agent and in vivo response
to an antimicrobial do not coincide. For example, despite the fact

that the typhoid bacillus shows equal susceptibility to tetracycline and chloramphenicol in vitro, the clinical response in man to the two antibiotics is quite different. As is well known, the response of patients with typhoid fever treated with chloramphenicol is predictable; most patients become afebrile after three to five days of therapy; in contrast, patients treated with tetracycline show either no response or a very slow response.

A number of other drugs show excellent in vitro activity against Salmonella typhosa and yet no effect, or at best poor results, in the treatment of human beings with typhoid fever (Hook 1970). These drugs include, in addition to the tetracyclines, cephaloridine, streptomycin, kanamycin, the polymyxins, gentamicin, nalidixic acid, paromomycin, the sulfonamides, and penicillin G in small doses. Furzolidone can probably be added to this list, although it has shown more promise than most of these other drugs.

Ampicillin, amoxicillin, and co-trimoxazole, on the other hand, all exhibit impressive antisalmonella activity in vitro and are effective in the therapy of enteric fever in man (Hornick 1973, Hook 1974). It is interesting that despite greater in vitro activity of ampicillin than chloramphenicol against Salmonella typhosa, the clinical response is slower in patients treated with ampicillin than in patients treated with chlorampenicol.

In view of these observations, it is obvious that all antibacterial agents with strong in vitro activity against salmonella will have to be tested in man at the present time if we are to have definitive information on efficacy.

A model of enteric fever in an animal that paralleled the disease in man in pathogenesis and response to antimicrobial therapy would be of great potential value. A model would perhaps permit an attack on problems as that just cited regarding the discrepancy between in vitro and in vivo effects as well as play a role in the selection of certain drugs for further study in man.

Thus, with the two most common salmonella syndromes, there are important questions which might be studied if relatively economical, practical animal models were available which mimicked the syndromes seen in man. Salmonella species are, of course, widespread throughout the animal kingdom, and a wide sprectrum of disease has been described. Some animals do have intestinal infections with diarrhea whereas others have widespread dissemination of microorganisms from the gut to regional lymph nodes, and subsequently to blood, spleen, liver and other organs. Infection can be initiated by oral, peritoneal, intravenous, conjunctival and subcutaneous routes, and perhaps by other means. Although some of these infections, at least from a microbiologic standpoint, resemble enteric fever (a good example, of course, is "mouse typhoid," Salmonella typhimurium infection in

mice), the parallels, especially with respect to clinical manifestations, are vague and distant (Carter and Collins 1974).

The pathophysiology and microbiology of salmonella-induced
diarrhea has been studied in rats, rabbits, guinea pigs and other
rodents. The relevance of the diseases produced in these rodent
models to intestinal infection in man is uncertain, but a more
promising model appears to be salmonella diarrhea in the rhesus
monkey (Rout et al 1974). Salmonellosis in the monkey, a natural
host of this disease, appears to resemble gastroenteritis as it
occurs in man more closely than does salmonellosis in the various
rodent models.

Monkeys fed large numbers of viable Salmonella typhimurium by
stomach tube develop mild to severe diarrhea which is at its peak
48 to 72 hours after infection; the illness is brief, but lasts
several days. Rout et al (1974) studied fluid and electrolyte
transport in infected monkeys with diarrhea. Control, non-infected
monkeys show water and electrolyte absorption in the jejunum, ileum
and colon. In contrast, monkeys with salmonellosis have a marked
decrease in water absorption in the jejunum and ileum; in animals
with severe diarrhea, there is a striking reversal of net water
transport from absorption to secretion. Sodium and chloride
transport parallel net water transport in both magnitude and
direction.

In addition to observations on transport of water and electrolytes, the growth of salmonella and histopathology were studied in
segments of jejunum, ileum and colon (Rout et al 1974). In general,
the number of organisms increased progressively from jejunum to
colon. There was a correlation between the number of intraluminal
salmonella, the magnitude of water-electrolyte transport abnormality,
and the severity of diarrhea. The animals showed striking mor-
phologic changes in the gut, varying in proportion to the severity
of the diarrhea; pathologic changes were most marked in the ileum
and colon.

Salmonella induced-diarrhea, "salmonella gastroenteritis," in
the rhesus monkey is due to transport alterations in the small
intestine and colon induced by multiplication and epithelial penetration of salmonellae in the intestine. Recovery is prompt in the
absence of therapy even though organisms persist in the intestine
for some time after clinical recovery. To what extent these
findings in monkeys can be extrapolated to human salmonellosis is
uncertain but the model does appear to be quite similar to salmonella
gastroenteritis in man. Inability to compare the pathophysiology
of the diseases in man and monkey is attributable to the fact that
little is known in human salmonellosis about intestinal transport
and its relation to changes in intestinal morphology and bacteriology.

The monkey model of salmonella gastroenteritis certainly seems worthy of study with respect to potential use in assessment of antimicrobial therapy. To my knowledge, such studies have not been done.

There is also an animal model of enteric fever which mimics the syndrome as observed in man but there are enormous problems with it. Edsall and colleagues demonstrated that a disease resembling typhoid fever could be induced by feeding live Salmonella typhosa to young chimpanzees, thus confirming reports of Grunbaum and of Metchnikoff and Besredka which were made just after the turn of the century (Edsall et al 1960). Although the illness observed in chimpanzees resembles to some extent typhoid fever in man, major differences are apparent. The principal difference between typhoid fever in chimpanzees and man is the clinical course of the disease, which is mild and self-limited in chimpanzees, as compared to the prolonged, debilitating course in man. The pathological changes in chimpanzees, although typical of mild typhoid in man, do not include ulceration of Peyer's patches or any of the other complications of typhoid fever. Perhaps it is best that the chimpanzee model didn't work out so well; I am told that chimpanzees cost about $2000 each at present and I guess they are somewhat difficult to obtain!

In summary, animal models for assessment of antimicrobial agents in salmonella infections have been inadequately studied. Although there is no adequate model of enteric fever in animals, the monkey gastroenteritis model has many similarities to human salmonellosis and deserves further study as a potential means for evaluating antimicrobial effectiveness. It is possible that factors accounting for antimicrobial failure in salmonella gastroenteritis in man could be identified in animal models. However, at the present time, evaluation of clinical efficacy of new antimicrobials which show in vitro activity against salmonella will have to continue to be accomplished in man.

REFERENCES

Carter, P. B. and Collins F. M. (1974), Journal of Experimental Medicine, 139, 1189.

Edsall, G., Gaines, S., Landy, M., Tigertt, W.D., Sprinz, H., Trapani, R. J., Mandell, A. D. and Benenson, A.S. (1960), Journal of Experimental Medicine, 112, 143.

Hook, E. W. (1970), Journal of the Egyptian Public Health Association, 45, 206.

Hook, E. W. (1974), American Journal of Tropical Medicine and Hygiene, 23, 771.

Hook, E. W.   (1975), In Beeson, P. B. and McDermott (eds.), Textbook of Medicine, 14th ed., Philadelphia, W. B. Saunders, Chapter 213, p. 364.

Hornick, R. B.   (1973), Transactions of the American Clinical and Climatological Association, 85, 164.

Mandell, G. L. and Hook, E. W.   (1971), Archives of Internal Medicine, 127, 137.

Rout, W. R., Formal, S. B., Dammin, G. J. and Giannella, R. A. (1974), Gastroenterology, 67, 59.

ANIMAL MODELS AND PHARMACOKINETICS

G.E. Mawer

Professor of Clinical Pharmacology

Medical School, University of Manchester, England

Experimental models of human infections may help us to design treatment schedules which make more effective use of available antibacterial drugs. At the present time we determine the minimum inhibitory concentration of an antibiotic against a particular organism under conditions of steady antibiotic concentration. Yet in the treated patient the antibiotic concentration is never steady. Practical treatment schedules almost invariably involve a series of doses repeated at intervals of several hours. After each dose the concentration of antibiotic in the body fluids rises, reaches a more or less transient peak and then falls to a trough value immediately before or shortly after the next dose. We do not know how to relate the in vitro inhibitory concentration to this continuously changing antibiotic concentration in vivo.

The shape of the plasma concentration/time curve is determined largely by the characteristics of the drug and the patient. Highly water soluble drugs like the aminoglycosides tend to have a distribution volume Vd which approximates to the extracellular water volume, say 15000ml; thus each dose goes into a relatively small space and the plasma antibiotic concentration attains a high peak value. Then follows a period of rapid decay. The plasma elimination clearance Ce approximates to the rate of glomerular filtration in the kidney, say 100 ml/min and the half time for the decay is given by the expression

$$T_{\frac{1}{2}} = 0.693 \times \frac{Vd}{Ce} \quad \text{or} \quad 0.693 \times \frac{15000}{100} = 104 \text{ min}$$

Since the doses are often spaced at intervals of 4 or more half times the trough concentrations are negligible. The plasma concentration therefore swings over a wide range and the concentration/time curve is a series of spikes.

The same pattern is seen with the penicillins for although they have a larger distribution volume than the aminoglycosides, they are cleared much more rapidly. This is because the penicillins which are relatively strong acids are almost completely ionised at the plasma pH and the penicillin anion is actively secreted by the kidney tubule.

The concentration/time pattern with more lipid soluble drugs like doxycycline, lincomycin or rifampicin tends on the other hand to be much flatter; the peaks are less prominent, the elimination half time is longer and the troughs are higher. These drugs can penetrate tissue cells and the distribution volume is large. They are also readily reabsorbed across the epithelium of the kidney tubule and the clearance by the kidney is small. They are therefore dependent largely upon the liver for elimination.

These contrasting plasma concentration/time patterns are also modified in different ways by disease states. Impairment of kidney function prolongs the half time of the relatively water soluble antibiotics whereas the elimination of lipid soluble antibiotics is affected more by impairment of liver function.

Although the shape of the plasma concentration/time curve is largely determined by the characteristics of the drug and the patient, the prescribing physician has some measure of control. The rate of rise of concentration can be increased by giving the antibacterial agent by intravenous injection and the height of the peak can be increased by giving a larger dose. The height of the trough concentration can be increased by reducing the interval between doses.

Unfortunately we do not know the influence of such changes in the treatment schedule on the bacteriological response. We do not know whether the exposed bacteria respond mainly to the rate of rise of concentration, to the peak height or to the average

TABLE 1

Species differences in the half times* of drugs with different modes of elimination

plasma concentration half time* in hours

	mode of elimination	horse	man	monkey	dog	rabbit	rat	mouse	references
gentamicin	renal excretion		1-2	1-2	1-2			0.5	1,2
tobramycin	renal excretion		1-2	1-2	1-2		1-2		3
cephaloridine	renal excretion		1-2	1-2	0.5-1	0.5-1		0.5	4
isoniazide	N-acetylation		1-4	1-2	2-3		0.5		5
antipyrine	C-hydroxylation		12	1-2	1-2	1	2-3	0.5	6
phenylbutazone	C-hydroxylation	6	72	8	6	3	6		6

1   Gingell, Chisholm, Calnan & Waterworth, 1968.

2   Heifetz, Chodubski, Pearson, Silverman & Fisher, 1963.

3   De Rosa, Buoncristiani, Capitanucci & Frongillo, 1974.

4   Fare, Actor, Sachs, Phillips, Joloza, Pauls & Weisbach, 1974.

5   Smith, 1966.

6   Burns, 1966.

*   These values take no account of the effects of disease states or drug interactions.

concentration. Investigators may state that a particular peak concentration is necessary for therapeutic success; for example Dr. Noone and his colleagues (Noone, Parsons, Pattison, Slack, Garfield-Davies & Hughes, 1974) reported that peak plasma gentamicin concentrations above 5 or even 8 µg/ml were necessary for the successful treatment of severe Gram negative infections. The selection of this particular parameter is quite arbitrary however and the bacteriological response may be related more to the average concentration or some other parameter.

We will probably not know the answer to this type of question until we have made systematic studies in suitable animal or in vitro models. It may be of course that the relevant parameter of the concentration/time curve is different for different antibacterial agents and even for different pathogens.

The most suitable animal species for these systematic studies will probably also vary with the drug and with the pathogen. If we are to simulate the antibiotic concentration/time curves of man we require animal species with similar plasma concentration half times. These may not be difficult to find for drugs which are eliminated mainly by the kidney; aminoglycoside antibiotics for example have similar half times in man, dog and rat (Table 1). Isoniazide, which is mainly eliminated by N-acetylation, also has half times similar to man in several species. Drugs which are mainly eliminated by C-hydroxylation in the liver however show very large species differences in half time. This phenomenon is clearly shown in the data for antipyrine and phenylbutazone and we must expect to encounter similar variation when studying those antibacterial agents which are eliminated mainly by metabolism. It will be noted from Table 1 that there are no grounds for expecting a close resemblance to man in the drug metabolism of the non-human primates. There is no general rule by which a suitable species can be selected. It is necessary to study the pharmaco-kinetics of the relevant drug in a variety of eligible species before selecting one for more detailed study.

It must also be our objective to produce plasma antibiotic concentrations in the experimental animal which are of the same order as those produced in treated patients. Very often in published animal studies this is not the case. Enormous doses are given to the animal in order to produce a desired effect. For example in a recent study of aminoglycoside toxicity in guinea pigs the doses of gentamicin and tobramycin given per kilo were 10-50 times greater than the doses given to man (Brummett, Hines, Saine & Vernon, 1972). Such doses may be appropriate for certain types of toxicity study but they cannot give information which is directly applicable to the human situation. Drug distribution volumes in smaller animals tend to represent a relatively larger proportion of the body weight. Thus some increase in dose on a weight basis is often appropriate. De Rosa and his colleagues (1974) for example found that tobramycin doses of 10 mg/kg in the rat gave concentrations similar to those produced by 2 mg/kg in man. Once again there is no general rule which can be used to predict doses for similar concentrations in different species. Equivalent doses can only be determined by trial and error.

There are obvious practical reasons why there is a tendency for animal investigators to administer doses of antibiotics on a once daily basis. With certain lipid soluble drugs like doxycycline this is acceptable because it simulates what happens in man but with many drugs this is not so; a single daily dose of an amino-glycoside for example gives one peak and leaves the animal effectively untreated for long periods. This may be acceptable when studying the response of the tubercle bacillus but for the majority of acute infections this does not simulate the conditions of treatment in man.

Pharmacokinetic properties and bacterial response have too often been studied independently but the need for parallel study is now appreciated. Fare and his coworkers (1974) compared the pharmacokinetic properties of six cephalosporins with their ability to protect mice against lethal intraperitoneal doses of E. coli; the in vivo antibacterial potency correlated positively with both the peak plasma concentration and the half time. Hunter, Rolinson & Witting (1973) compared the pharmacokinetic properties of ampicillin and amoxycillin with their ability to protect mice against doses of Gram negative organisms injected into the thigh muscles; the greater in vivo potency of amoxycillin was not explained by differences in the plasma concentration/time curves.

Future studies of this kind will I hope teach us the relation-ships between in vivo drug concentrations and antibacterial effect and eventually enable us to design more effective treatment schedules for man.

REFERENCES

Brummett, R.E., Himes, D., Saine, B. & Vernon, J. A comparative study of the ototoxicity of tobramycin and gentamicin. Arch. Otolaryng. 1972, 96, 505-512.

Burns, J.J. Prepared discussion. Proceedings of conference of non-human primate toxicology. Ed. Miller, Dept. of Health, Education and Welfare. Food and Drug Administration. Warrenton, Virginia. 1966, 66-68.

De Rosa, F., Buoncristiani, U., Capitanucci, P. & Frongillo, R.F. Tobramycin; toxicological and pharmacological studies in animals and pharmacokinetic research in patients with varying degrees of renal impairment. Journal of international medical research. 1974, 2, 100.

Fare, L.R., Actor, P., Sachs, C., Phillips, L., Joloza, Mac D., Pauls, J.F. & Weisbach, J.A. Comparative serum levels and protective activity of parenterally administered cephalosporins in experimental animals. Antimicrob. Ag. Chemother. 1974, 6, 150-155.

Gingell, J.C., Chisholm, G.D., Calnan, J.S. & Waterworth, P.M. The dose, distribution and excretion of gentamicin with special reference to renal failure. J. infect. Dis. 1969, 119, 396-401.

Heifetz, C.L., Chodubski, J.A., Pearson, I.A., Silverman, C.A. & Fisher, M.W. Butirosin compared with gentamicin in vitro and in vivo. Antimicrob. Ag. Chemother. 1974, 6, 124-134.

Hunter, P.A., Rolinson, G.N. & Witting, D.A. Comparative activity of amoxycillin and ampicillin in an experimental bacterial infection in mice. Antimicrob. Ag. Chemother. 1973, 4, 285-293.

Noone, P., Parsons, T.M.C., Pattison, J.R., Slack, R.C.B., Garfield-Davies, D. & Hughes, K. Experience in monitoring gentamicin therapy during treatment of serious Gram-negative sepsis. Brit. med. J. 1974, i, 477-481.

Smith, C.C. Role of non-human primate in predicting metabolic disposition of drugs in man. Proceedings of conference on non-human primate toxicology. Ed. Miller. Dept. of Health, Education & Welfare. Food & Drug Administration, Warrenton, Virginia. 1966, 57-66.

USE OF AN IN VITRO MODEL OF THE URINARY BLADDER IN THE INVESTIGATION

OF BACTERIAL RESPONSE TO ANTIBIOTICS

D. GREENWOOD

DEPARTMENT OF MICROBIOLOGY
UNIVERSITY OF NOTTINGHAM
CITY HOSPITAL, NOTTINGHAM NG5 1PH

Conventional in vitro tests of antibacterial activity offer a simple means of assessing microbial sensitivity in the diagnostic laboratory, but the conditions of exposure of bacteria to antibiotic in such tests are remote from those encountered in vivo. In acknowledgement of this a number of experimental models have been designed utilizing laboratory animals, in which the therapeutic efficacy of new drugs or treatment regimens may be assessed. Unfortunately, animal models of infection also possess inherent limitations in terms of the treatment of human disease. One problem is that, because of anatomical and physiological differences, the conditions in which bacteria and antibiotic interact in the experimental animal differ from those encountered in man. Furthermore, it is difficult to establish the precise factors governing therapeutic efficacy in in vivo models because of their inherent complexity.

In order to gain a deeper understanding of drug/germ interactions, therefore, a third approach has been tried which seeks to simulate in vitro particular aspects of the in vivo situation. One fundamental way in which the in vivo circumstances differ from those of conventional tests is that antibiotic is presented to the infecting bacteria in conditions in which the concentrations of both drug and germ are constantly changing and in which the inhibitory or destructive effects of antibiotic are complemented by those of intrinsic defence mechanisms. Perhaps the clearest example of this is found in the urinary bladder in bacterial cystitis in which the antibiotic concentration in the urine varies with the drug, the dosage, the efficiency of the kidneys and the micturition pattern, and in which the concentration of bacteria is affected both by antibiotic action and by discharge during

241

micturition.   These conditions have been simulated in a mechanical
model.

THE MODEL

Details of the design and operation of the model have been
presented elsewhere (Mackintosh et al, 1973; O'Grady et al, 1973;
Greenwood and O'Grady, 1974).   Briefly, an overnight broth culture
of bacteria is diluted with fresh broth at a rate equivalent to
the ureteric urine flow rate; at intervals determined by an
automatically resetting clock, the system is emptied of the
accumulated broth, leaving a standard residual volume, simulating
the act of micturition.   For most experiments an inflow rate of
1 ml per minute (approximating to the normal diurnal rate of
secretion of urine) or 2 ml per minute (simulating the state of
diuresis) is used.   The residual volume after 'micturition' is
held at 20 ml and 'micturition' episodes occur hourly, 2 hourly or
4 hourly.   A simple photometric device (Watson et al, 1969;
Mackintosh et al, 1973) enables the turbidity of the culture to be
continuously monitored.

USES OF THE MODEL

The model provides information on three major aspects of
drug-organism interaction: (1) the effect of antibiotics on
extremely dense bacterial populations.   This is made possible by
the dilution effect of the model which may reveal antibacterial
effects undetectable in static systems. (2) the influence on
drug/germ interaction of parameters such as length of exposure
time to antibiotics, metabolic state of the bacteria at the time
of exposure, etc.   As an extension of this antibiotic may be
presented to the culture in fluctuating concentrations such as
occur in vivo and the efficacy of different antibiotic regimens
can be compared. (3) recovery of cultures from antibiotic effects
may be studied as dilution and 'micturition' reduce the antibiotic
level to below inhibitory levels.

THE MODEL IN USE

Results obtained in the bladder model have been reported in a
number of previous communications (O'Grady et al, 1973; Greenwood
and O'Grady, 1974a, b; 1975a, b, Greenwood, Teoh and O'Grady,
1975a).   The general form of the growth/dilution response in the
absence of antibiotic is shown in Fig. 1. This shows the result of
diluting an overnight broth culture of Escherichia coli at 1 ml/min,
with a 'micturition' episode occurring at 1 hr intervals leaving a
residual volume of 20 ml.   The effect of adding a β-lactam
antibiotic, such as ampicillin or cephaloridine, to such a culture

is shown in Fig. 2. These antibiotics cause rapid lysis of the culture shown by a precipitous fall in opacity, but recovery occurs as the antibiotic concentration declines and 'persisters' re-establish the bacterial population. Slow-acting β-lactam agents of the cephalexin type do not cause much alteration in opacity during the first hour and regrowth tends to occur sooner than with rapidly lytic agents (Fig. 3). The time to regrowth following exposure to β-lactam antibiotics is governed not only by the lytic activity of the drug, but also by its stability to β-lactamase (Greenwood and O'Grady, 1973, 1974b, 1975b). Even ampicillin sensitive strains of E. coli characteristically exhibit 'slow' β-lactamase activity which slowly hydrolyses cephalosporins, but not penicillins (Greenwood and O'Grady, 1973). Consequently penicillins appear superior to cephalosporins when tested in the model against such strains in a way which could not be predicted on the basis of conventional tests (Greenwood and O'Grady, 1974a). Furthermore, ampicillin resistant strains generally owe their resistance to β-lactamase which has considerable activity against cephalosporins despite the appearance of sensitivity when such strains are tested by conventional methods (Greenwood and O'Grady, 1975c; Greenwood, Teoh and O'Grady, 1975b). Examples of these differences are shown in Table 1.

It might be predicted that the performance of antibiotics _in vivo_ would be greatly influenced by the length of time to which bacteria are exposed to their action. Such predictions may be tested in the model by comparing the times taken for cultures to regrow following exposure to antibiotics under different conditions

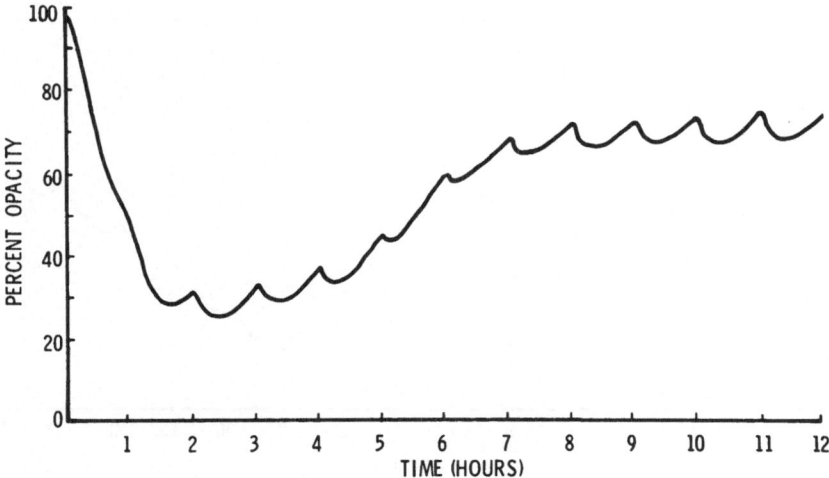

Figure 1 General form of results obtained in the bladder model with antibiotic free cultures of Escherichia coli.

of 'diuresis' and 'frequency of micturition'. A comparison of the
effectiveness of some bactericidal and bacteristatic agents in
conditions where the antibiotic concentration is maintained
(dilution rate 1 ml/min; 'micturition' 4 hourly) and rapidly
depleted (dilution rate 2 ml/min; 'micturition' hourly), is shown
in table 2. It can be seen that rapidly bactericidal antibiotics
such as ampicillin and polymyxin B are virtually unaffected by the
increased hydrokinetic washout effect of diuresis, whereas bacteristatic agents such as chloramphenicol and tetracycline are
strikingly affected. This suggests that high dose therapy aimed at
maintaining a high urinary level of rapidly excreted antibiotics
such as penicillins may not be of any great benefit as far as the

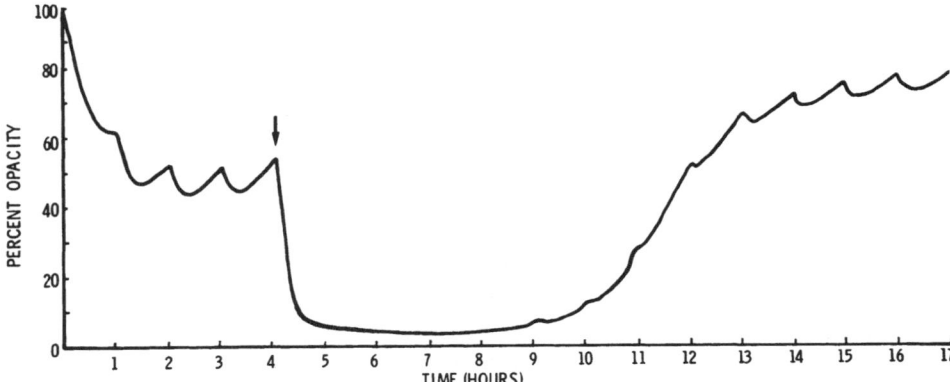

Figure 2 A typical result obtained by addition of ampicillin or
cephaloridine after 4 cycles of dilution and hourly 'micturition'.

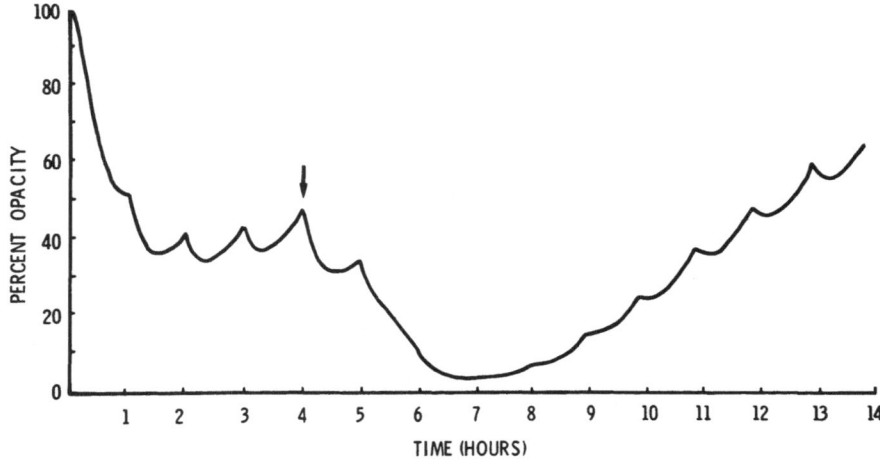

Figure 3 Characteristic result obtained after addition of cephalexin
after 4 cycles of dilution and hourly 'micturition'.

Table 1 Comparison of MICs with regrowth times in bladder model for 4 β-lactam antibiotics and 2 strains of E. coli.

	ampicillin sensitive Escherichia coli		ampicillin resistant Escherichia coli	
Antibiotic	MIC* (μg/ml)	time (hr) to regrowth[+]	MIC* (μg/ml)	time (hr) to regrowth[+]
Ampicillin	4	10	RESISTANT	
Benzylpenicillin	64	8		
Cephalothin	16	6.5	16	4
Cephalexin	32	6	16	3.5

* = MIC judged by conventional titration using a low bacterial inoculum.

+ = time taken for opacity to reattain original level following addition of a single pulse of antibiotic to achieve initial concentration of 500 μg per ml.

Table 2 Comparison of effectiveness of some bactericidal and bacteristatic antibiotics under different conditions of dilution and discharge.

		Time (hr) following antibiotic addition* for opacity to reattain 50 per cent level.	
Antibiotic	MIC (μg/ml)	Inflow 1 ml/min discharge 4 hrly	Inflow 2 ml/min discharge hourly
Ampicillin	4	9	8
Polymyxin B	1	9	8.5
Chloramphenicol	16	10	3
Tetracycline	2	11	6

* pulse of antibiotic to achieve an initial concentration of 50 μg per ml.

destructive capacity of the agent is concerned, although maintenance of adequate concentrations of such agents may serve to suppress the bacteristatically affected 'persister' fraction of the population during therapy (O'Grady et al, 1973). These results also underline the important contribution to the effectiveness of predominantly bacteristatic agents made by relatively slow,

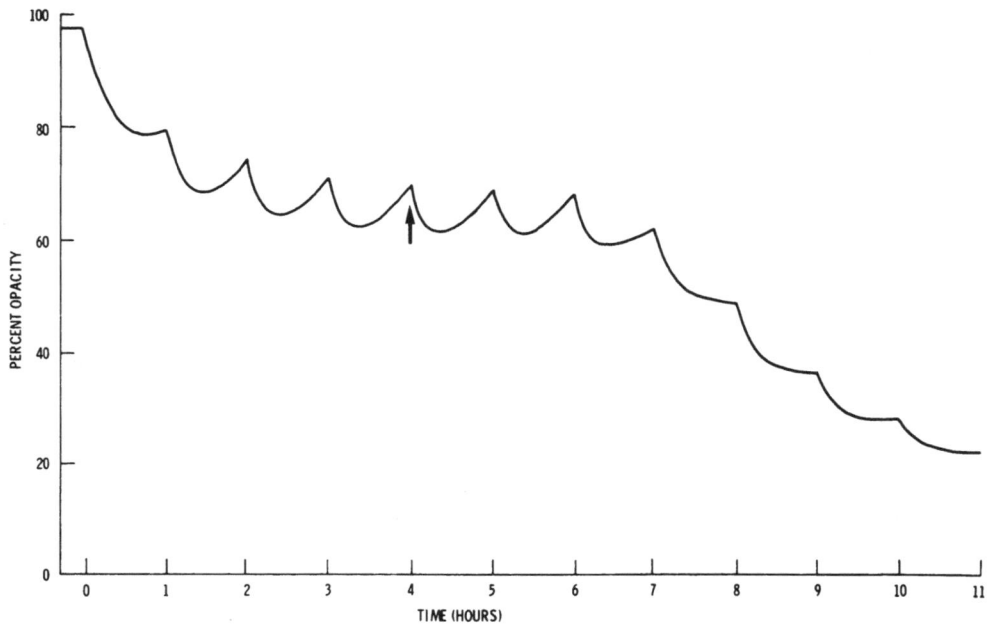

Figure 4 Antibacterial effect of a low concentration of sulphamethoxazole on a dense population of E. coli demonstrated in the
bladder model. After 4 cycles of dilution and hourly 'micturition',
dilution was continued with broth containing 5 μg sulphamethox-
azole/ml.

prolonged excretion rates, which serve to maintain inhibitory levels
in support of hydrokinetic and other clearance mechanisms, and help
to explain the virtually identical success rates obtained in the
treatment of urinary tract infection with bactericidal and
bacteristatic antibiotics.

Similar considerations may help to explain the efficiency of
sulphonamides in the treatment of urinary tract infection, despite
their well-known apparent ineffectiveness when tested against high
inocula of otherwise sensitive bacteria. Bacterial concentrations
in urine are frequently found to be in excess of 10^8 organisms/ml;
when such a dense bacterial population is exposed to a pulse of
sulphamethoxazole in the bladder model, a concentration as high as
500 μg/ml fails to evoke a detectable response. If the culture is
infused with broth containing sulphamethoxazole, however, an
antibacterial effect is induced after a lag of several hours
(presumably as the intracellular folate pool is diluted by bacterial
division) and is subsequently maintained throughout the infusion
period. This response is obtained even when the concentration of
sulphonamide in the infusion is less than the conventionally

determined MIC (Fig. 4) because the MIC value includes a factor attributable to adaptation of bacteria to otherwise inhibitory concentrations of drug during the incubation period (Greenwood and O'Grady, manuscript in preparation). These results suggest that the massive inoculum effect, so easily demonstrated in _in vitro_ tests of sulphonamide activity is irrelevant to the treatment of urinary tract infection with representatives of this group of agents which are excreted into the urine slowly over long periods of time.

The bladder model has already proved to be a valuable tool in the investigation of bacterial response to antibiotics. Adaptation and development of the model to monitor parameters other than opacity and to simulate other circumstances in which bacteria and drug interact in the body should help towards establishing optimum therapeutic regimens, which are frequently defined at present in disturbingly arbitrary terms.

REFERENCES

Greenwood, D. and O'Grady, F. (1973) J. infect. Dis. 128: 211.

Greenwood, D. and O'Grady, F. (1974a) Brit. J. exp. Path. 55: 245.

Greenwood, D. and O'Grady, F. (1974b). J. Clin. Path. 27: 192.

Greenwood, D. and O'Grady, F. (1975a). Brit. J. exp. Path. 56: 167.

Greenwood, D. and O'Grady, F. (1975b). Chemotherapy (in the press).

Greenwood, D. and O'Grady, F. (1975c). J. infect. Dis. (in the press)

Greenwood, D., Teoh, C.H.C. and O'Grady, F. (1975a) Antimicrob. Ag. Chemother. 7: 191.

Greenwood, D., Teoh, C.H.C. and O'Grady, F. (1975b) Antimicrob. Ag. Chemother. 7: 693.

Mackintosh, I.P., Watson, B.W. and O'Grady, F. (1973). Phys. Med. Biol. 18: 265.

O'Grady, F., Mackintosh, I.P., Greenwood, D. and Watson, B.W. (1973) Brit. J. exp. Path. 54: 283.

Watson, B.W., Gauci, C.L., Blache, L. and O'Grady, F. (1969) Phys. Med. Biol. 14: 555.

EXPERIMENTAL INTRA-ABDOMINAL SEPSIS

J.G. Bartlett, A.B. Onderdonk, T. Louie,
and S.L. Gorbach

Infectious Disease Service, Veterans Administration
Hospital, Boston, Mass. U.S.A.
and
Tufts-New England Medical Center, Boston, Mass. U.S.A.

INTRODUCTION

Intra-abdominal sepsis usually involves multiple different bacterial species derived from the normal colonic flora. In most instances both aerobes and anaerobes are present, and the problem is to determine which of the several constituents represent true pathogens. Are these to be considered aerobic or anaerobic infections? Alternatively, there may be bacterial synergy in which both microbial types are contributing to the pathologic events. These distinctions have important implications in the area of chemotherapeutics. For practical clinical purposes, a key question concerns the necessity to treat all microbial components at the infected site. If selective antimicrobial therapy is possible, which microorganisms should receive the thrust of the attack?

Clinical studies have not provided conclusive answers to these queries. In most studies of human infections there are vast differences in the hosts, variations in disease states and no untreated controls. Moreover, surgical intervention often represents the most important therapeutic modality.

We have developed an animal model of intra-abdominal sepsis in order to better understand the pathophysiology of infectious complications of bowel perforation (1,2). This report summarises our studies on the natural history of this experimental model and the results with several chemotherapeutic regimens.

THE MODEL

Animals. Male Wistar rats (Simonsen Laboratories, Palo Alto, Ca.)
weighing 160-180 grams were used in all studies. Initially,
animals were caged in groups of 10: following surgical procedures
they were housed in individual cages. All animals received rat
chow (Ralston Purina) and water ad lib.

Inoculum. All animals received an identical challenged made by
pooling the large bowels of 15 meat fed rats in the following
manner: The abdomen of each rat was aseptically opened and the
large intestine was clamped, excised, and immediately entered
into an anaerobic glovebox. Intestinal contents were carefully
extruded into a sterile beaker and the tissue was mascerated. An
equal volume of pre-reduced peptone-yeast glucose broth (PYG) was
added to this material and vigorously mixed. The resultant slurry
was filtered through two layers of surgical gauze into a second
sterile beaker in order to remove large particulate matter and
tissue. Ten percent weight/volume sterile barium sulfate was
added and the inoculum was then divided into small aliquots of
approximately 5 ml which were placed in glass vials fitted with
rubber stoppers and screw caps. The closed vials were removed
from the chamber, immediately immersed in liquid nitrogen for
4 minutes and stored at -40°C until used.

Quantitative bacteriology was performed on the quick frozen
inoculum by preparing serial 100-fold dilutions in the anaerobic
chamber for plating on appropriate aerobic and anaerobic media.
After incubation, colony types were enumerated, isolated and identified. This analysis revealed a total of 22 bacterial species
including 13 anaerobes and 9 aerobes (Table 1) (2)

In highest concentration were 2 species of Eubacterium
which were present at levels of $10^{7.5}$/ml. These organisms outnumbered the most frequent aerobe in the inoculum by more than
two logs. The next most frequent organisms were an anaerobic
pleomorphic Gram-negative bacillus and an anaerobic non-sporulating
Gram-positive bacillus. These organisms did not fit conventional
classification schemes and could not be speciated. Several
Clostridia species, Bacteroides fragilis, peptococci and Fusobac-
terium varium were present in concentrations of 10^5 - $10^6.1$/ml.
Enterococci and E.coli were the predominant aerobic isolates,
occurring in concentrations of $10^{5.4}$ and $10^{5.2}$/ml respectively.
Several other facultative isolates were also present including
Lactobacillus, Micrococcus, Corynebacterium, Proteus, α-hemolytic
streptococcus and Morazella. Thus the inoculum contained a polymicrobial flora in which anaerobes outnumber aerobes by a factor
of 100:1. Intestinal studies in man have shown similar bacterial
populations in terms of the ratio of aerobes to anaerobes and the
major bacterial species (3).

TABLE 1

BACTERIOLOGY OF THE INOCULUM

Anaerobes	Log cfu/ml	Aerobes	Log cfu/ml
Eubacterium tenue	7.5	Enterococcus	5.4
Eubacterium aerofaciens	7.5	Escherichia coli	5.2
Pleomorphic Gram-negative rod	7.0	Lactobacillus sp.	5.0
		Micrococcus sp.	4.5
Non-spore forming Gram-positive rod	6.3	Corynebacterium sp.	4.4
		α-hemolytic streptococcus	4.0
Clostridium perfringens	6.1	Proteus mirabilis	4.0
Clostridium para-putrificum	6.0	Proteus morganii	3.9
		Moraxella sp.	3.1
Clostridium species	6.0		
Bacteroides fragilis	5.8		
Peptococcus prevotii	5.8		
Peptococcus morbillorum	5.7		
Fusobacterium varium	5.2		
Clostridium sartago-formum	5.2		
Clostridium tyro-butyricum	5.0		

Bacteriological studies were also performed on an inoculum prepared from grain-fed rats. In this inoculum, however, aerobes actually outnumbered anaerobes and the major isolates were quite different than those in the human intestine (3). Consequently, all experimental studies were performed with the inoculum pre-prepared from meat-fed rats.

Implantation of inocula. The frozen inoculum obtained from meat-fed rats was thawed in the anaerobic chamber. One-half ml was placed in a sterile gelatin capsule, removed from the chamber and immediately implanted into rats anaesthetised by intraperitoneal injection of 0.15 ml of Sodium Nembutal (50 mg/ml). The abdomen of each animal was shaved, cleaned twice with 1% iodine, and a 1.5 cm anterior midline incision was made through the abdominal wall and peritoneum. The capsule was then inserted into the pelvic region of each rat. The incision was closed with three or four interrupted 3-0 silk sutures and the animals returned to separate cages.

Anatomical studies. Deaths which occur within 4 hours are ascribed to anaesthesia or to surgery and these animals were eliminated from the study. All animals were observed at 8 hour interval throughout the test period. Rats which survived 10 days were sacrificed and autopsies were performed. The criterion for peritonitis was free-flowing peritoneal exudate; for intra-abdominal abscess it was a localised purulent collection.

Bacteriological studies. Quantitative bacteriology was performed on specimens obtained from the infected site of randomly selected rats immediately following sacrifice. Specimens were obtained with a tuberculin syringe and passed immediately into the anaerobic chamber for processing. A 0.1 ml sample of purulent material was placed in 9.9 ml of pre-reduced VPI dilution salts for serial 100-fold dilutions. Aliquots of 0.1 ml of each dilution were then spread on both pre-reduced and aerobic plating media to give final dilutions of 10^{-3}, 10^{-5}, 10^{-7} and 10^{-9} ml. Anaerobic media including pre-reduced brucella agar base containing 6% sheep's blood and 10 mcg/ml menadione (BMB); BMB containing 100 mcg/ml neomycin sulfate; and laked blood agar containing 75 mcg/ml kenamycin and 7.5 mcg/ml vanomycin. These three media were incubated at 37°C inside the anaerobic chamber and held for 3-5 days. The following media were employed for aerobic and facultative isolates: blood agar plates incubated with increased CO_2; MacConkey's agar and Pfizer Selective Enterococcus Agar. These plates were incubated at 37°C for 24-28 hours. After incubation, colony types were enumerated, isolated and identified. Anaerobic isolates were identified according to the procedures outlined by the VPI Anaerobe Laboratory Manual (4). Enterobacteriaceae and other aerobic isolates are identified by established procedures (5).

NATURAL COURSE OF INFECTION IN UNTREATED ANIMALS

Initial studies concerned the sequential bacteriologic and pathologic changes in 106 untreated rats. Three control groups consisted of animals implanted with an autoclaved (sterile) inoculum, $BaSO_4$ alone and $BaSO_4$ plus sterile inoculum. The animals were observed daily and all rats which succumbed were autopsied for gross anatomical studies. In order to define the natural history of this infection, surviving rats were randomly sacrificed for autopsy examination at intervals of 4-14 days.

Among the 106 animals which received the inoculum, 7 died between 8 and 16 hours, and 21 (19.8%) were dead before 24 hours. Autopsy of these animals revealed that the gelatin capsules began to dissolve shortly after insertion, but even at 8 hours the inoculum was usually still localised in the pelvis. Within 24 hours a suppurative infection and ileus developed, and 0.2-0.5 c.c of peritonitis fluid had accumulated. The fur appeared ruffled, and the animals were lethargic and cold. At 48 hours, peritoneal adhesions began to appear anteriorly and loosely attached collections of purulent material were noted. By 3 days 41 (39%) of the

animals had died, and, at 4 days, 43% (46/106) of the animals had
expired. There were no further natural deaths after this time.
After 7 days a well-formed abscess was usually palpated inferiorly
along the anterior abdominal wall. The surgical incision was well
healed and peritoneal fluid was seldom present. All animals sacrificed at 7 days or later had multiple localised purulent collections distributed throughout the abdominal cavity. Abscess cavi-
ties continued to enlarge and by 2 weeks contained 0.2-0.5 cc
of pus.

Control animals which received the sterile inoculum in gelatin
capsules showed no signs of toxicity. At 14 days the animals were
sacrificed and no pathologic changes could be found. The barium
sulfate alone or the combination of $BaSO_4$ and sterile inoculum
produced a similar clinical picture. At autopsy the only findings
in these animals were multiple sterile granulomas.

Bacteriological studies of infected sites were performed on
20 animals. Samples were obtained at various intervals for up to
2 weeks following implantation. These specimens consistently
yielded a complex mixed aerobic-anaerobic flora. There was a mean
of 6.2 bacterial species/case including 3.2 aerobes and 3.0
anaerobes. Four organisms were uniformly present and numerically
dominant: E.coli, enterococci, Bacteroides fragilis and Fusobac-
terium varium. Comparison of relative concentrations of these
organisms in peritonitis exudate and abscess contents showed that
the 2 facultative species outranked the 2 anaerobes during the
peritonitis stage while the reverse applied to the abscess stage.
According to rank order analysis these differences are highly
significant.

Blood cultures were obtained from randomly selected animals
at 1-3 days, 7 days and 14 days. All 10 animals sampled in the
acute peritonitis stage had bacteremia, and many had polymicrobial
bacteremia. Blood culture isolates in these 10 animals were E.coli
(9 rats), Proteus mirabilis (5), B.fragilis (2) and enterococci (1).
At 7 days bacteremia was less frequent and at 14 days the blood
cultures failed to yield any pathogens.

These experiments show that several important goals for a
suitable experimental model were satisfied. The standardised fecal
implant produced a predictable disease which followed a biphasic
course. Initially, there was acute, often lethal, peritonitis.
This was followed by the formation of intra-abdominal abscesses
at 5-7 days in all surviving animals. The pathologic changes and
the organisms most frequently isolated from infected sites were
similar to observations in human infections. Additionally, mortality and abscess were well defined objective criteria to judge
different stages of the disease in future experiments.

Of particular interest were the sequential bacteriological changes which occurred during evolution of the disease. Starting with a complex inoculum containing at least 22 identifiable bacterial species, there was a simplification of this flora at the infected site. All specimens yielded a mixture of aerobes and anaerobes, but the relative concentrations of these 2 bacterial types changed during the course of the disease. Aerobes were predominant during initial peritonitis, a stage associated with E.coli bacteremia and high mortality. Surviving animals uniformly developed localised intra-abdominal abscesses in which the numerically dominant organisms were anaerobes, principally B.fragilis and F.varium.

ANTIMICROBIAL PROBES

Several antimicrobial regimens have been tested in this model. Agents used initially were clindamycin and gentamicin due to their selective activity against aerobic and anaerobic components of the infection (6). Gentamicin is highly active against coliform bacteria but had little effect on anaerobes. Clindamycin has the opposite effect, excellent activity against anaerobes but virtually no effect on coliforms.

There were four experimental groups of 60 animals each: 1) gentamicin alone, 2) clindamycin alone, 3) gentamicin and clindamycin in combination and 4) untreated controls.

Antimicrobial dosage was based on our preliminary results of serum level assays using various doses in rats. Rat blood was obtained by cardiac puncture at 1 hr (peak level) and $7\frac{1}{2}$ hrs after intramuscular administration. Gentamicin serum levels were measured using a bioassay with Bacillus globigii as described by Winters et al (7). Doses of 8.0 mg/kg in 4 animals produced mean peak levels of 6.9 mcg/ml with trough levels of less than 1.3 mcg/ml. After 2 weeks of therapy there was no significant increase in serum concentrations and renal function tests (creatinine and BUN) remained normal. Clindamycin levels were measured using a bioassay with a sensitive Staphylococcus epidermidis as described by Alcid and Seligman (8). Intramuscular administration of 80 mg/kg in 4 rats produced mean peak concentrations of 5.5 mcg/ml. There was no significant increase in serum levels during the course of treatment.

Antimicrobials were administered intramuscularly in the above doses every 8 hours for 10 days beginning 4 hours after implantation. All survivors were sacrificed at the end of the 10 day treatment. Autopsy exams included a careful inspection of the abdominal cavity for evidence of peritonitis or abscesses. Quantitative bacteriological analysis was performed on a sample population of randomly selected animals with abscesses from each group.

TABLE 2

RESULTS WITH GENTAMICIN AND CLINDAMYCIN

Agent	No. tested	Mortality	Abscesses in survivors
Untreated animals	60	22/60 (37%)	38/38 (100%)
Gentamicin	57	2/57 (4%)	54/55 (98%)
Clindamycin	60	21/60 (35%)	2/39 (5%)
Gentamicin plus clindamycin	58	5/58 (7%)	3/53 (6%)

Results of these experiments are summarised in Table 2. The untreated animals followed a course similar to that described previously. The mortality in this group was 37% and all surviving animals had localised intra-abdominal abscesses. Animals given gentamicin had a significantly lower mortality (4%), but 98% of survivors had abscesses. Animals given clindamycin had a mortality rate which was not significantly different from untreated controls; however, autopsies at 10 days revealed abscesses in only w animals (5%). The combination of clindamycin and gentamicin produced the salutary effects of each agent - mortality was 7% and only 6% had abscesses. These results support the impression that coliforms are primarily responsible for the early mortality in this model while anaerobic bacteria appear to play a critical role in abscess formation.

Another chemotherapeutic trial was studied using penicillin G and amikacin. These agents were of interest for two reasons: First, penicillin is relatively inactive against Bacteroides fragilis, but in vitro testing shows that most strains are susceptible to levels which can be attained with high parenteral doses (9). Thus, it has been suggested that penicillin is adequate treatment for infections involving B.fragilis. The second reason to study these agents concerns the enterococcus. This organism is not susceptible to clindamycin or gentamicin, and it was frequently recovered from infected sites. Amikacin is an aminoglycoside similar to gentamicin which, when combined with penicillin, is active against the enterococcus.

The design of this study was identical to that described with clindamycin and gentamicin except there were 30 animals in each group. Doses of antimicrobials were selected which gave peak serum levels of 25 mcg/ml for amikacin and 150 mcg/ml for penicillin.

TABLE 3

RESULTS WITH PENICILLIN AND AMIKACIN

Agent	No. tested	Mortality	Abscesses in survivors
Controls	30	11/30 (37%)	19/19 (100%)
Penicillin	30	5/30 (18%)	23/25 (92%)
Amikacin	30	2/30 (7%)	27/28 (97%)
Penicillin and Amikacin	30	0/30	23/30 (73%)

Results are summarised in Table 3.   Mortality rates were reduced with all 3 therapeutic regimens.   This observation is con-sonant with the activity of amikacin and high dose penicillin ver-sus coliform bacteria.   However, 92% of the animals receiving penicillin which survived had localised abscesses on autopsy exam-ination at 10 days.   Moreover, 6 of these abscesses were cultured and B.fragilis was present in every instance.   It should be noted that the strain of B.fragilis used in these experiments is sus-ceptible to 8 mcg/ml of penicillin.   Thus, this organism was not eliminated despite penicillin blood levels well in excess of the minimum inhibitory concentration.

Using penicillin and amikacin directed against the entero-coccus, all animals survived, but 73% had abscesses at autopsy examination after 10 days.   Cultures of the abscesses showed that the enterococcus was eliminated in this experimental group. These results for mortality and abscess formation are not significantly different from those using amikacin alone.

SUMMARY

These studies show that there is a biphasic disease in this experimental model of intra-abdominal sepsis.   Aerobic and anaer-obic bacteria appear to play distinctive roles in the sequence of pathological events.

During the first 5 days following the fecal implant there is acute peritonitis and a 35-45% mortality rate.   Coliforms, espec-ially E.coli, appear to be primarily responsible.   There are several observations to support this conclusion.   First, quanti-tative cultures of peritonitis exudate show that facultative organisms outrank anaerobes despite the numerical dominance of the anaerobes in the implant.   Second, blood cultures during this

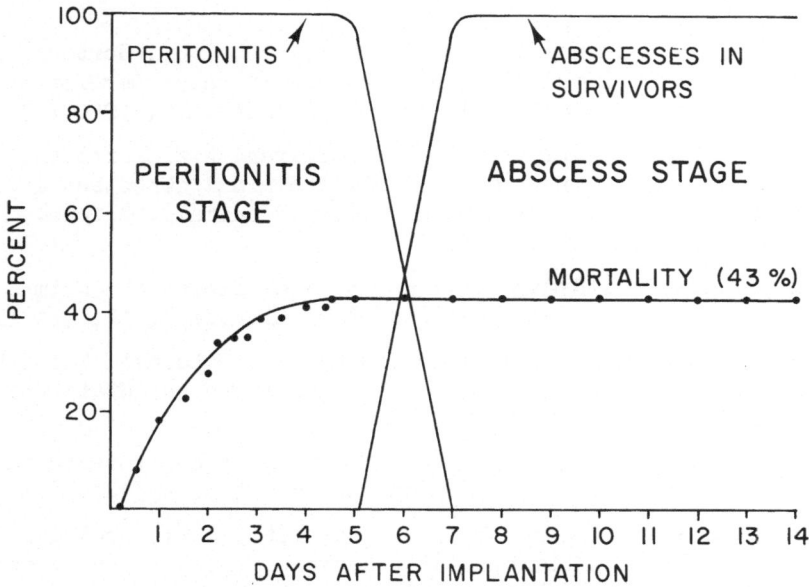

Figure 1

period show a high incidence of E.coli bacteremia. Finally, anti-microbials directed against coliforms generally prevented the lethality associated with this stage of the disease.

The second stage consists of intra-abdominal abscess forma-tion 5-7 days after the fecal implant. Here, anaerobic bacteria appear to play a critical role. These organisms outrank faculta-tive bacteria in quantitative cultures of abscesses. It was also shown that clindamycin therapy directed against anaerobes sig-nificantly reduced the incidence of abscesses. Finally, it should be noted that we have never encountered an abscess in these experi-ments which failed to yield an anaerobe.

With regard to the enterococcus, this organism does not appear to play an important role in the early mortality since it was seldom recovered from blood cultures, and therapy direct against coliforms was successful in preventing lethality. Enterococci could often be recovered from abscesses but anaerobes were invar-iably present as well. Moreover, antimicrobial therapy directed against the enterococcus failed to significantly reduce the inci-dence of abscess formation.

REFERENCES

1. Weinstein, W.M., Onderdonk, A.B., Bartlett, J.G., Gorbach, S.L.,
    Experimental intra-abdominal abscess in rats: Development
    of an experimental model. Infect.Immunity, 10, 1250 (1974).

2. Onderdonk, A.B., Weinstein, W.M., Sullivan, N.M. Bartlett, J.G.,
    Gorbach, S.L. Experimental intraabdominal abscesses in rats:
    Quantitative bacteriology of infected animals. Infect.
    Immunity, 10, 1256 (1974).

3. Moore, W.E.C., Holdeman, L.V. Human fecal flora; the normal
    flora of 20 Japanese-Hawaiian. Appl.Microbiol, 27, 961 (1974).

4. Anaerobe Laboratory Manual. Edited by L.V. Holdeman, W.E.C.Moore.
    Blacksburg. Virginia Polytechnic Institute and State Univer-
    sity Anaerobe Laboratory (1972).

5. Edwards, P.R., Ewing, W.H. Identification of Enterobacteriaceae
    3rd ed. Burgess Pub.Co., Minneapolis, Minn. (1972).

6. Weinstein, W.M., Onderdonk, A.B., Bartlett, J.B., Louis, T.E.,
    Gorbach, S.L. Antimicrobial treatment of experimental intra-
    abdominal sepsis. I.Infect.Dis. (in press).

7. Winters, R.E., Litwack, K., Hewitt, W.L. Relation between dose
    and levels of gentamicin in blood. J.Infect.Dis.,124,Suppl.
    590 (1971).

8. Alcid, D., Seligman, S.J. Simplified assay for gentamicin in
    the presence of other antibiotics. Antimicrob.Ag.Chemother.,
    3, 559, (1973).

9. Tally, F.P., Jacobus, N.V., Bartlett, J.G., Gorbach, S.L. In
    vitro activity of penicillins against anaerobes. Anti-
    microbial Ag.Chem., 7, 413, (1975).

COMPARATIVE EFFECTS OF AMOXYCILLIN AND AMPICILLIN IN THE TREATMENT OF EXPERIMENTAL MOUSE INFECTIONS

K. R. Comber, C. D. Osborne, R. Sutherland

Beecham Pharmaceuticals Research Division

Brockham Park, Betchworth, Surrey, England

SUMMARY

Amoxycillin was significantly more effective than ampicillin in the parenteral treatment of intraperitoneal mouse infections. After subcutaneous injection, antibiotic blood concentrations were the same for both compounds, but amoxycillin was more effective than ampicillin in reducing bacterial counts in the peritoneal cavity and in the blood of infected mice. Amoxycillin also produced greater bactericidal effects than ampicillin _in vivo_ after intraperitoneal injection and consequently was more effective by this route in the treatment of infection. The results of these studies show that the superior activity of amoxycillin in the mouse when given by injection was due to its higher level of bactericidal activity _in vivo_ compared with ampicillin and to differences in the distribution of the two penicillins in the infected animal.

Amoxycillin shows a spectrum and general level of antibacterial activity in vitro similar to that of ampicillin (Sutherland and Rolinson, 1971) but initial chemotherapeutic studies showed that amoxycillin was significantly more effective than ampicillin in the treatment of a variety of experimental mouse infections (Acred et al, 1971). The superior activity of amoxycillin by the oral route was attributed to the higher blood concentrations produced by amoxycillin in mice by this route, but this was not the case for parenteral administration where the serum concentrations produced by amoxycillin in experimental animals were no greater

than those of ampicillin (Acred et al, 1971). Similar findings
were reported by Hunter et al (1973) who concluded that amoxycillin
produced greater bactericidal effects in vivo than did ampicillin.

In the studies reported here the effects of amoxycillin and
ampicillin given by injection in the treatment of intraperitoneal
mouse infections have been compared by measurement of levels and
bacterial growth in the blood and peritoneal cavity of infected
mice and correlation of these data with effectiveness of treatment,
(Comber et al, 1975).

METHODS

Mouse protection tests. Albino mice (CSI or Olac strain)
weighing 18-22g were infected intraperitoneally with 0.5ml of a
suspension in hog gastric mucin of an overnight broth culture of
the test organism, standardised to give an infective inoculum of
100-1000 Median Lethal Doses. The penicillins were administered
immediately after infection as a single dose, 0.2ml/20g, and the
numbers of animals surviving four days after infection were
recorded, (Comber et al, 1975).

Bactericidal activity in vivo. Mice were infected intraperitoneally with Escherichia coli 8 and dosed with a single
injection of amoxycillin or ampicillin immediately after infection.
Groups of five mice were killed at intervals during the 8 hour
period after infection and samples of blood and peritoneal washings
were collected. The bacterial counts of the specimens were
determined by plating 0.1ml volumes of suitable dilutions on
nutrient agar plates and counting colonies formed after overnight
incubation at 37°C.

Assay of antibiotic levels. Specimens of blood and peritoneal
washings from mice infected intraperitoneally with E. coli 8 were
collected as described above and assayed for amoxycillin and
ampicillin content by large plate diffusion assay with Sarcina
lutea NCTC 8340 as assay organism.

RESULTS

Activity against Various Intraperitoneal Infections

Amoxycillin was significantly more active than ampicillin
$(p < 0.01)$ by the subcutaneous route in the treatment of experimental
infections due to sensitive strains of Escherichia coli, Salmonella
typhimurium, Klebsiella edwardsii, Proteus mirabilis, but there
was no significant difference between the compounds against the

staphylococcal and streptococcal infections (p⟩0.1) (Table 1).
All six test organisms were equally sensitive _in vitro_ to both
penicillins.

TABLE 1. Relative activities of amoxycillin and ampicillin
against intraperitoneal mouse infections.

Organism	M.I.C. (μg/ml)	No. of tests	Mean CD/50 (mg/kg) subcutaneous	
			Amoxycillin	Ampicillin
E. coli (8)	5.0	40	19.7	63.7
Salm. typhimurium (10)	0.5	33	11.0	24.0
K. edwardsii (18)	2.5	31	9.5	27.0
P. mirabilis (13)	1.25	12	22.2	38.2
S. aureus (Smith)	0.05	39	0.27	0.33
Str. pyogenes CN10	0.01	7	0.19	0.19

TABLE 2. Relative activities of amoxycillin and ampicillin by
the subcutaneous route against Escherichia coli 8.

Dose (mg/kg)	Amoxycillin		Ampicillin	
	No. survivors	CD 50 (mg/kg)	No. survivors	CD 50 (mg/kg)
200	24		22	
100	23		19	
50	20	21.0	14	48.0
25	14		6	
12.5	10	(14.3-30.9)	2	(32.6-70.6)
6.25	3		4	
3.12	7		1	
0	0		0	

+ 25 mice per group

Effects of Subcutaneous Treatment of Infection due to E. coli 8

Activity. Data in Table 2 illustrate the effects of a single
subcutaneous dose of amoxycillin or ampicillin in the treatment
of an intraperitoneal infection due to <u>E. coli</u> 8. Groups of
25 mice were treated at each dose level and it can be seen that
amoxycillin was significantly more active than ampicillin ($p < 0.05$).

<u>Antibiotic Levels in Blood and Peritoneal Washings</u>. Both
penicillins produced similar blood levels in mice infected with
<u>E. coli</u> 8 after a single subcutaneous dose of 12.5mg/kg, the
concentrations falling rapidly from a peak level of 8.5µg/ml at
10 minutes to 0.5µg/ml at 2 hours (Fig. 1).

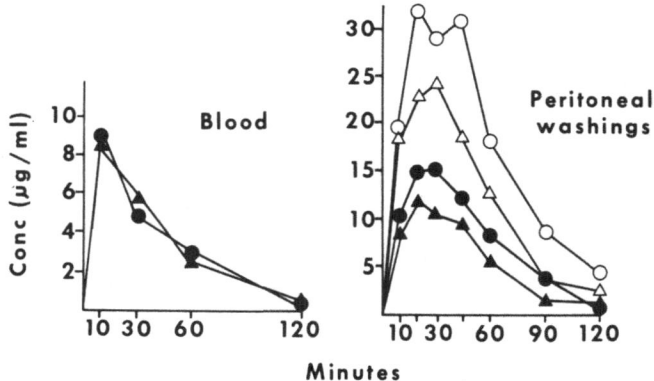

FIG. 1.   Antibiotic concentrations in mice after
                subcutaneous injection
        Amoxycillin : ● , 12.5mg/kg
                      ○ , 25   mg/kg
        Ampicillin : ▲ , 12.5mg/kg
                      △ , 25   mg/kg

In peritoneal washings, the antibiotic concentrations reached
peak values within 20 minutes and fell to relatively low levels
at 2 hours. The levels obtained with amoxycillin were higher
than those of ampicillin at both doses shown, 12.5mg/kg and
25mg/kg, but the differences were less than two-fold.

<u>Bactericidal Effects in Blood and Peritoneal Washings</u>. In
untreated mice infected with <u>E. coli</u> 8 bacterial counts rose
rapidly in the peritoneal cavity after intraperitoneal injection
of the organism, and there was a similar rapid rise in the bacterial
blood count (Fig. 2). Administration of a single subcutaneous dose
(12.5mg/kg) of the penicillins resulted in an initial fall in the

bacterial peritoneal count and the bactericidal effect of
amoxycillin was notably greater than that of ampicillin.
Amoxycillin also had a greater effect than ampicillin on the
blood count and the blood count was lower in amoxycillin-treated
mice, barely exceeding 10 cells/ml over the first 4 hour period.
Similarly, the lower dose level (3.1mg/kg) of amoxycillin was
again more effective than ampicillin in reducing the bacterial
counts in blood and peritoneal washings. The superior bactericidal
effects of amoxycillin were reflected in the greater effectiveness
of amoxycillin in protecting the infected mice as can be seen from
Fig. 2.

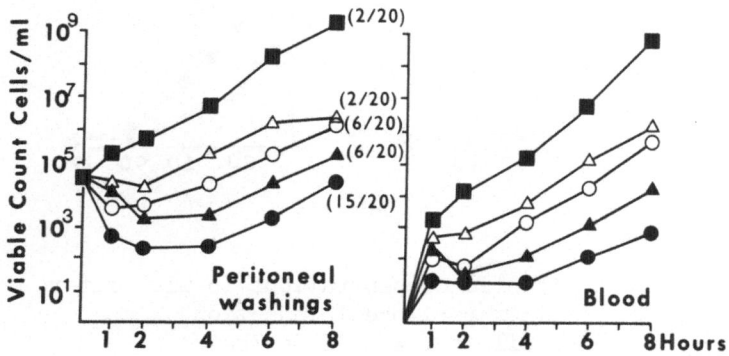

FIG. 2.   Bactericidal activity in mice after
          subcutaneous injection
          Untreated Controls : ■
          Amoxycillin   : O , 3.1mg/kg
                               ● ,12.5mg/kg
          Ampicillin   : △ , 3.1mg/kg
                               ▲ ,12.5mg/kg

Effects of Intraperitoneal Treatment of Infection due to E. coli 8

  Antibiotic levels in blood and peritoneal washings. The
penicillin concentrations measured in the peritoneal washings of
mice infected with E. coli 8 after a single intraperitoneal dose
of amoxycillin and ampicillin were the same for both compounds,
whereas, in blood, amoxycillin concentrations were twice as high
as those found with ampicillin (Fig. 3).

  Activity. Amoxycillin was significantly more active (p<0.05)
than ampicillin by intraperitoneal injection against an infection
due to E. coli 8 (Table 3) and viable count studies showed that
amoxycillin was markedly more effective than ampicillin in reducing
the bacterial counts in the peritoneal cavity of infected mice

treated by the intraperitoneal route (Fig. 4) although the antibiotic concentrations in the peritoneal cavity were the same for both compounds.

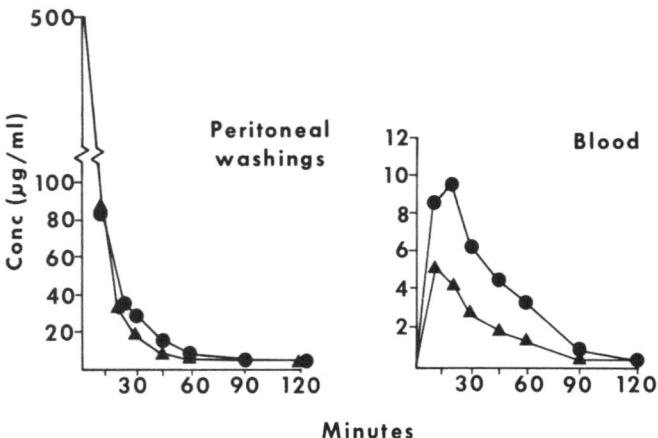

FIG. 3.   Antibiotic concentrations in mice after
intraperitoneal injection
Amoxycillin : ● , 12.5mg/kg
Ampicillin : ▲ , 12.5mg/kg

TABLE 3.   Relative activities of amoxycillin and ampicillin
by the intraperitoneal route against Escherichia coli 8.

Dose (mg/kg)	Amoxycillin		Ampicillin	
	No. survivors[+]	CD 50 (mg/kg)	No. survivors	CD 50 (mg/kg)
200	19		19	
100	19		17	
50	18	12.5	13	24.5
25	11		6	
12.5	13	(8.0–19.3)	6	(15.3–39.2)
6.25	9		3	
3.12	4		6	
0	0		0	

+ 20 mice per group

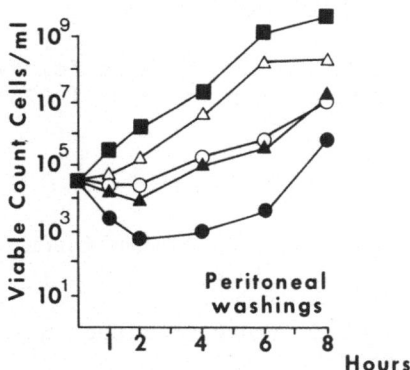

FIG. 4.   Bactericidal activity in mice after
          subcutaneous injection
          Untreated Controls : ■
          Amoxycillin   : ○ , 3.1mg/kg
                                 ● ,12.5mg/kg
          Ampicillin   : △ , 3.1mg/kg
                                 ▲ ,12.5mg/kg

DISCUSSION

     After injection, amoxycillin was more effective than ampicillin
in reducing bacterial growth in the peritoneal cavity of mice
infected intraperitoneally with E. coli. This was in turn
reflected in the blood bacterial counts which resulted in greater
protection of the infected mice by amoxycillin than with ampicillin.
The superior bactericidal activity of amoxycillin in the peritoneal
cavity can only be explained in part by differences in the
peritoneal concentrations of amoxycillin and ampicillin and it
would appear that amoxycillin was producing greater bactericidal
effects than ampicillin in vivo in this intraperitoneal infection,
as has been reported by Hunter et al (1973) in a different
experimental model.

     These results show that amoxycillin is more effective by
parenteral administration than ampicillin in the treatment of
experimental mouse infections as a result of superior in vivo
bactericidal activity combined with better distribution
characteristics in the infected animal, and it is possible that
amoxycillin might prove to be more effective in the clinical
situation than would be predicted from knowledge of in vitro
activity and antibiotic blood concentrations.

ACKNOWLEDGMENT

We thank the American Society of Microbiology for permission to reproduce certain data from Comber et al (1975).

REFERENCES

Acred, P., Hunter, P. A., Mizen, L. and Rolinson, G. N. 1971. Antimicrob.Ag.Chemother., 1970, p. 416.

Comber, K. R., Osborne, C. D. and Sutherland, R. 1975. Antimicrob.Ag.Chemother., 7, 179.

Hunter, P. A., Rolinson, G. N. and Witting, D. A. 1973. Antimicrob.Ag.Chemother., 4, 285.

Sutherland, R. and Rolinson, G. N. 1971. Antimicrob.Ag.Chemother., 1970, p. 411.

Model of Pleuropneumonia in Rats

Krüger,Ch., Commichau,R. and Henkel,W.

Med. Hochsch., Lübeck, Abt. Inn. Med.

2400 Lübeck, Ratzeburger Allee 160, F.R.G.

Summary:
Intrapleural instillation of a suspension of E. coli
(0 25:19:12) results in a double sided pulmonary pleuropneumonial and peribronchial inflammation in albino
Wistar rats. This infection lasts at least for 3
weeks when being facilitated by estradiolundecylate
(10 mg/rat, weekly) and seems therefore to be a suitable model for testing antimicrobial drugs.

Up to now testing of antimicrobial substances in vivo
occurs preferably on experimental pyelonephritis.
These infections being facilitated mainly by obstructive methods e.g. ligature of the ureter (Prát et al.
1959).

In analogy to hormonally induced pyelonephritis (Commichau 1971) – an interstitial chronic inflammation
lasting at least for three months (Sack et al. 1971)
– we choose estradiolundecylate to keep up pulmonary
infection since without hormone the inflammation tends
to heal spontaneously within short time.

Experimental models in animals to provoke bronchial
asthma, pulmonary edema or emphysema with secondary
bronchitis have been described by Preuner (1951),
Dieke and Richter (1946), Lulling (1968) and others.
However, there exists no standardized procedure to
induce unspecific pneumonia in animals. In preliminary tests we investigated several strains

of E. coli for its potency to start a pulmonary infection. For this purpose the infection was facilitated by methylprednisolone (Urbason-Depot, Hoechst,
Frankfurt) and not by estradiol. We found that only
serum resistant strains of E. coli were virulent enough
to induce an inflammation spreading throughout the organ (Henkel 1971)(tab. 1).

Tab. 1: Rate of pulmonary infection with different serum resistant and-sensitive strains of E. coli (Facilitation of infection: methylprednisolone 6 mg/kg,
i.m., 14 days).

	serum resistant		serum sensitive	
Strains of E. coli	O 25	O 15	O 15	O 111
Total number of lungs	36	34	38	40
Infected lungs	34	33	19	3

These results agree very well with the experimental data
on infections of other organs with the same strains (Henkel et al. 1974).

For further experiments the serum resistant strain E.
coli O 25:19:12 was chosen. As a laboratory strain it
is easily to identify serologically at the end of the
test period and has a good sensitivity to most antibiotics inclusively those being commonly used in pulmonary infections in man.
Estradiol has an advantage over prednisolone, because
the facilitation of infection is not as brisk.

Estradiolundecylate 0.5 mg/kg or 10 mg/rat was i.m.
applicated weekly to female albino Wistar rats. On the
7th day instillation of 0.5 ml of a suspension of E.
coli after setting a right sided partial pneumothorax.
Bacterial concentration 10^8 - 10^9/ml. Dissection of
animals and homogenisation of lungs for quantitative

evaluation of the bacterial count after 7, 14 or 21 days post infectionem. Therapeutics were given twice daily over a period of one week, starting at the 4th day after infection. Statistical work up: Wilcoxon- and X^2-test.

Initially the optimal dose of estradiol had to be determined to maintain inflammatory activity of the pulmonary process during three weeks or longer (tab. 2).

Tab. 2: Rate (in %) of infected lungs and mean log. number of bacteria/lung under treatment with estradiolundecylate in different doses in comparison to a control (without hormone) within a period of 3 weeks.

Estradiol	7 days	14 days	21 days
10 mg/rat i.m., 7 d.	100 % 3.9	95 % 2.5	75 % 1.9
0.5 mg/kg i.m., 7 d.	100 % 4.0	83 % 1.7	61 % 1.0
Control	100 % 4.0	89 % 1.7	29 % 0.6

Intrapleural infection without hormonal facilitation tends to heal within 21 days. Only 29 % of the lungs were infected with a very low bacterial concentration (mean log. no. of bact./lung = 0.6). Estradiol in a very low dose (0.5 mg/kg, i.m., weekly) elevates the activity of inflammation significantly within a longer test period (after 3 weeks rate of infection 61 %, mean log. no. of bact./lung = 1.0) but investigations after shorter intervals reveal no difference to the control.

A relatively high dose of estradiol (10 mg/rat, weekly) leads to a significant elevation of the inflammatory activity even after 14 days after infection (17 out of 18 lungs were infected, mean log. no. of bact./lung = 2.5) (fig. 1 and 2).

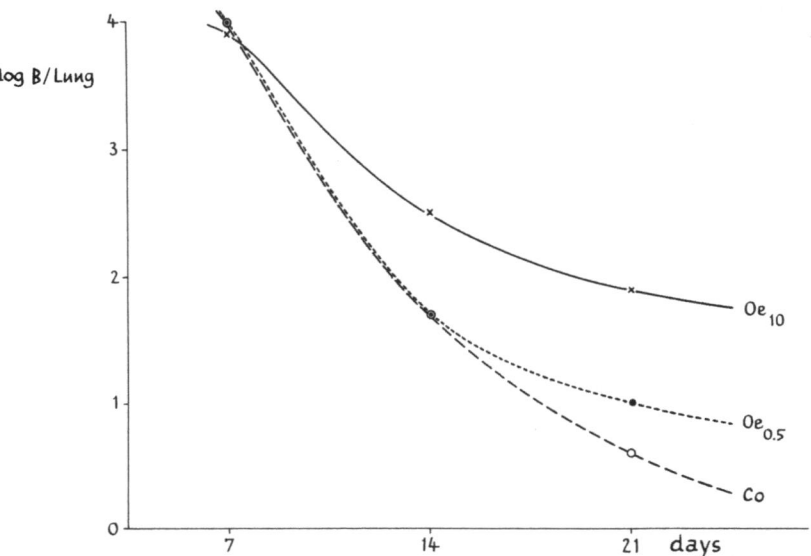

Fig. 1: Dosage dependant hormonal facilitation of pulmonary infection by different doses of estradiol within a course of 3 weeks (Oe 0.5 = 0.5 mg estradiol-undecylate/kg, i.m., weekly, Oe 10 = 10 mg/rat, weekly). Comparison of mean log. no. of bacteria/lung.

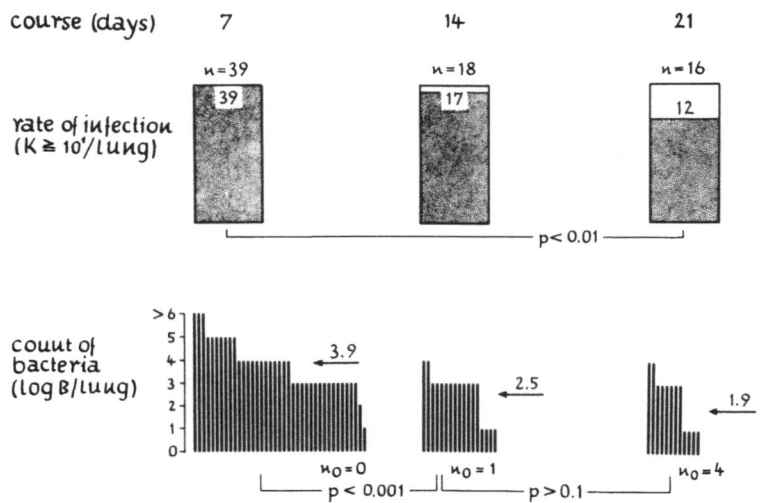

Fig. 2: Course of experimental pulmonary infection in female albino Wistar rats after intrapleural instillation of E. coli O 25:19:12 under facilitation of infection with 10 mg estradiolundecylate, i.m., weekly. B = number of bacteria. n_o = B $<$ 10^1/lung. ← = mean log. no. of bacteria/lung.

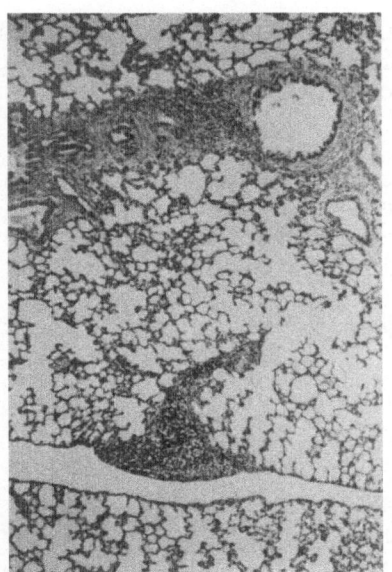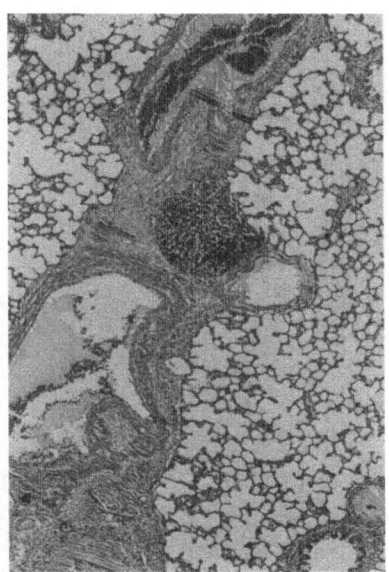

Fig. 3: Histologically right lungs are predominantly
affected by pleuropneumonial inflammation (left). Whereas
left lungs show nearly exclusively peribronchial inflammatory areas (right).

Tab. 3: Efficacy of ampicillin (2 x 150 mg/kg, i.m.,
daily), cyclacillin (2 x 150 mg/kg, p.o., daily) and
gentamicin (2 x 3 mg/kg, i.m., daily) on experimental
hormonally (10 mg estradiolundecylate/kg, i.m., weekly)
facilitated pulmonary infection in rats with E. coli
O 25:19:12.

	Control	Ampicillin	Cyclacillin	Gentamicin
Total number of lungs	18	18	18	20
infected lungs	17	14	14	16
Mean log. no. of bact./lung	2.5	1.7	1.8	1.9
	$p < 0.05$			

At this time histologically pleuropneumonial (predominantly right lungs) and dissiminated peribronchial (preferably left lungs) infiltrations could be stated (fig.
3).

Tendency to change into abscessing pneumonia are seen
after 21 days, therefore the period of 14 days was
chosen **for** therapeutic aim. An example of suppression
of infective activity by ampicillin, cyclacillin and
gentamicin is given in tab. 3. The mean log. no. of
bact./lung could be reduced significantly from 2.5 to
1.7 e.g. with ampicillin.

References:

COMMICHAU,R. (1971), Fortschr. Med., 89, 1095.
DIEKE,S.H. and RICHTER,C.P. (1946), Proc. Soc. exp.
        Biol. (N.J.), 62, 22.
HENKEL,W. (1971), Z. med. Mikrobiol. u. Immunol. 156,
        284.
HENKEL,W., FREIESLEBEN,H., WÖHRMANN,W., KRÜGER,CH. and
        COMMICHAU,R. (1974), Zbl. Bakt. Hyg., I. Abt.
        Orig. A, 227, 306.
LULLING,J., PRIGNOT,J. and LIEVENS,P. (1968), Nanyn-
        Schmiedebergs Arch. Pharmak. u. exp. Path.,
        261, 1.
PRÁT,V., BENEŠOVÁ,D., PÁVKOVÁ,L. and CERVINKA,F. (1959),
        Acta med. Scand., 165, 305.
PREUNER,R. (1951), Arzneimittel-Forsch., 1, 301.
SACK,K., HENKEL,W. and COMMICHAU,R. (1971), Virchows
Arch. Abt. A. Path. Anat., 352, 219.

For technical assistance we thank Mrs. Ch. Mohr.

MURINE MENINGOENCEPHALITIS CAUSED BY PS. AERUGINOSA OR KL. PNEUMONIAE AS AN EXPERIMENTAL CHEMOTHERAPEUTIC MODEL

E.N. Padeiskaya, S.N. Kutchak, G.N. Perchin

S. Ordzhonikidze All-Union Chemical-Pharmaceutical Research Institute
Moscow, USSR

The treatment of secondary purulent bacterial meningitis particularly meningitis caused by Ps. aeruginosa or Kl.pneumoniae offers significant difficulty. A large number of antibacterial agents developed up to the present time has not solved the problem which is complicated by the peculiarities of localization of pathological process. Investigation of new drugs and their approbation on the models characterized by changes in tissue and brain membranes typical for purulent meningoencephalitis are necessary. A study of such models is of great practical importance. At the 5th International Congress of Infection Diseases (Vienna, 1970) we reported about models of experimental purulent meningitis of rabbits provoked by Ps.aeruginosa or Kl.pneumoniae. Peculiarities of the infections depending on the pathogene as well as the methods of evaluating the antibacterial compounds were demonstrated.

In this paper we present the results of reproduction and approbation of meningitis models, caused by the same strains of bacteria in experimental mice. Availability of these animals for numerous trials is an important factor in chemotherapeutic investigation. Experiments were carried out on 2,800 white mice.

The infection was reproduced by intracerebrally inoculation into the region of middle line of the cranium 2-3 mm over eye-socket. A needle with a special

nozzle preventing a deep penetration into the brain has
been used (2 mm end of needle is free from the nozzle).
The mice were injected intracerebrally with 0.05 ml of
the suspension of bacterial culture in saline. At the
same time we compared the peculiarities of the development of the infection at intraperitoneal or intranasal
injection.

The results were evaluated at different period after
inoculation according to the clinical picture, the
survival of the animals from 10 to 30 days, the bacteriological and pathomorphological observation of
killed or dead animals. We specially investigated brain,
blood and inner organs. Efficiency of the compounds
was evaluated by the same indicators.

Mice very well tolerate a prick or an injection of
0.05ml sterile non-infected material into the area
mentioned above. In these cases pathomorphological
investigation does not reveal purulent inflammation
of brain membranes or tissue.

Ps.aeruginosa injected intracerebrally (1×10^3 -
5×10^6 bacterial cells) produces a development of purulent meningoencephalitis, accompanied by generalization
of infection at infective doses 1×10^6 bacterial cells
and higher. The severity of the process depends on the
amount of the infective dose. Already one or two hours
after the beginning of the experiment we can observe
constant isolation of Ps.aeruginosa from brain tissue
applying all the infective doses. Death from 80 to 100%
of mice after inoculation with 1×10^6 bacterial cells
and higher took place. As a rule, the generalization
of the infection and death of the animals at lower infective doses are not observed. It is interesting to
note that survived mice on the second or third day
after inoculation displayed disturbance of motor co-
ordination (circular stereotypic motions, lateral
position of body and head). Elucidation of pathogenesis
of this symptom is of great interest.

During the trials with Kl.pneumoniae high sensitivity of mice to inoculation with this type of bacteria
have been demonstrated. We must mention the development
of meningoencephalitis after the injection of extremly
low infective doses. Generalization of the infection
and death of the animals 48-72 hours after the
inoculation take place in 96% of cases at infective
dose 250 bacterial cells. The increase of the infective dose intensifies the course of the process.

If we compare Ps.aeruginosa with Kl.pneumoniae we can
see that the latter begins to constantly isolate 24
hours after the injection; the isolation of Kl.pneu-
moniae from blood and inner organs takes place still
later. There were no clinical manifestations of
meningoencephalitis typical for this infection.

Pathomorphologic observation reveals differences
in the character of lesions depending on the pathogene.

Ps.aeruginosa provokes purulent meningoencephalitis
with diffusive thickening and dense infiltration of
brain membrane with segmentnuclear leucocytes and the
development of purulent ventriculitis, periventriculitis and ependimatitis (Fig.I). As to more severe
cases we observe microabscesses accompanied by sharp
brain oedema (Fig.2). The degree and the severity of
above changes depend on the amount of infective dose. Kl.
pneumoniae gives purulent-haemorrhagic or haemorragic meningoencephalitis with persistent injury of blood vessel
walls followed by serious vascular lesions. Leucocytic
reaction is often suppressed and oedematious membranes
contain large quantity of erythrocytes and Kl.pneumoniae.
We constantly observed enhanced permeability of the
wall of blood vessels in form of the swelling of endo-
thelium, homogenization of the wall and the appearance
of circular haemorrhages (Fig.3). Sometimes necroses
of the vessel wall may take place. The grave lesions
described above are observed apply low infective doses.

Both infections are not neurotropic. Primarily
the brain membranes and intermediate tissue are injured.
The injury of the elements of nervous system takes place
afterwards. The lesions of neurocytes and neuroglia are
non-specific and bear hypoxic or ischemic character;
rarer - sever toxic one.

We have observed the following processes: oedema
and cytolisis of neurocytes, lysis of tigroid, cary-
opycnosis, caryolisis, diffusive and focal reaction
of glia (nodes near the vessels from astrocytes with
histiocytes), proliferation and hyperthrophia of
astrogliocytes, olygodendroglia and microglia; the
appearance of drainage forms ofolygodendroglia.

Rapid dissemination of the infection in brain
membranes and tissue is probably dependent on natural
routes of communication between perivascular, intrapial
and subarachnoidal spaces. This supposition indirectly

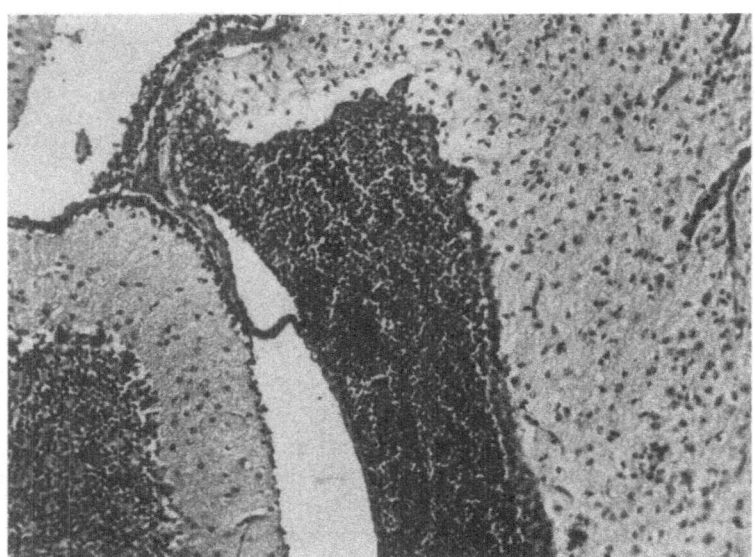

Fig. 1 Purulent ventriculitis, periventriculitis;
       desquamation of ependima; purulent exudate in
       the ventriculus; leucocytic infiltration of
       plexus chorioideus ventriculi. Surrounding
       brain tissue, proliferation of glia is observed.

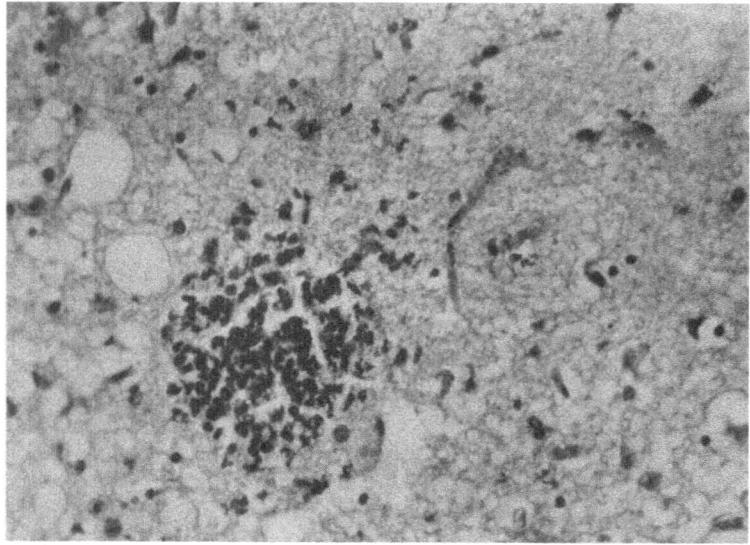

Fig. 2 Microabscess in brain tissue; focal accumulation
       of leucocytes; brain tissue oedematous.

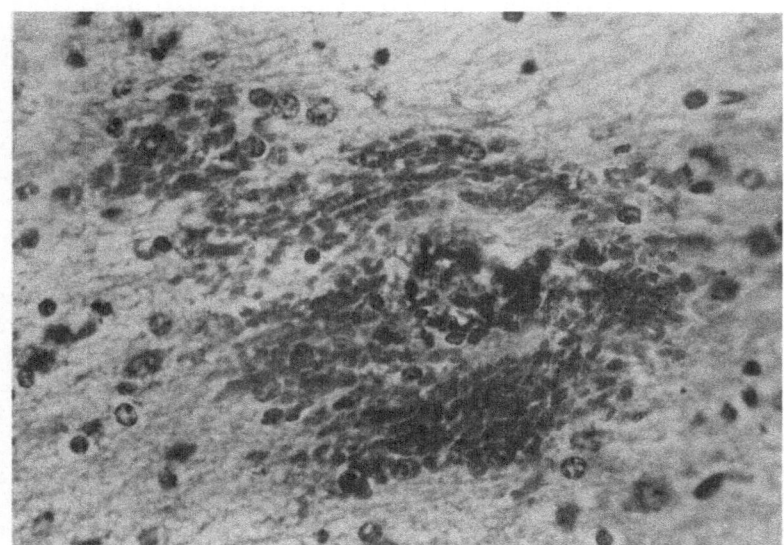

Fig. 3 Circular haemorrhage. In the centre- blood
        vessel with homogenized wall, surrounded with
        zone of plasma and extra-zone of erythrocytes.

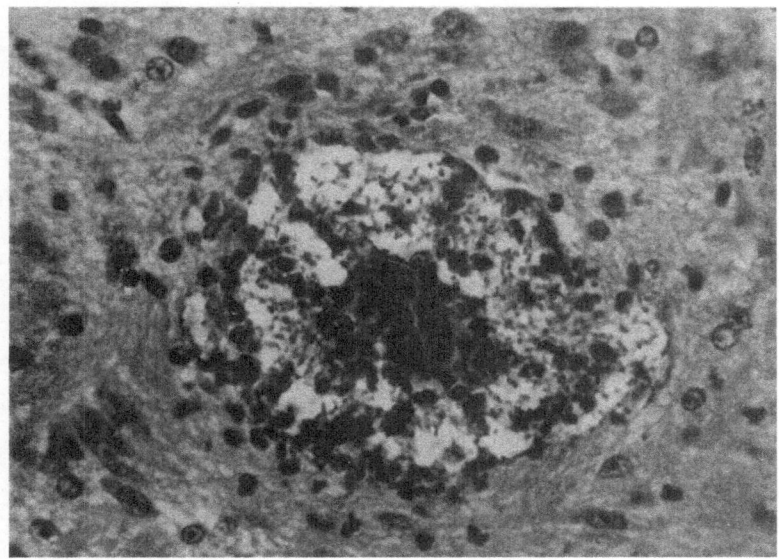

Fig. 4 Expension of perivascular space (space of
        Virchov-Roben) containing large number of
        Kl.pneumoniae.

testified by persistant sharp expansion of perivascular
spaces (the space of Virchov-Roben) with a large amount
of Kl.pneumoniae (Fig.4).

Elucidation of the role of endotoxines in patho-
genese of the infection is of special interest. With
this aim in view it is expedient to study the character of the changes in brain tissue following the
injection of killed bacterial cells.

The purulent meningoencephalitis is not developed
at intraperitoneal or intranasal inoculation of mice
in the case of the generalization of the infection,
the development of bacteriemia and isolation of
pathogene from brain tissue, as during the trials with
simultaneous trauma of the brain (the prick with a
needle). Pathomorphological observation reveals only
the traces of trauma: limited haemorrhages into the
tissue and membranes of brain, rarefication and death
of single cells along the canal of the needle.

The worked out models allow us to evaluate the
activity of the drugs at oral and parenteral administration. It is recommended to use infective doses
which provoke severe lethal meningoencephalitis. While
experimenting we studied the activity of Dioxidine
I,4-di-N-oxide 2,3-bishydroxymethylquinoxaline),
Quinoxidine (I,4-di-N-oxide 2,3-bisacetoxymethylquin-
oxaline) and Chloramphenicol.

In the experiments with Ps. aeruginosa Dioxidine
(100 mg/kg p.o. or s.c.) and Quinoxidine (500 mg/kg p.o.)
in a single dose immediately following the infection
prevent the death of mice and the development of
severe changes in brain tissue. No foci of necrosis,
purulent ventriculitis, microabscesses are found;
inflammatory infiltration of membranes decreases
(Fig. 5). After a three day administration of drugs
we succeeded in obtaining a sterilizing effect.

In the experiments with Kl.pneumoniae a single
injection of the drugs at dose 500 mg/kg shortly after
the inoculation practically prevents completely the
development of the infection and the pathological
changes in brain membranes and tissue. If the treatment begins 4 or 24 hours following the inoculation
we can observe a high chemotherapeutic effect after
a three day administration of the drugs.

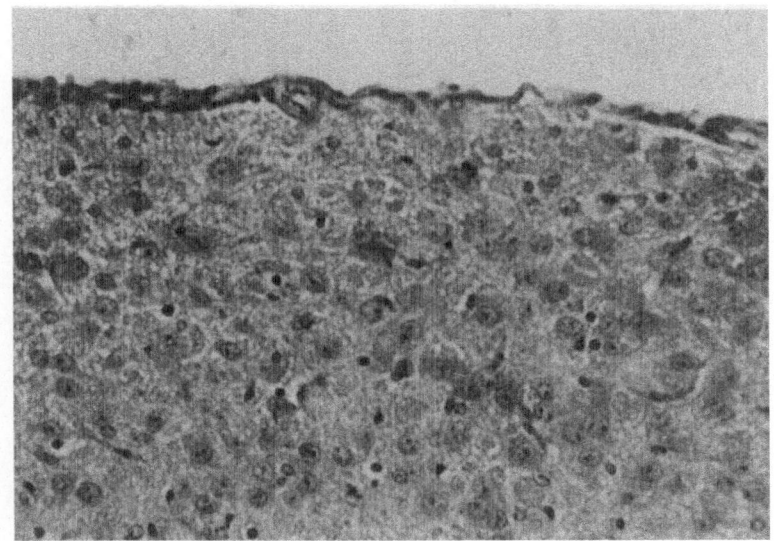

Fig. 5. Brain membrane and brain tissue of mice
        infected with Ps.aeruginosa, after the treat-
        ment of Dioxidine. Residual symptoms.

        Dioxidine was more active than Quinoxidine.
Both drugs exceeded chloramphenicol or chloramphenicol
sodium succinate by their effectiveness. The investigations demonstrate the possibility of the reproduction
of murine purulent bacterial meningoencephalitis with
characteristic pathomorphological picture depending
on the type of pathogene. The value of these models
for chemotherapeutic trials is evident.

ANIMAL EXPERIMENTS ON CURRENT ANTIBIOTICS

Ritzerfeld, W., Koschmieder,R., Drees,W.

Hygiene-Institut der Universität

44 Münster/W., Germany

Summary

Our experiments were carried out on acute,obstructive pyelonephritis in the rat (caused by various Gram-negative rods) and staphylococcal osteomyelitis in the pig. The former model was used to investigate the bacterialreducing action of, amongst others, epicillin, the penicillin derivatives BAY f 1353 and BAY e 6905, sisomycin, tobramycin, and cefazolin and cefradine. Prophylaxis and therapy of experimental osteomyelitis was investigated by the addition of gentamicin to polymethylmethacrylate. Summary reports of the results of the individual test series are presented.

Our research team investigated repeatedly and by means of various methods the anti-bacterial activity of new derivatives of three groups of active substances: penicillins, cephalosporins and aminoglycosides. For in vitro experiments we used diffusion and dilution tests together with the measurement of the O_2 consumption of micro-organisms under the influence of these agents. In the animal experiments we used mainly the therapy and infection model of acute obstructive pyelonephritis. A report on the systematic investigation of a new substance - cephazolin - by appropriate methods was delivered at the 8th. International Congress of Chemotherapy in Athens in 1973 (Ritzerfeld and Loew 1974). The present paper is an account of results obtained with a number

of recent antibiotics * - the emphasis being on animal
experiments - pyelonephritis and osteomyelitis.

First the report on the activity of certain new
penicillin derivatives. At the 14th. Interscience Conference in San Francisco in 1974 the two wide-spectrum
penicillins BAY f 1353 and BAY e 6905 were introduced
for the first time (Metzger 1974, König et al.1974).
While the former is said to influence primarily enterobacteriaceae, BAY e 6905 is characterised mainly by its
effect on pseudomonas. Our own first in vitro experiments
more or less confirm the manufacturers' claims, though
varying degrees of sensitivity were detected within
individual groups of bacteria. The effectiveness of the
substance was further clarified through the animal experiment (pyelonephritis in rats). Treatment of this
pyelonephritis according to the experimental procedure
laid down by Prat and his research team is as follows:
1 hour after removal of temporary ligature from ureters
(left kidney previously damaged) intraurethral injection
of 1 ml suspension 1,5 x 10^9 living bacteria. Therapy
commenced 6 hours later and medication continued over 3
days. After a further 2 days, animals were killed and bacteriological, cultural examination of pre-damaged left
and undamaged right kidney, together with urine test.
Criterion of effect of antibiotics: reduction of bacteria
after therapy; in addition control groups without agents;
statistical signifance were done with the help of Wilcoxon test.

Fig. 1 shows results obtained with BAY f 1353 after
proteus mirabilis infection and dosage of 3 x 150 mg/kg/
die i.m..Ampicillin administered in the same doses and
by the same method was used to provide a comparison. The
diagram clearly shows the anti-bacterial effect of the
substances as compared to the control group (constant,
significant reduction of bacteria). The activity of
ampicillin was greater than that of BAY f 1353, but this
superiority could not be verified by means of the significance calculations. In a second series of experiments
the infection strain was E.coli and the rats were treated
by the same method.Similar noticeable effect of both substances as compared with untreated control group. No difference between effects of the two substances.

---

*Substances were made available by: Farbenfabriken Bayer
GmbH, Leverkusen; Sandoz AG, Nürnberg; Eli Lilly GmbH,
Bad Homburg; Boehringer Mannheim GmbH, Mannheim; Heyden,
München; E.Merck, Darmstadt, Hoechst, Frankfurt.

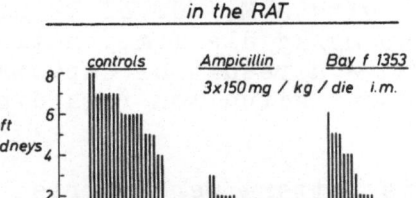

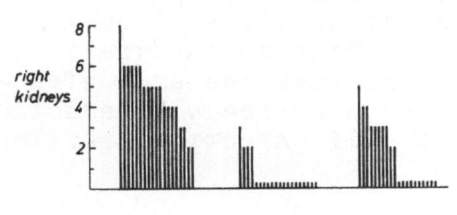

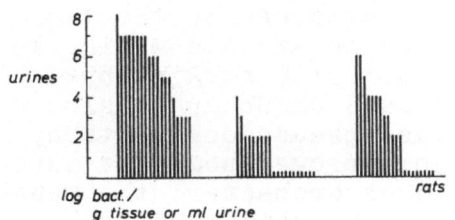

Fig. 1:
results (number
of bacteria)
with BAY f 1353
after proteus
mirabilis infection

Fig. 2:
results (number
of bacteria)
with BAY e 6905
after pseudomonas
aeruginosa
infection

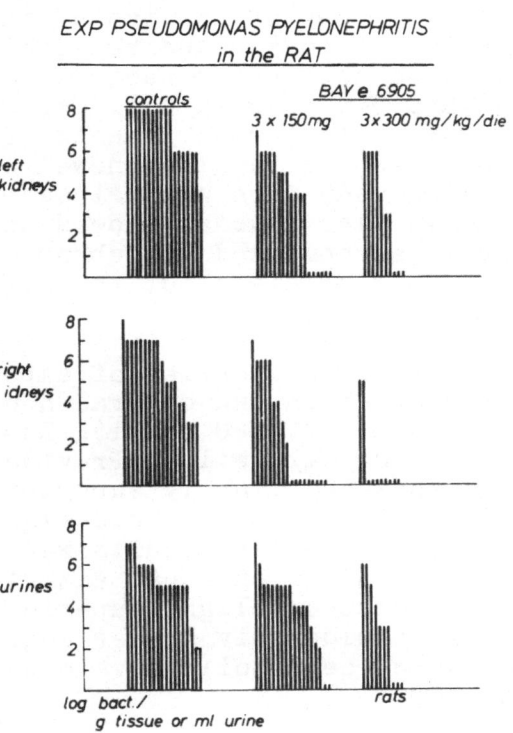

We investigated the effectiveness of BAY e 6905 on
pseudomonas aeruginosa (Fig. 2) with a M.I.C. of 32 μg/ml.
Reduction of bacteria by 3 x 150 mg/kg/die i.m., notice-
ably greater when dosage doubled - a result of especial
importance, considering the present situation regarding
pseudomonas infections.

Further experiments on this pattern were carried
out using epicillin. The anti-bacterial spectrum of the
substance is similar to that of ampicillin; the medic-
ament was recommended to be used in smallish doses -
a recommendation which we would criticise. In experiments we found that both substances have the same effectiveness when used in equal doses: a noticeable reduction
of bacteria in treatment of an E.coli infection, particularly in kidney tissue.

Recently importance has been attached to the two
aminoglycoside antibiotics tobramycin and sisomycin. In
vitro experiments on over 1300 bacterial strains by
means of a plate diffusion test have shown an equal
level of activity against proteus, pseudomonas, staphylococci and enterococci. Sisomycin proved somewhat superior in its effect on E.coli and enterobacter; the measurement of M.I.C. values revealed the same tendency.
Fig. 3 shows an in vivo comparison of results with tobramycin, sisomycin and kanamycin. Only kanamycin failed to
produce noticeable bacterial reduction. The dosage was
always 3 x 3 mg/kg/die i.m. over 3 days. The effect was
stronger in tissue than in urine. The same experiment
on proteus mirabilis showed similar results, though bacterial reduction was not as pronounced as with E.coli.
The in vivo studies showed that the activity of sisomycin as compared to tobramycin was somewhat greater
for both species, but the differences were not statistically significant.

A further series of experiments tested the effect
of cephazolin and cephradin on a resistant enterobacter
strain(M.I.C. 160 μg/ml). Dosage: 3 x 100 respectively
3 x 50 mg/kg/die i.m. Previous experiments with E.coli
had shown a slightly superior effect on the part of
cephazolin, but this was significant only in undamaged
kidneys. Similar results were obtained with the enterobacter infection:equal activity on the part of both
substances or slight superiority of cephazolin. In spite
of a considerably higher degree of combination with
albumin, cephazolin developed the same anti-bacterial
effect.

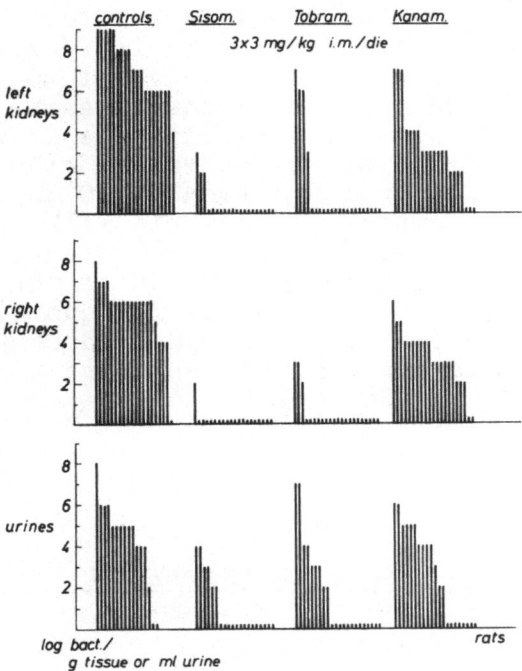

Fig.3: results (number of bacteria) with tobramycin, sisomycin, kanamycin after E.coli infection.

In the animal experiment we further tested the therapeutic effect of gentamicin with the addition of polymethylmethacrylate on staphylococcal osteomyelitis in pigs. This combination is recommended at present for infectional prophylaxis in the fitting of artificial alloplastic joints. It is questionable whether sufficient quantities of the antibiotic are released to combat the development of bacterial resistance or a secondary infection. Our own first experiments, in which we administered 500 mg of gentamicin to 60 gm of polymethylmethacrylate, showed a post-operational secretion level which would be expected to result in noticeable antibacterial effect (3 μg/ml and over) up to the 10th. day (Koschmieder et al. 1973). For the model infection (M.I.C. value of staph. aureus: 0.5 μg/ml) 2×10^8 bacteria/ml were deposited, following an operation, in the ventricles of the femora of a pig, and the type of bacteria and their quantity in the resulting secretion were measured daily. The addition of gentamicin reduced

significantly the numbers of bacteria, while the values
remained constant in the untreated femur. Nevertheless
the bacterium reappeared 3 - 4 days after the operation,
together with other types of bacteria, notably E.coli,
proteus and enterococci (Koschmieder et al. 1975).
In a further series of experiments (5 animals) the gentamicin dose was doubled. The results are shown in the
last diagrams. Fig. 4 shows the values obtained with
staph. aureus alone over a period of 20 days. In the
top half are the numbers of bacteria without gentamicin,
in the bottom half those registered after dosage with
1 gm gentamicin. The powerful effect of the antibiotic
throughout the period is evident. The quantity of staphylococci in the untreated femur remained constant.
Basically the same results were obtained with other
animals.

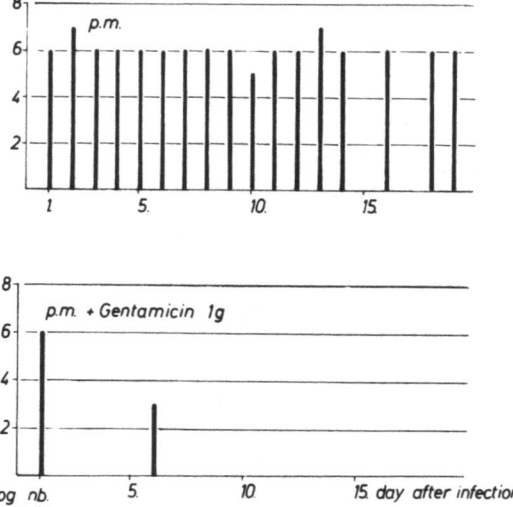

STAPH.AUREUS in EXP. OSTEOMYELITIS

p.m. = polymethyl methacrylate

Fig. 4: results (number of bacteria) after
       staph. aureus infection.

Finally the values for staphylococci together with those of other bacterial species, for which another animal was used. Here too there is evidence of the powerful effect on staph. aureus. At the same time other bacteria are present both after treatment with gentamicin and without any treatment, particularly enterococci. In general the staphylococcal osteomyelitis, which could also be traced histologically was easily combated, but other bacteria were greatly in evidence. This fact is partly due to the animal model in question; on the other hand similar phenomena are under discussion by clinical practitioners. Thus further experiments will have to be carried out on the use of a combination of polymethylmethacrylate and gentamicin as an infectional prophylaxis and possible cure for osteomyelitis.

References

König, H.B., Metzger, K.G. and Offe, H.A. (1974), Abstract 14th. Interscience Conference on Antimicrobial Agents and Chemotherapy No 372.

Koschmieder, R., Ritzerfeld, W. and Kleymann, H. (1973) Z. Orthop. 111, 244

Koschmieder, R., Ritzerfeld, W. and Homeyer, L. (1975) Z. Orthop. 113, 147

Metzger, K. (1974) Abstract 14th. Interscience Conference on Antimicrobial Agents and Chemotherapy No 371

Ritzerfeld, W. and Loew, H. (1974) Proceedings of the 8th. Int. Congress of Chemotherapy, Athens, 289.

EFFECT OF CARBENICILLIN ON PSEUDOMONAS INFECTION

P. A. Hunter, G. N. Rolinson and D. A. Witting

Beecham Pharmaceuticals Research Division

Brockham Park, Betchworth, Surrey, England

Using a mouse thigh lesion model, studies have been made on the effects of carbenicillin on a localized Pseudomonas aeruginosa infection. The infective model used was based on the original work by Selbie and Simon (1952).

Carbenicillin had a minimum inhibitory concentration of 50 μg/ml against the strain of Pseudomonas used in these studies. Mice were infected intramuscularly with a dilution of an overnight broth of the infecting organism containing $2-5 \times 10^6$ CFU. Multiplication takes place resulting in enlargement of the infected thighs. The percentage protection afforded by various doses of carbenicillin was determined by calculating the reduction in thigh size of the treated groups relative to the infected non-treated group.

Using this technique a good correlation was seen between the size of the dose and the number of doses of carbenicillin required to produce a good therapeutic effect.

When one dose was given at the time of infection, this had to be extremely high to produce any effect at all (Fig. 1). If the number of doses was increased, even relatively low doses had a therapeutic effect. However, the timing of these subsequent doses was critical; if the interval extended beyond 2 hours, a drop in effectiveness was seen (Fig. 2). For example, 500 mg/kg given at 0 and 2 hours produced 80% protection; when given at 0 and 3 hours less effect was seen, and when the interval was 4 hours very little effect was seen. The optimum dosage regime in this system was found to be 500 mg/kg at 0, 2 and 4 hours post-infection, this resulted in a consistent cure. Lower doses produced erratic results even when repeated frequently.

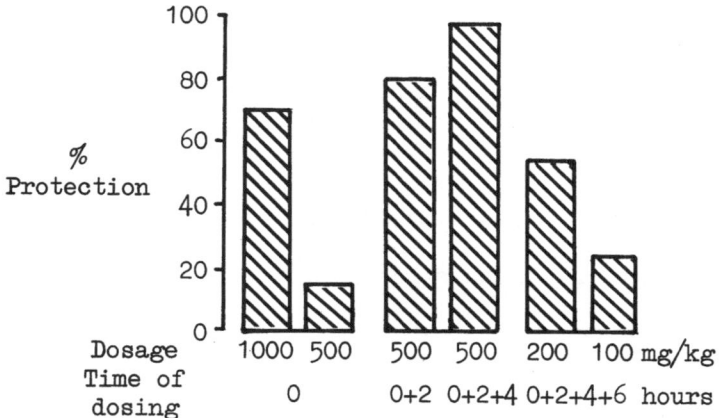

FIG. 1. Effect of varying dosage regimens of carbenicillin
administered subcutaneously.

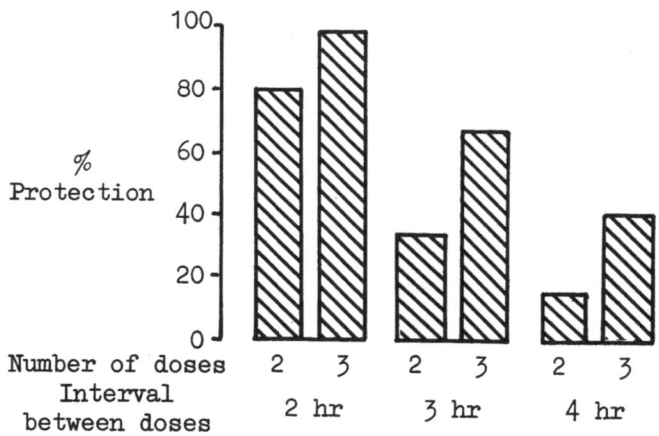

FIG. 2. Effect of carying the interval between doses of
carbenicillin administered subcutaneously at 500 mg/kg.

Using 500 mg/kg the growth of the infecting organisms was
followed by performing viable counts on the infected thigh tissue.
The concentration of carbenicillin present in the blood was also
determined at the same time.   500 mg/kg resulted in a rapid fall
in the numbers of infecting organisms up to 2 hours following
dosing (Fig. 3).   After $2\frac{1}{2}$ hours, when no carbenicillin was
detected in the blood, regrowth occurred and numbers rapidly rose
to equal those of the untreated controls.   However, if further
doses were given at 2 hours and 4 hours the numbers continued to
fall until they were subsequently eliminated completely by the
animal (Fig. 4).   If the interval between these subsequent doses
was greater than 2 hours, regorwth occurred between doses,
decreasing their overall effectiveness (Fig. 5).

When the effect of carbenicillin on this strain of Pseudomonas
was studied _in vitro_, it was found that removal of carbenicillin
(by the addition of β-lactamase) resulted in rapid regrowth of the
organisms such as was seen _in vivo_ when the dosing interval was
3 hours (Fig. 6).

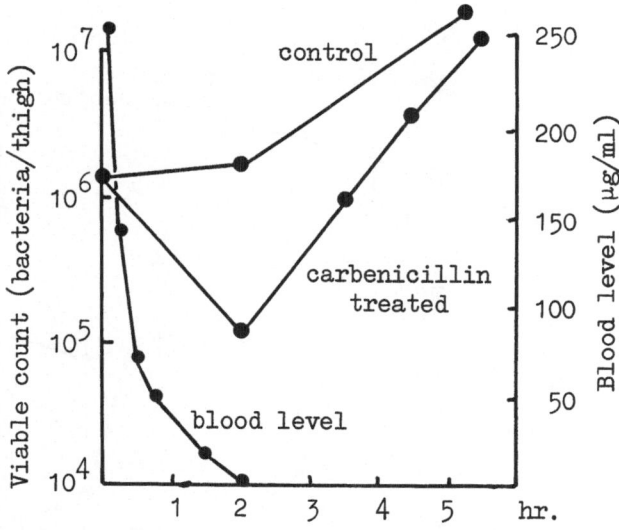

FIG. 3.   Effect of carbenicillin administered subcutaneously
    at a dose of 500 mg/kg at the time of infection only

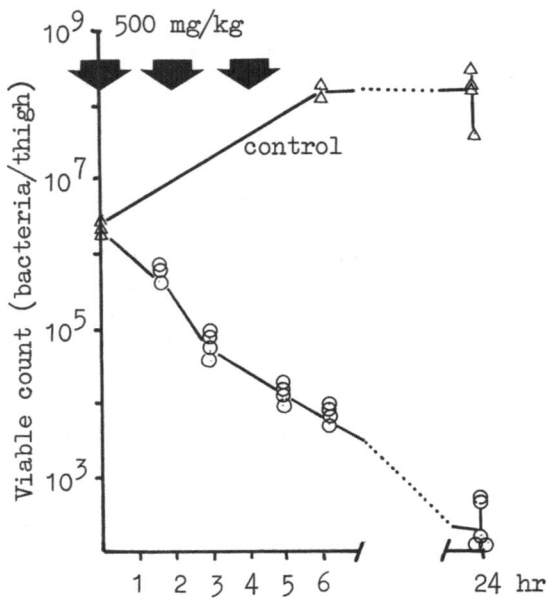

FIG. 4. Effect of carbenicillin administered subcutaneously
at 500 mg/kg at 0, 2 and 4 hours after infection.

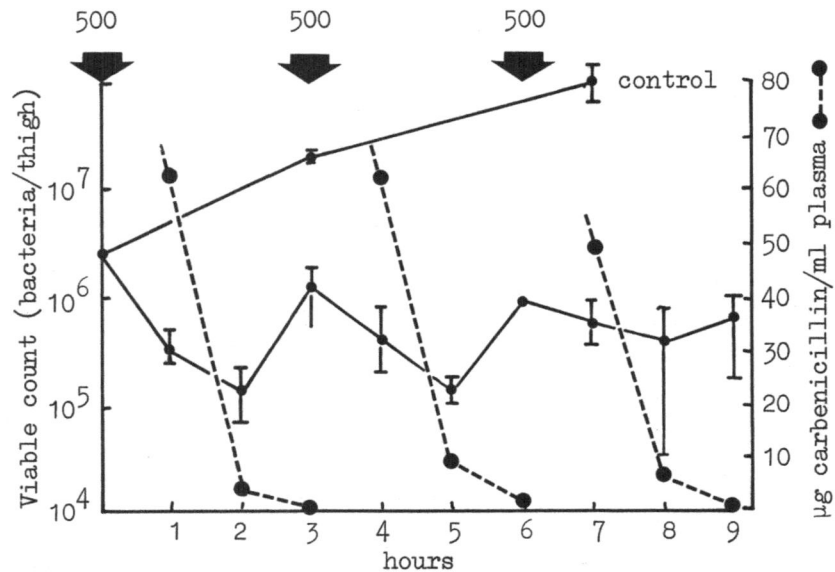

FIG. 5. Effect of carbenicillin administered subcutaneously
at 500 mg/kg at 0, 3 and 6 hours after infection.

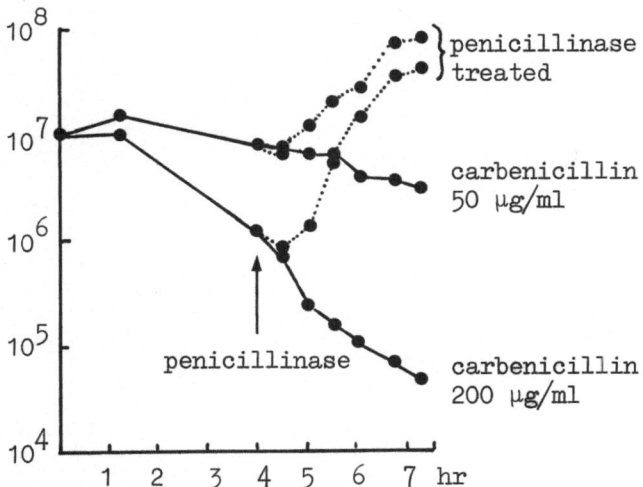

FIG. 6. Effect of exposure of Pseudomonas to carbenicillin
          followed by removal of the drug after 4 hours.

    In conclusion, using a mouse thigh lesion test system,
carbenicillin could be shown to be effective both in suppressing
the development of a lesion, and in reducing the numbers of
organisms present.   A dosing schedule was used which resulted in
high initial concentrations in the blood and allowed a minimum
period between doses when no detectable levels were present.

                        REFERENCE

Selbie, F. R. and Simon, R. D.   1952.   Brit.J.exp.Path., 33, 315.

COMPARISON OF CARFECILLIN AND CARBENICILLIN ON EXPERIMENTAL URINARY TRACT INFECTION

Hatala M., Morávek J., Schück O., Prát V.,
Liška M., Spousta J.
Institute for Clinical and Experimental
Medicine (Director Prof. MUDr. P. Málek, DrSc.)
Budějovická 800, Praha 4 – Krč, Czechoslovakia

The effect of carfecillin and carbenicillin in experiments on rats is compared.

The first part describes pharmacokinetics of the two drugs. However, following administration of carfecillin the serum concentrations of carbenicillin in urine were high.

The antimicrobial efficacy of the two antibiotics was tested in two model infections, i.e. on the model of renal infection and of the lower urinary tract inflammation. In the therapy of renal infection both carfecillin and carbenicillin produced a significant effect only after a prolonged therapy. In the therapy of lower urinary tract infections, carfecillin proved highly efficacious, its effect being distinctly better compared with carbenicillin even when given over a shorter period of time.

The antibacterial therapy of kidney and urinary tract infections continues to be one of the major clinical problems. At screening new antibacterial substances in therapeutical experiments on model urinary tract infections a new drug, carfecillin, was evaluated. It is phenyl-ester of carbenicillin. However, unlike the latter, carfecillin given orally is well absorbed from the gastrointestinal tract and is recommended by the manufacturer for the treatment of cystitis, pyelonephritis and asymptomatic bacteriuria. Both carfecillin

(Uticillin[R]) and carbenicillin (Pyopen[R]) were obtained
by the offices of Beecham Ltd.

The first series of experiments was undertaken to
study the pharmacokinetics of oral carfecillin in rats.
it will be noted from Fig. 1 that serum concentrations
of carbenicillin, obtained by hydrolysis of carfecillin,
were not particularly high. After 250 mg/kg the highest
concentration amounted to 6.7 mcg/ml, a double amount
of the therapeutical dose (500 mg/kg) produced a maximum serum concentration of 22 mcg/ml. Serum concentrations after the same dosage of intramuscular carbenicillin were several time higher.

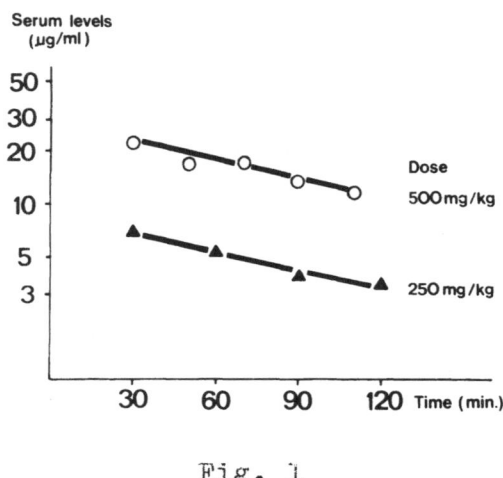

Fig. 1

Mean carbenicillin concentrations in urine after
250 mg/kg of carfecillin were high and significantly
exceeded MIC for the strains used to produce experimental infection (Fig. 2).

The antimicrobial efficacy of carfecillin and carbenicillin was tested on two different models of urinary tract infections in rats:
1) Model of renal tissue infection after a direct
microbial injection into three sites of the kidney characterised by infection lasting several weeks and associated with focal fibrosis of the kidney (Hatala et al.
1974);

URINE CONCENTRATION OF CARBENICILLIN IN RATS
(250 mg OF CARFECILLIN ; 3 TIMES A DAY)

Time (hr)	Total volume of urine (ml)	Urine concen. of PY(ug/ml)	Amount of PY excreted (%)
0-8	1,37	777	17,85
8-16	4,5	207	15,58
16-24	1,37	680	13,86

Fig. 2

2) Model of lower urinary tract infection marked by prolonged (2 months at the least) significant bacteriuria without involvement of the kidney. The latter infection was produced by microbial suspension injected into the urinary bladder marred on the anterior wall by a scar after incision (Prát et al. 1973).

To induce experimental infection, Proteus mirabilis and Pseudomonas aeruginosa strains were used in both models. MIC of carbenicillin for the two strains was 1.56 and 25.0 mcg/ml, respectively. Therapy of the infection started 24 hours after application of the infection agent lasted 5 or 10 days. Drugs were administered three times a day at 8 hour intervals – carfecillin (250 mg/kg) was administered via a gastric tube, carbenicillin (125 mg/kg) was given intramuscularly. Given in identical doses, serum concentrations after carbenicillin are reported (Barrera and Ortega 1973, Modr and Dvořáček 1969, Modr and Dvořáček in press) to exceed approximately twofold those after carfecillin, therefore the above dosage ratio was chosen. Forty-eight hours after the last dose the rats were sacrificed, their urine collected and the kidneys were removed. The results of the 5- or 10-day therapy were evaluated by comparing the number of microbes in homogenised renal tissue or in the urine with that found in untreated rats. The difference was statisti-

cally evaluated using the non-parametrical Wilcoxon
test.

    In the first series of therapeutical experiments
we evaluated the results of treatment with the two antibiotics in experimental renal infection. Fig. 3 shows

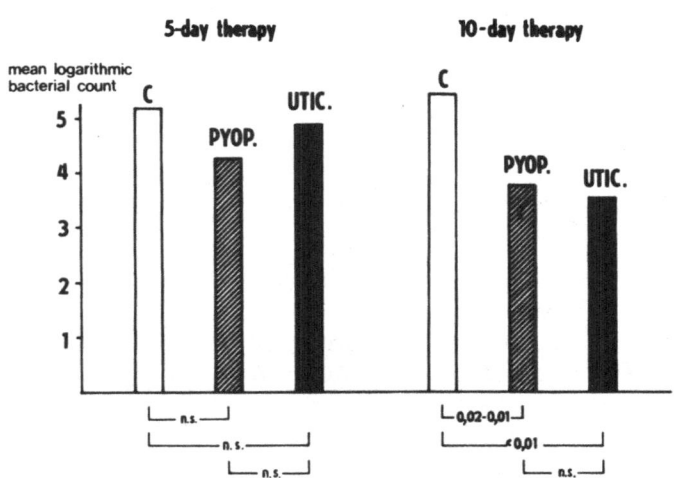

Fig. 3

the results of therapy on the model of Proteus renal
infection. The values are mean logarithmic numbers per
1 g of renal tissue. The groups were composed of 10 to
12 animals each. Administered for 5 day, both antibiotics produced an insignificant therapeutical effect. On
the other hand, after therapy of 10 days microbial number in renal tissue was at all times significantly lower, however at no time was the renal tissue entirely
microbe-free. Essentially, both antibiotics had a uniform efficacy.

    In the second series of experiments we compared
efficacy of the antibiotics tested on the same model,
using however Pseudomonas infection. Only the 10-day
therapy was evaluated. The results roughly agreed with
those obtained in the first series (Fig. 4).

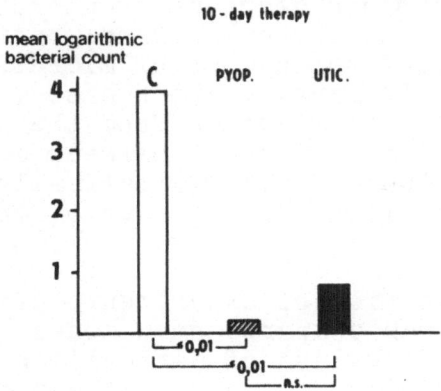

Fig. 4

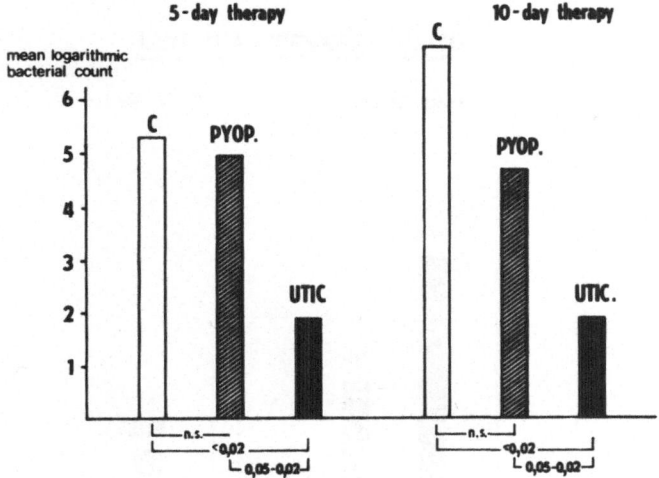

Fig. 5

In the third series of experiments we compared efficacy of the two drugs on a model of cystitis with chronic bacteriuria. Fig. 5 shows the results obtained in
Proteus infection. In that case carbenicillin therapy
produced an appreciable effect neither at 5- nor 10-day
therapy, despite a minor decrease in microbial count
found in the urine. On the other hand, carfecillin
significantly reduced the number of microbes in urine
as early as 5 days therapy. In both cases, carfecillin
therapy utterly cleared microbes from the urine in 50
per cent of rats. The difference between carfecillin
and carbenicillin therapy was statistically significant
in favour of carfecillin irrespective of the duration
of therapy.

In the last series of experiments efficacy of the
above antibiotics was compared on a model of Pseudomonas-
induced cystitis. Five days of carfecillin therapy resulted in a significant decrease in the number of microbes in urine. Despite that bacteriuria decreased
after carbenicillin therapy, the decrease was statistically insignificant. The 10-day therapy with the two
drugs led to a significant decrease in the number of
microbes in urine, while after carfecillin the urine
was sterile in 90 per cent of rats (Fig. 6).

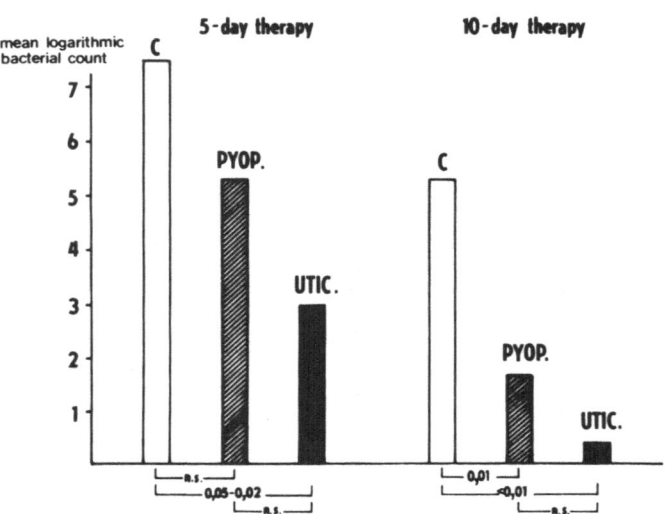

Fig. 6

The following conclusions may be drawn from our results:
1) The serum concentration of carbenicillin were low after carfecillin application, however, they markedly exceeded MIC for the strains used to induce infection.
2) In the treatment of renal infection both carfecillin and carbenicillin were found to have a significant effect only after a prolonged therapy.
3) Carfecillin was highly efficacious in the treatment of lower urinary tract infections. In that case, its effect was significantly higher even at 5-day therapy, as compared with carbenicillin.

References

Barrera, A.M. and Ortega, F.F. (1973), Revista Medicina, 53, 344.
Hatala, M., Prát, V., Liška, M., Koníčková, L. and Slugeň, I. (1974), Zbl. Bakt. Hyg., I. Abt. Orig. A, 230, 466.
Modr, Z. and Dvořáček, K. (1969), Int. J. clin. Pharmacol. Supplement Pyopen, 21.
Modr, Z. and Dvořáček, K., Progr. in Chemotherapy (1975), in press.
Prát, V., Mohr, H.J., Hatala, M. and Koníčková, L. (1973), Beitr. Path., 150, 55.

Model of Experimental Cystitis

in Albino Wistar Rats

KRÜGER,CH.,FREIESLEBEN,H.,SACK,K.,and COMMICHAU,R.

Med. Hochsch., Lübeck, Abt. Inn. Med.
2400 Lübeck, Ratzeburger Allee 160, F.R.G.

Summary:
Progesterone capronate facilitates vesical inflammation in albino Wistar rats after transurethral infection with a serum resistant strain of E. coli. This hormone has an anticholinergic side reaction and leads to dilatation and incomplete voiding of the bladder which has a mainly parasympathetic innervation. That effect of hormonal treatment is probably responsible for the high rate of bladder infections - the prerequisite to test antimicrobial drugs.

Pyelonephritis is given more interest in urinary tract infections than cystitis though bladder infections often cause pyelonephritis. Mechanisms leading to acute or chronic bladder infections are as yet not well understood. Experimentally the instillation of a bacterial suspension into the intact bladder does not establish infection. However, several authors succeeded by previous damaging the bladder in different ways in analogy to obstructive urinary tract infection. Besides chemical irritations of the mucous membrane with terpentine, alcoholic salicylic acid solution or xylol (Uebel 1965), mainly mechanical factors inducing a subacute to chronic disease were preferred (Rényi-Vámos and Horváth 1961; Prát et al. 1969).

In continuation of the findings of our team that esters of estradiol and progesterone were effective in facilitating renal infection in rats (Commichau 1971) we now investigated the hormonal influence on bladder infections. We found that progesterone kept up vesical

inflammatory activity at least for 3 weeks, a prerequisite to test the therapeutic effect of antimicrobial drugs.

Method:
Female albino Wistar rats (Wistar AF/Han.), average
weight about 200 g; Food: "altromin-R". Facilitation of infection with estradiolundecylate (Progy-
non Depot, Schering, Berlin: 0.5 mg/kg, i.m., weekly) and hydroxyprogesterone capronate (Proluton-
Depot, Schering, Berlin: 200 mg/kg, i.m., weekly).
The hormones were applied one week before infection
and then in weekly intervals. Bacterial infection
with 1 ml suspension of the serum resistant E. coli
strain O 25:19:12, concentration 10^8 - 10^9 bact./ml
(Henkel 1971).

Hematogenous infection once into the dorsal vein of
the tail. After 7 days dissection in pentobarbital
narcosis under aseptical conditions and homogenisation of the bladder wall. Evaluation of the homogenates by quantitative bacterial culture. Besides
application of hormones additional facilitations of
infection were employed: forced saluresis with fu-
rosemid (Lasix, Hoechst, Frankfurt: 5 mg/rat together with 2 ml of water i.p.) under constant urethral clamping for 2 1/2 hours prior to intravenous
injection of the bacteria, or transurethral instill-
lation of 1 ml of saline 2 hours prior to intravenous infection.

Transurethral infection twice in weekly intervals
with 1 ml of a bacterial suspension. Fourteen days
later dissection and homogenisation of the kidneys
and bladders after rinsing vesical cavity with saline.

Quantitative bacterial cultures of the kidneys, blad-
der and urine.
Histology: Hemalaun eosin stain.
Statistical evaluation: Wilcoxon test.

Results:
In analogy to experimental hormonally induced pyelonephritis (Commichau 1971) only serum resistant
strains of E. coli were virulent enough to initiate
and maintain a severe bladder inflammation after

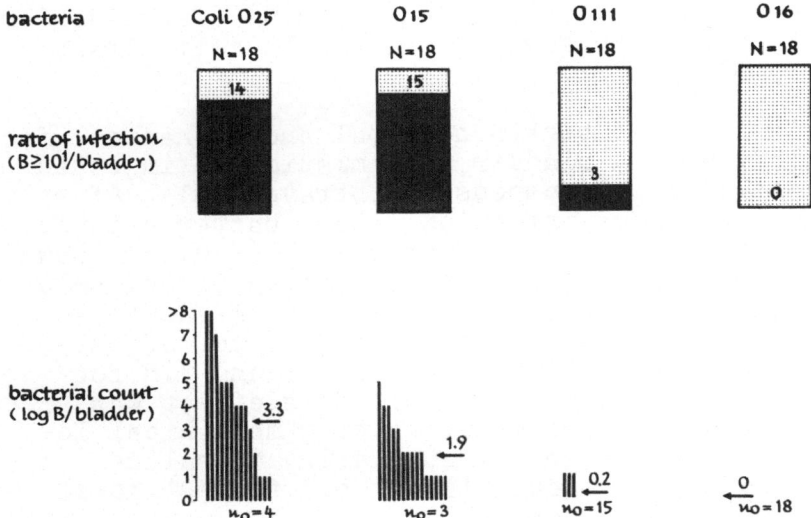

Fig. 1: Rate of infection and bacterial count (log. no. of bact./bladder) in homogenates of the bladder after application of serum resistant (025, 015) and serum sensitive (0 111, 0 16) strains of E. coli.

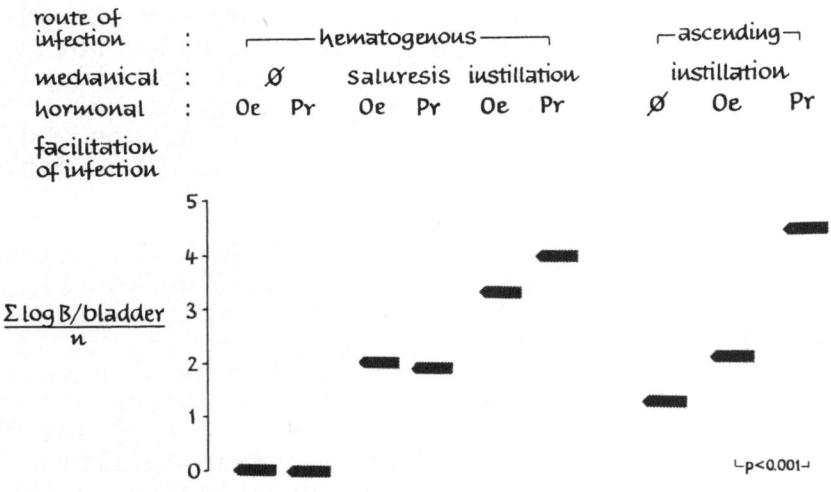

Fig. 2: Bacterial count (mean log. no. of bact./bladder) in vesical walls under different mechanical and hormonal facilitation and different route of infection.

transurethral infection (Henkel 1971) (fig. 1). For
further experiments we choose the E. coli strain
O 25:19:12.

In order to investigate hormonal and mechanical factors influencing bladder inflammation we injected
1 ml of bacterial suspension intravenously. After
this hematogenous infection alone, bacteria could
not be detected in the bladder wall (fig. 2). However overdistension of the bladder by forced saluresis with intermittant urethral block caused a
significant infection (the mean log. no. of bac-
teria/bladder was 2.0 for estradiol and 1.8 for
progesterone treated animals). This effect was
even more pronounced after setting mechanical lesions by transurethral instillation of saline
(mean log no. of bact./bladder 3.3 for estradiol
and 4.0 for progesterone).

These results demonstrate, that on this condition
mechanical factors were neccessary to establish an
infection. Significant differences between both
hormones could not be found in this experimental
scheme. Transurethral infection, however, revealed
a significantly higher induction of bladder infection for progesterone (mean log. no. of bact./
bladder = 4.2) than for estradiol (2.1). (fig.3)
Bacterial counts in the kidneys (fig. 4) in experiments with ascending route of infection showed
no difference in inflammatory activity under both
hormones after a period of 2 weeks post infectionem. This means, that the primary infection has
been similar effective in both hormonal groups and
the control and that progesterone has an additional
effect on the bladder.

This hormonally induced ascending bladder infection
with progesterone lasts at least over 3 weeks (fig.
5). At this time 13 out of 20 organs were still infected (mean log no. of bact./bladder = 1.3). A
sufficient bacterial concentration for testing antimicrobial substances was found after a course of
14 days (mean log no. of bact./bladder = 3.3). At this
time histology revealed marked leucocyte infiltrations in the bladder wall which corresponded to the
high bacterial counts (fig. 6).

In order to explain the different hormonal effect of
both hormones on bladder infection we refer to their
different pharmacological actions on the autonomic

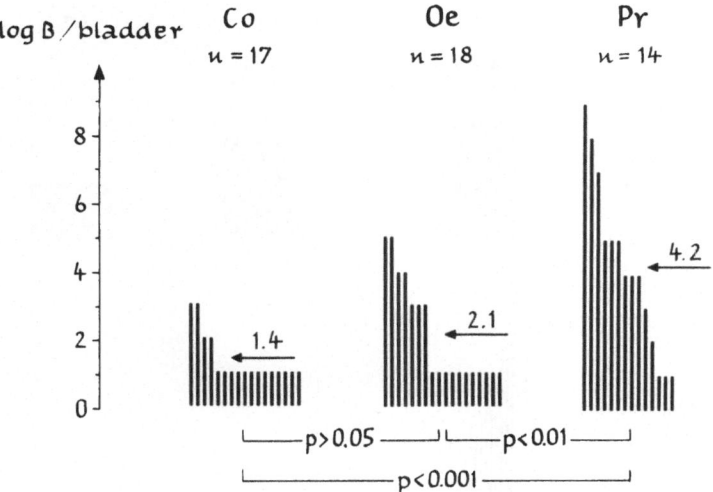

Fig. 3: Bacterial count (log. no. of. bact./bladder) in vesical homogenates of female albino Wistar rats. Facilitation of infection: estradiolundecylate (10 mg/ kg, i.m. weekly), progesterone capronate (200 mg/kg, i.m. weekly) in comparison to a control.

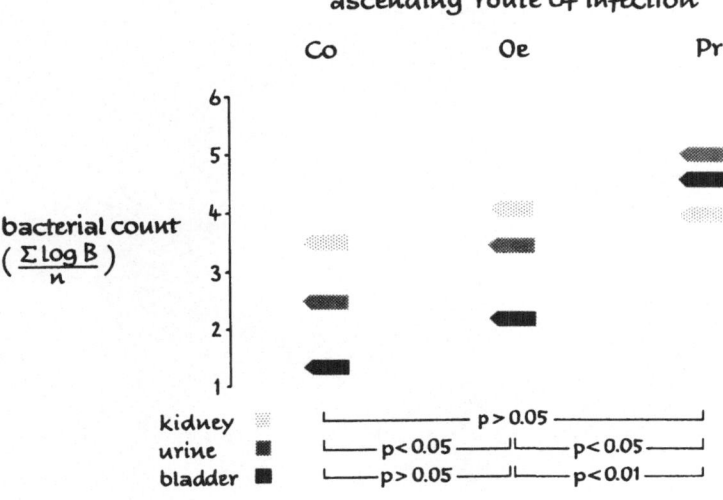

Fig. 4: Bacterial count (mean log no. of bact./bladder) in homogenates of kidneys and bladders and in the urine under facilitation of infection by estradiol and progesterone in comparison to a control.

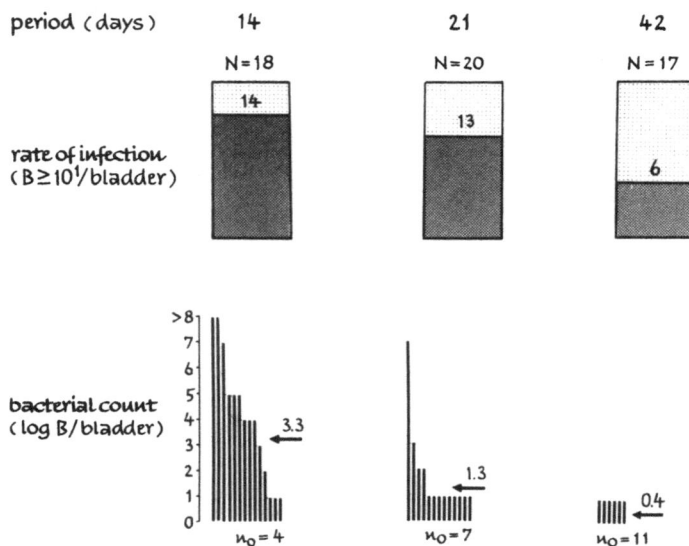

Fig. 5: Rate of infection and bacterial count after twice transurethral infection with E. coli O 25:19:12 during a course of 42 days.

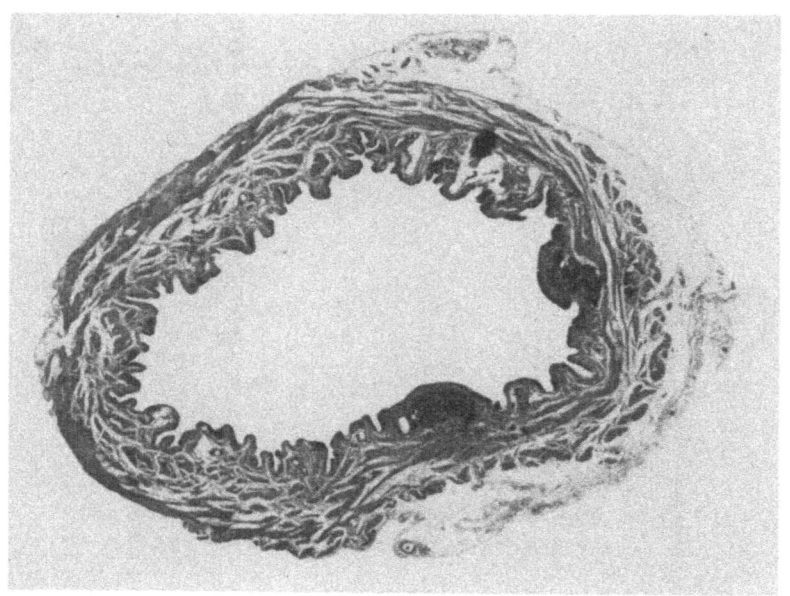

Fig. 6: Histology of the bladder wall: Massive leucocyte infiltrations under facilitation of infection with progesterone after a course of 14 days.

nervous system. Progesterone has an anticholinergic effect while that of estrogen is adrenolytic (Artner 1954, Wagner 1958).

The predominant parasympathetic innervation of the distal ureter and bladder (Diemer 1971) is inhibited by progesterone - a fact which might explain dilatation of the bladder under hormonal influence (Commichau 1971). Dilatation causes formation of residual urine in the bladder and thus facilitation of infection. The infection inducing effect of estradiol is only relevant for pyelonephritis because its adrenolytic action causes distension of the proximal ureter and the pyelon.

References:

ARTNER,J. (1954), Geburtsh. u. Frauenheilk., 14, 677.
COMMICHAU,R. (1971), Fortschr. Med., 89, 1095.
DIEMER,K.-F. (1971), in: Ureterdynamik, Thieme-Verlag, Stuttgart, 17.
HENKEL,W. (1971), Z. med. Mikrobiol. u. Immunol., 156, 284.
PRÁT,V., KONICKOWA,L., HATALA,M. and ROSSMANN,P. (1969), Ärztl. Forsch. 23, 376.
RÉNYI-VÁMOS,F. and HORVÁTH,L. (1961), Z. Ges. exp. Med., 135, 216.
UEBEL,H. (1965) in Handbuch exp. Pharmakol., Springer-Verlag, Berlin, 16, 315.
WAGNER,H. (1958), in: Hormone und Psyche, Springer-Verlag, Berlin, 314.

For technical assistance we thank Mrs. Ch. Mohr.

PATHOGENESIS OF AN EXPERIMENTAL PYELONEPHRITIS MODEL IN THE MOUSE

AND ITS USE IN THE EVALUATION OF ANTIBIOTICS

K. R. Comber

Beecham Pharmaceuticals Research Division

Brockham Park, Betchworth, Surrey, England

SUMMARY

Intravenous inoculation of Escherichia coli, Proteus morganii
and Pseudomonas aeruginosa into healthy mice failed to produce
infections of the kidneys. Large inocula of cells caused death
of the animals without obvious involvement of the kidneys while
small inocula were cleared rapidly from the renal tract. The
renal virulence of the organisms was markedly enhanced by
concomitant administration of ferric sorbitol citrate which
resulted in extensive growth of the bacteria in the kidneys and
development of a progressive pyelonephritis. Therapy with
appropriate penicillins prevented development of infection and in
the studies reported here a combination of ampicillin and
cloxacillin demonstrated marked synergy against an infection
caused by an ampicillin-resistant strain of E. coli.

Establishment of infection in the intact kidneys of healthy
laboratory animals by intravenous inoculation of Gram-negative
bacilli is difficult because of the need to inject large numbers
of bacteria resulting either in endotoxic death of the animal or
septicaemia long before development of pyelonephritis, or in the
disappearance of the bacteria from the kidney without giving rise
to an inflammatory response. However, it has been reported that
concomitant administration of low molecular weight iron can
enhance the renal virulence of Gram-negative bacteria for rats
and mice without increasing the incidence of generalised infection
(Fletcher and Goldstein, 1970). Stimulation of growth of bacteria

in the kidney by parenterally administered iron would appear to offer a simple method for the production of experimental renal infection. Accordingly, this study was undertaken to measure the effect of iron sorbitol citrate on the virulence of Gram-negative bacteria for the kidneys of mice and the effect of therapy with appropriate penicillins on the infections produced in this way.

METHODS

Production of pyelonephritis. Mice (18-20g, C.S.I. strain) were infected intravenously with 0.2ml of a culture of the test organism suitably diluted in double strength veal infusion broth (Difco). The mice were injected with approximately 10^8 cells of Escherichia coli (JT415) 2 to 5 x 10^8 cells of Proteus morganii (14) or 2 to 5 x 10^6 cells of Pseudomonas aeruginosa (11). Iron sorbitol citrate (Jectofer, Astra Chemicals Ltd.) was administered by the intramsucular route 18, 42, 66 and 90 hours after infection. In tests to study the development of infection, groups of mice were killed by dislocation of the neck at intervals up to 7 weeks after infection, the kidneys were removed aseptically and examined for macroscopic abscesses, and viable counts were made of kidney homogenates.

Therapy. Mice were infected intravenously and treated with 30mg Jectofer/kg as described above. Treatment with subcutaneous injection of the penicillins was started 19 hours after infection and continued 4 times a day at 2 hourly intervals for 4 days. Groups of five mice were killed 7 days and 14 days after infection, the kidneys were examined for abscesses and bacterial counts were performed on homogenates of the infected kidneys.

RESULTS AND DISCUSSION

Effect of iron on renal virulence. Results in Table 1 show the effects of intravenous inoculation of E. coli, P. morganii and Ps. aeruginosa in untreated mice. It can be seen that large inocula of E. coli and Ps. aeruginosa killed 80-100% of the animals infected without producing a significant number of kidney lesions, while smaller inocula of the bacteria had little effect on the animals. The strain of P. morganii was relatively avirulent in these tests. Injection of iron sorbitol citrate (Jectofer) produced a marked enhancement of renal virulence and results in Table 2 illustrate the increase in incidence of kidney lesions that developed as a result of iron treatment. With all three bacteria the inocula tested produced a very low incidence of kidney lesions, but following treatment with 10-15mg/kg iron sorbitol citrate, up to 50% of the mice had visible kidney lesions and at a dose level of 30mg/Jectofer/kg, 80-90% of of the mice showed evidence of obvious kidney infection. The abscesses were distributed throughout the kidney and were observed in the cortex, medulla and pelvis.

TABLE 1. Effect of intravenous inoculation of gram-negative bacteria into mice

Organism	Inoculum No. orgs/mouse x 10^6	% Dead	% survivors with kidney lesions
E. coli (JT415)	260 52	80 10	0–20 0
P. morganii (14)	200–500	0–5	0
Ps. aeruginosa aeruginosa (11)	340 34 3.4	100 80 4	– 100 0

TABLE 2. Effect of intramuscularly-dosed iron sorbitol citrate on the incidence of kidney lesions in mice infected intravenously

Organism	Inoculum No. orgs/mouse x 10^6	Dose* Fe^{+++} mg/kg	No. with abscesses / No. of mice	% mice with kidney lesions
E. coli JT415	82	0 10 30	0/18 10/18 15/18	0 56 83
P. morganii 14	880	0 15 30	0/18 8/18 16/18	0 44 89
Ps. aeruginosa 11	5	0 15 30	2/12 6/12 11/12	17 50 83

* Iron sorbitol citrate (Jectofer)

The effect of iron on bacterial growth in the kidneys of mice infected with E. coli JT415 is illustrated in Fig. 1. A non-lethal intravenous inoculum resulted in no significant proliferation

of the bacteria in the kidneys of untreated mice although bacteria
persisted at low levels in the kidneys for more than 56 days.
In contrast, injection of ferric sorbitol citrate caused a marked
increase in the kidney counts, the effects being greater with a
dose of 30mg/kg than with a dose of 10mg/Jectofer/kg. The
infection appeared to be self-limiting and the counts gradually
fell to levels of 10^2 to 10^3 cells/ml of kidney homogenate
56 days after infection. These effects were reflected in the
macroscopic appearance of the kidneys and lesions were observed
in the majority of mice during the duration of the test.

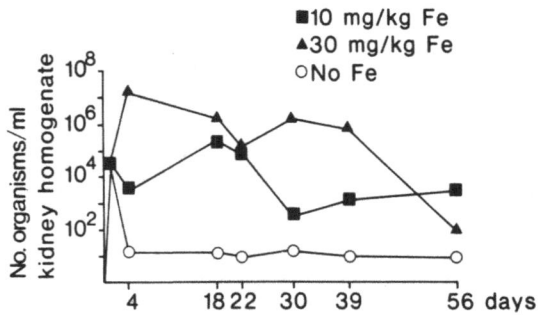

FIG. 1. The effect of iron sorbitol citrate on the growth of
E. coli (JT415) in the mouse kidney

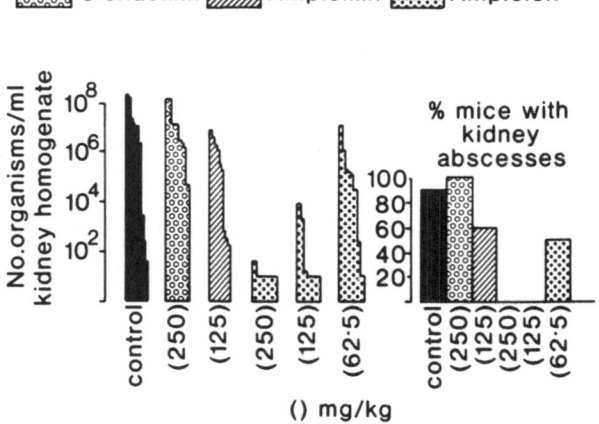

FIG. 2. Activity of subcutaneously dosed ampicillin, cloxacillin
and ampiclox against E. coli (JT415) in an experimental mouse
pyelonephritis model.

Therapy of experimental pyelonephritis. The effect of treatment of a pyelonephritis infection produced by E. coli (JT415) is illustrated in Fig. 2. This strain was relatively resistant to ampicillin in vitro (M.I.C. 250μg/ml) and to cloxacillin (M.I.C. >500μg/ml) but was sensitive to a combination of ampicillin and cloxacillin containing 12.5μg ampicillin/ml and 12.5μg cloxacillin/ml. In untreated infected mice, 90% of the kidneys showed macroscopic lesions and 60-70% of animals treated with ampicillin (125mg/kg) and 70-100% of those given cloxacillin (250mg/kg) were similarly infected. Treatment with the combination of equal parts of ampicillin and cloxacillin resulted in significant reductions in the numbers of animals with kidney abscesses (0-20%). The bacterial counts of kidney homogenates were in agreement with these findings and high counts (10^5 to $>10^8$ organisms/ml of homogenate) were found in untreated animals or animals treated with ampicillin or cloxacillin, whereas the bacterial counts were significantly lower in the animals treated with combinations of equal parts of ampicillin and cloxacillin.

The results reported demonstrate that a small molecular weight iron complex, iron sorbitol citrate (Jectofer), which is capable of crossing the glomerulus enhances the growth of strains of E. coli, P. morganii and Ps. aeruginosa in the kidneys of mice, using a non-lethal inoculum which does not result in the establishment of kidney infection in the absence of iron treatment. The effect of the iron is limited to the kidneys and does not affect the clearance of the organisms from other organs or blood.

The mechanism of action of the iron in this experimental model is unknown. It may act by supplying an essential growth factor as iron stimulates the growth in serum in vitro of a wide spectrum of micro-organisms, including species of Candida, Clostridium, Escherichia, Myco-bacterium (Schade, A. L. 1964; Rogers, H. J. 1967; Bullen, J. J. and Rogers, H. J. 1969; Brubaker, R. R. 1972). Another possibility is that it may depress host resistance within the kidney as inhibition in vivo of immune mehcanisms has been reported following iron injections (Bullen, J. J. et al, 1968).

These results illustrate that enhancement of the virulence of intravenously-inoculated Gram-negative bacteria by parentally-administered iron offers a simple model for the production of pyelonephritis in the mouse, and is suitable for the study of therapy with appropriate penicillins.

REFERENCES

Brubaker, R. R. 1972. Nature, (Lond) 57, 111.

Bullen, J. J. and Rogers, H. J.   1969.   Nature, (Lond), <u>224</u>, 380.

Bullen, J. J., Wilson, A. B., Cushnie, G. H. and Rogers, H. J.
    1968.   Immunology, <u>14</u>, 889.

Fletcher, J. and Goldstein, E.   1970.   Brit.J.Exp.Path., <u>51</u>. 280.

Rogers, H. J.   1967.   Immunology, <u>12</u>, 285.

Schade, A. L.   1964.   Journal of Investigative Dermatology.,
    <u>42</u>, 415.

Chronic E.coli Nephritis in Rats:

Model for Assessment of Activity of Antimicrobial Agents

COMMICHAU, R., H. FREIESLEBEN, K. SACK,
CH. KRÜGER, W. HENKEL
Abteilung für Innere Medizin und Abteilung für Med.
Mikrobiologie der Medizinischen Hochschule Lübeck,   F.R.G.

Summary :
Antibacterial activity of chemotherapeutic drugs is preferably tested in
acute animal infections. In contrast, the prevailing clinical problem is
therapy of chronic local infections. For this reason an animal model
has been developed which takes a chronic course for months by cautious
impairment of systemic and local defence mechanisms, and thus allows
delayed therapy of a well established infection. Results of experimental chemotherapy of hormonally induced chronic E.coli nephritis in rats
are domonstrated to be significantly inferior to results with immediate
treatment of acute renal infections. The method of this animal model
and its applicability for the assessment of antimicrobial agents are presented.

Animal experiments, besides being used for exploration of properties of
bacteria and of host defence mechanisms, were preferably applied for
assessment of the effectiveness of chemotherapeutic drugs. For this purpose renal infection models have gained more and more interest and
preference in the past years. As far as the mode of infection causes a
massive impairment of the urinary tract (Prát et al. 1968) or even of
the kidneys (Miller and Robinson 1973) difficulties arise if prolonged
observation of the experiments is intended: this means, those infections
tend to heal spontaneously or,- mostly due to superinfections - tend to
kill the animals. Therefore it turned out to be neccessary in all these
types of animal models to start with therapy very early in the course
of infection, i.e. in the acute phase of infection.

The model of hormonally facilitated pyelonephritis developed in our group doesn't give rise to disadvantages mentioned above. This procedure has proved to be of great value for investigations of pathogenetic relationships, and especially for therapeutic studies in infections already persistant.

Methods:

As previously reported (Commichau et al. 1972), female albino Wistar rats with an average weight of 200 g were given 0.5 mg/kg of estradiolundecylate by weekly i.m. injection. After the first week a suspension of the E.coli test strain was instilled into the bladders. This instillation was repeated 7 days later. 10 days after the second infection chemotherapy was started. The antibiotics were given twice daily for one week. Four days after discontinuation of therapy the animals were sacrificed. Results of therapy were assessed by quantitative culture of the homogenized kidneys.

Results and discussion:

Using this way of discreet facilitation of infection, depending firstly on a hormone induced widening of the distal parts of the urinary tract - thus impairing local defence (Commichau et al. 1973)- and, furthermore, on a weakening of general defence mechanism (e.g. inhibition of leucocyte emigration and intracellular killing: Freiesleben et al. 1974) the virulence of the infecting agent is of substantial importance. The virulence can be estimated in advance by the criterion of serum resistance in vitro (Henkel and Commichau 1971). Only serum resistant strains turned out to be able to cause higher rates of infection.

Table 1: Ratio (in %) of infected Kidneys 4 Weeks after Challenge with E.coli Strains of Different in vitro Virulence

Strain	In vitro Serum Resistence	Kidneys with $\geqslant 10^2$ bacteria/g
2: 1: 4	+++	73 %
22:13: 1	+++	76 %
15:14: 4	+++	92 %
25:19:12	+++	75 %
16: 1: .	+	26 %
111: 58: 2	+	23 %

At the end of experiment both kidneys show small scars predominantly near the medulla. The histological picture shows focal, uniformly scattered infiltrations, but massive abscesses never occured(Sack et al. 1971).

Besides estradiol the facilitation of the infection also is possible with prednisolon and progesteron with dosages of 6 mg/kg/week and 200 mg/kg/week, respectively. With the three hormones similar results can be obtained after five weeks even if the evaluation is based upon the mean logarithms of the bacterial count in the kidneys, which were found to be between 3.6 and 3.8. The different mechanisms of pathogenicity hereby concerned including consequences for prognosis and therapy have been reported elsewhere (Henkel et al. 1974).

The facilitation of infection with estradiol enables to get a chronic infection for more than 5 weeks. Even after a 12-week period of observation 50 % of the kidneys turned out to be infected.

The reproducibility of the results is remarkably reliable. In table 2 the results of a series of 10 control experiments has been compiled. The rate of infected kidneys was 71 % on the average, whereas the mean logarithm of the bacterial count was 2.91.

Table 2: Results of a series of 10 control experiments

test series	no. of kidneys		infected kidneys in %	bacteria/g kidney (mean log no.)
	total	infected		
1	40	29	73	2.75
2	38	24	63	2.39
3	40	30	75	2.80
4	38	20	68	2.92
5	48	35	73	2.63
6	30	24	80	3.27
7	38	29	76	3.29
8	38	28	74	3.16
9	42	30	71	2.95
10	40	28	70	2.93
total	392	277		
mean			71	2.91 $\pm$ 0.28 (S.D.)

Corresponding to clinical conditions we start therapy after the acute phase of infection has decreased, that is 17 days after the first infection. Under these conditions our therapeutic results naturally turned out to be successful, compared to therapeutic experiments of other authors who employed obstructively induced pyelonephritis models in rats and started medication immediately after infection. Comparative investigations have been reported by us elsewhere (Koch et al. 1971).

The dosage of the chemotherapeutics was determined according to the following criteria: The MIC of the test strain, the serum concentration achievable in the rat, and the threshold dose of nephrotoxicity estimated according to the method of Sack.

The evaluation of the therapeutic experiments in the case of unambiguous results may be accomplished by the "curative effect", which is indicated by the decrease of the ratio of infected kidneys with a bacterial count per gram tissue of 10^2 or more, statistically assessed by the x^2-test. For both less successful therapy and comparative investigations of substances with only slight differences in effect the evaluation by the "suppressive effect" is preferred, this is assessed then by the mean logarithm of the bacterial count per kidney established at the end of an experiment, and statistically evaluated by the U-test. In figure 1, both possibilities of analysis are shown.

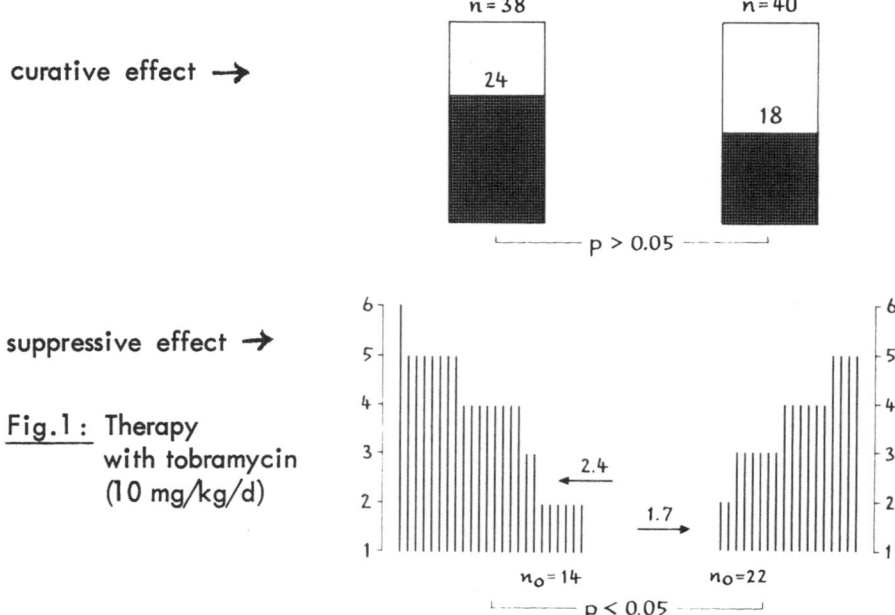

curative effect →

suppressive effect →

Fig.1 : Therapy with tobramycin (10 mg/kg/d)

The presented model, characterized by its chronicity and thus
allowing delayed start of treatment, generally yields less successful
curing rates compared to other models.For most antimicrobial drugs
the curing rates were in the range of about 50 %. This limited
success corresponds to clinical experiences with human chronic infections. The model provides facilities for screening of efficient combinations of therapeutics and, furthermore, an opportunity to study the
relationships between pharmacokinetics and therapeutic effectivity.

Conclusion:

The advantages of the model for studies on pathogenesis of chronic
local infections are: the discreet damage of the urinary tract by
avoiding surgery in the infecting procedure; the transition to chronic
course with a well balanced host-parasite-interaction; the good condition of the infected animals (increasing weight); and the double-
sided disseminated involvement with the histologic characteristics of
chronic interstitial nephritis. The advantages of the model for assessment of antimicrobial agents are: the good reproducibility of severity
of the infectious process; no trend to spontaneous healing; the feasibility of delayed therapy (weeks after infection); and the evaluation
by quantitative reculture of the causitive bacteria.

References:

Commichau, R., Henkel, W., Koch, H.-G., and Sack, K. (1972),
    Pyelonephritis III, H. Losse, M. Kienitz, Thieme Verlag Stuttgart

Commichau, R., Krüger, Ch., Freiesleben, H., Sack, K., Henkel, W.
    (1973), Geburtsh. u. Frauenheilk. 33, 464

Freiesleben, H., Sack, K., Woermann, K., and Henkel, W. (1974),
    Zbl. Bakt. Hyg. I. Abt. Orig. A, 227, 314

Henkel, W., and Commichau, R. (1971), Z. med. Mikrobiol. Immunol.
    156, 297

Henkel, W., Freiesleben, H., Wöhrmann, W., Krüger, Ch., and
    Commichau, R. (1974), Zbl. Bakt. Hyg., I. Abt. Orig. A, 227,
    306

Koch, H.-G., Freiesleben, H., Henkel, W., and Commichau, R.
    (1971), Verhandlungen der Deutschen Gesellschaft für innere Medi-
    zin, 77, 1336

Miller, T.E., and Robinson, K.B. (1973), J. infect. Dis., 127, 307

Prāt, V., Koničková, L., Ritzerfeld, W., and Losse, H. (1968),
   Z. ges. exp. Med. 146, 115

Sack, K., Henkel, W., Commichau, R. (1971), Virchows Arch.
   Abt. A, 352, 219

COMBINED THERAPY OF ANTI-ENDOTOXIN(OEP) ANTIBODY AND GENTAMICIN

IN THE IMMUNOSUPPRESSED MICE WITH PSEUDOMONAS AERUGINOSA INFECTION

Katsuyuki HARANAKA, Kazuo SUGANE, Keimei MASHIMO

The Institute of Medical Science, The University of Tokyo

P.O. Takanawa, Tokyo, Japan

INTRODUCTION

Immunosuppressive treattment has been widely applied for various purposes, for example, organ transplantation, therapies for autoimmune disease and so on.

On the other hand, numerous antibiotics have been widely used and super-infections are caused by highly resistant gram negative bacilli frequently.

According to NIH of U.S.A. report, cases of more than 40 per cent of renal transplantation died from infections, of which sepsis was counted to be 31.1 per cent. In our hospital, 4 of 10 cases of renal transplantation succumbed to pneumonia and sepsis, from which Gram-negativ bacilli of conventional flora, especially Pseudomonas aeruginosa were found.

In such conditions, large dose of the antibiotic, such as gentamicin, is required, then various and serious side effects occurred frequently especially renal failure.

Treatment of "opportunistic infection" raises two tasks; protection of immune mechanism and eradication of causative organisms.

In this work, we studied the therapeutic effect of anti-protein moiety of endotoxin antibody in combination with or without an antibiotic, gentamicin, employed as the treatment of Pseudomonas aeruginosa infection in mice previously immunosuppressed by Co-60 irradiation, cyclophosphamide, azathioprine and cortisone acetate.

MATERIALS AND METHODS

We used DD-strain male mice which were four to six weeks old and weighing twenty to thirty gram.

323

Pseudomonas aeruginosa, NC-5 strain was inoculated intraperito-neally and its LD-50 was 2.86 X 10^3 together with 2.5 per cent of mucin.

Minimum inhibitory concentration(MIC) of gentamicin to the bacteria was 1.6 mcg per ml.

As specific antigen of Pseudomonas aeruginosa, we used Original endotoxin protein(OEP), the protein moiety of endotoxin, purificated by Y.J.Homma.

The mice were immunized with OEP.   Four injections of each 10 mcg of OEP were performed every two weeks.   The first two injections were made with Freund's incomplate adjuvant into two foot pads.   The second two booster injections were made intraperitone-ally without the adjuvant.   The serum haemaggulutin titer resulted in more than 10.000 units per ml.

We separated Ig G from this immunized serum by chromatography on DEAE cellulose column and made pepsin hydolysis by the modified Nisonoff's method.   The digested Ig G was applied onto a column of Sephadex G-200 and eluted with PBS at pH 7.2.

The first fraction of this sample contained $F(ab')_2$ and HA-titer against OEP was 4096 units per ml.

On the other hand, we examined effect of immunosuppressants for thymus and spleen lymphocytes.   We counted these populations and performed cytotoxicity test by using anti-θ antibody to examine the differential effect of the suppressants for T and B lymphocyte in spleen cells.

One hundred mg per kg of cyclophosphamide or 100 mg per kg of azathioprine was injected intramusculary or 100 mg per kg of corti-sone acetate was injected intraperitoneally to mice one day before the intraperitoneal inoculation of Pseudomonas aeruginosa.

Co-60 irradiation was performed seven days before the inocula-tion.   One hundred LD-50 of the bacillus was inoculated to every mouse in each experiment except Co-60 irradiated mice group.

In Co-60 irradiated mice , ten fold inoculation dose was used.

$F(ab')_2$ solution was given by intravenous injection into the tail vein just after the inoculation.

Gentamicin was injected into the femoral muscle just after the inoculation and every morning and evening for 4 days thereafter.

Evaluation of the therapeutic effect was made by the number of survived mice 4 days after the inoculations.

RESULT

1. Cortisone acetate injected group.

Thymus and spleen cells decreased to the lowest number, about 20 per cent loss, on the next day after the cortisone acetate injec-tion.   Cytotoxicity index was increased to 56.4 per cent, and it meant T cell loss mainly.

The bacterial inoculation was done at that time and its dose was 1.6 X 10^4.(Fig.1)

Complete protection of infected mice by anti-OEP-$F(ab')_2$ was

Table 1. Result of therapeutic effects in Cortisone acetate injected group

GM per mouse \ days	AOEPF 100 U.					AOEPF 20 U.					AOEPF 4 U.					NMSF					PBS				
	1	2	3	4	S	1	2	3	4	S	1	2	3	4	S	1	2	3	4	S	1	2	3	4	S
100 mcg					5/5					4/5					3/5					2/5					1/5
20					5/5					5/5					2/5					1/5					1/5
4					5/5					3/5					1/5					1/5					1/5
PBS					5/5					2/5					1/5					1/5					0/5

▨ - marker means servived mice.   Numbers of S-column show ratio of servived mice to inoculated mice on the 4th day.

(AOEPF): Anti-O E P-F(ab')$_2$,   (NMSF): Normal mouse serum F(ab')$_2$.

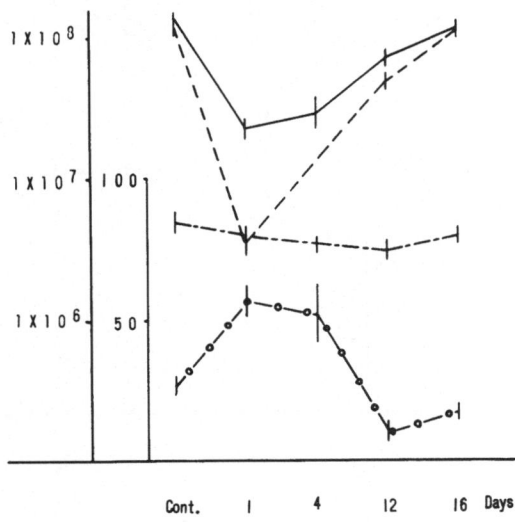

Fig. 1. Effects of Cortisone acetate on mouse lymphocytes (100 mg/kg, ip).

(———) : Spleen cell count, (— — —) : Thymus cell count
(—·—·—) : % lymphocytes (spleen), (●—○—●) : Cytotoxic index

Table 2. Result of therapeutic effects
in Cyclophosphamide injected group

G M per mouse days	AOEPF 100U.				AOEPF 20U.				AOEPF 4U.				NMSF				PBS			
	1	2	3	4	S	1	2	3	4	S	1	2	3	4	S	1	2	3	4	S	1	2	3	4	S
100 mcg					5/5					5/5					4/5					2/5					2/5
20					5/5					2/5					2/5					1/5					1/5
4					5/5					1/5					2/5					0/5					1/5
PBS					4/5					2/5					1/5					1/5					0/5

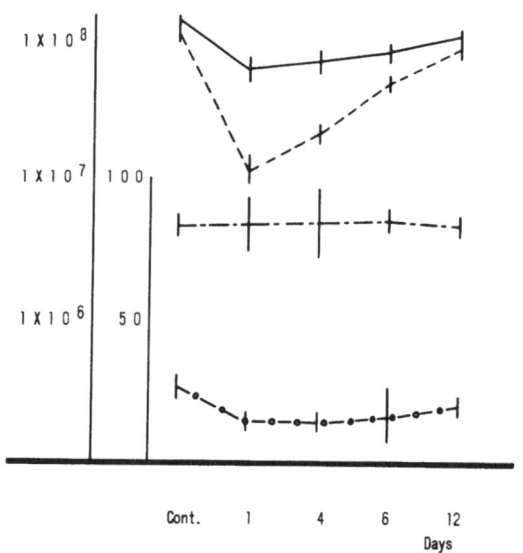

Fig. 2. Effects of Cyclophosphamide on
mouse lymphocytes (100 mg/kg, im).

Table 3. Result of therapeutic effects in Azathioprine injected group

GM per mouse / days	AOEPF 100U. 1 2 3 4	S	AOEPF 20U. 1 2 3 4	S	AOEPF 4U. 1 2 3 4	S	NMSF 1 2 3 4	S	PBS 1 2 3 4	S
100 mcg	▧▧▧▧	5/5	▧▧▧▧	5/5	▧▧▧▧	5/5	▧	1/5	▧	1/5
20	▧▧▧▧	5/5	▧▧▧▧	5/5	▧▧▧	4/5	▧	1/5	▧	1/5
4	▧▧▧▧	5/5	▧▧▧	3/5	▧▧	1/5		0/5		0/5
PBS	▧▧▧▧	5/5	▧▧	2/5	▧▧	1/5		0/5	▧	0/5

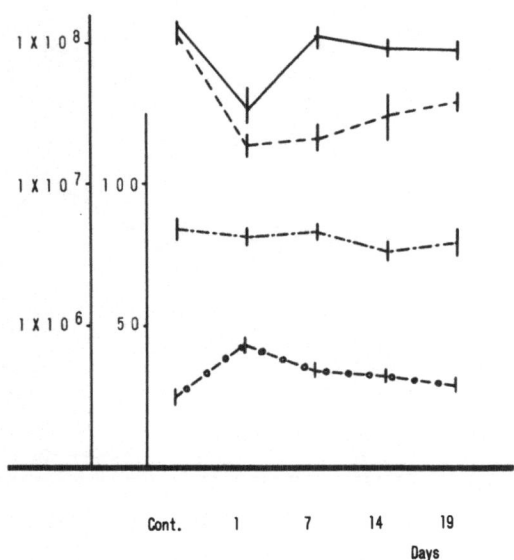

Fig. 3. Effects of Azathioprine on mouse lymphocytes (100 mg/kg, im).

Table 4. Result of therapeutic effects
in ^{60}Co irradiated group

G M per mouse days	AOEPF 100U.					AOEPF 20u.					AOEPF 4U.					NMSF					PBS				
	1	2	3	4	S	1	2	3	4	S	1	2	3	4	S	1	2	3	4	S	1	2	3	4	S
100 mcg					5/5					5/5					5/5					3/5					2/5
20					5/5					5/5					5/5					2/5					1/5
4					5/5					5/5					5/5					1/5					0/5
PBS					5/5					5/5					4/5					1/5					0/5

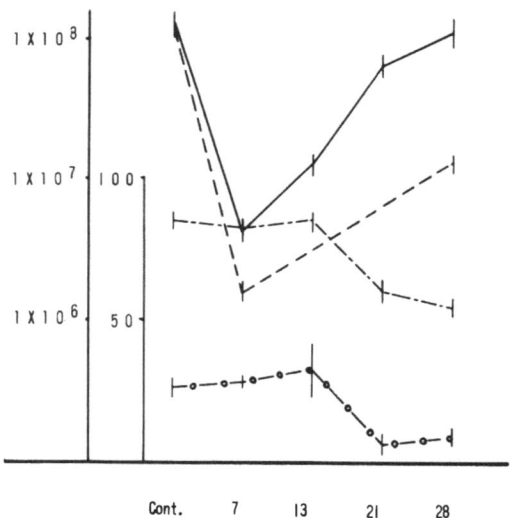

Fig. 4. Effects of ^{60}Co irradiation on
mouse lymphocytes (900 rad).

Table 5. Result of therapeutic effects
in non-immunosuppressed group

GM per mouse \ days	AOEPF 100U. 1 2 3 4	S	AOEPF 20U. 1 2 3 4	S	AOEPF 4U. 1 2 3 4	S	NMSF 1 2 3 4	S	PBS 1 2 3 4	S
100 mcg		5/5		5/5		4/5		2/5		3/5
20		5/5		4/5		3/5		0/5		2/5
4		5/5		5/5		2/5		0/5		1/5
PBS		4/5		4/5		2/5		1/5		0/5

evident in the 100 unit dose.   In 20 or 4 uint, therapeutic
effect was enhanced with combined use of gentamicin.

2. Cyclophsphamide injected group.
Thymus and spleen cells were decleased within 10 per cent.
Cytotoxicity index was 18.4 and it meant B cell loss mainly.
(Fig. 2)
The dose of bacterial inoculation was 1.4 X 10^4.
100 unit of antibody resulted in remarkable effect even in
abscence of the antibiotic.   20 or 4 unit antibody resulted
in more than 100 mcg of gentamicin.(Tab. 2)

3. Azathioprine injected group.
Thymus and spleen cells change was not significant.
Cytotoxicity index was 45.2 and it meant T_4 cell decrease.
The bacterial inoculated dose was 2.1 X 10^4.
All mice survived in 100 units.   20 or 4 unit of antibody
induced partial or complete protection in combination with appro-
priate dose of gentamicin.(Fig. 3 and Tab. 3)

4. Co-60 irradiated group.
Thymus and spleen cells decreased to the lowest number on
the 7th day after the irradiation.   Cytotoxicity index was 25.5
per cent and it meant both T and B cella loss.(Fig. 4)
The inoculated bacterial dose was 5.0 X 10^2.
Complete protection of infected mice by anti-OEP-F$(ab')_2$
was evident in all the groups.

5. Non-immunosuppressed(control)$_5$group.
The inoculated dose was 4.2 X 10^5.
In 100 and 20 units of anti-F(ab')$_2$, almost all mice
survived without gentamicin.   In 4 units, combined effect with
gentamicin was remarkable.

SUMMARY AND CONCLUSION

Therapeutic effect of anti-OEP-F(ab')$_2$ was remarkable,
particularly when the large dose, 100 units, of it was given.
It completely protected the immunosuppressed mice as well as
normal mice even without antibiotic from Pseudomonas aeruginosa
infection.   Small dose of the anti-OEP-F(ab')$_2$ induced partial
or complete protection and enhanced the therapeutic effect of
gentamicin.
It has been said that the antibody to the LPS of Pseudomonas
aeruginosa is contained exculusively in Ig M fraction, but we
have successfully obteined immune-specific Ig G-F(ab')$_2$ fragment,
because, it may be contained 13.8 per cent of nitrogen, and
shared a common antigen of Pseudomonas aeruginosa.
Intravenous injection of F(ab')$_2$ fragment of anti-OEP-Ig G
induced a remarkable and rapid therapeutic effect without serious
side effects.
The OEP is the protein moiety of endotoxin and it may be
existed in the plasma or its membrane of Pseudomonas aeruginosa.
It may be reasonable to suppose that the therapeutic effect
of anti-OEP-F(ab')$_2$ is due to the bacterial growth inhibition by
binding to it.
Immunosuppression by various products differed each other
in T and B lymphocyte population changes.   The therapeutic
effect of regard to anti-OEP-antibody, however, was found equally
in each experiment.

INVESTIGATIONS ON CIRCULATORY TOLERANCE OF DOXYCYCLINE (VIBRAVENOUS[R]) AND ROLITETRACYCLINE (REVERIN[R]) IN WAKING MINIPIGS

Tauberger, G., Schoog, M., Mehren, W.,
Mergler, G., Moussawi, M.
Pharmacological Institute of the University
of Bonn, Germany, and Department for Clinical
Research, Pfizer GmbH Karlsruhe, Germany

Summary: The antibiotics were infused at doses of 16, 24, and 32 mg/kg over 4, 6, and 8 min, each group including 6 minipigs. After 16 mg doxycycline or rolitetracycline/kg a slight increase of the blood pressure and an extension of the P-Q interval in the ECG were observed. These changes were transient and reversible. The positively pathological P-Q interval of 16o msec was observed in none of the cases treated with doxycycline, whereas rolitetracycline led to positively pathological P-Q intervals in 2/6 of the cases and to an AV block in 4/6 of the cases. The injection of 24 and 32 mg doxycycline and rolitetracycline/kg did not lead to an increase of effect as compared with the previous tests. This is probably due to the fact that the higher doses were infused over a prolonged period of time.

Previous studies performed on anaesthetized dogs, cats and rabbits showed that intravenous tetracyclines may cause both changes of the blood pressure and ECG disorders. It has not been clarified as yet to what extent these results are transferrable to human conditions as the side effects observed in the individual species differ both quantitatively and, partly, qualitatively. Neither has the influence of anaesthesia in this context been elucidated (Hergott and Ther 1958, Tauberger et al. 1971, Schölkens et al. 1974).

In the present study we are concerned with the circulatory tolerance of large doses of doxycycline

(Vibravenous[R]) and rolitetracycline (Reverin[R]) in minipigs. In various respects of circulatory relevance,
minipigs resemble man more than other species do. The
animals used in our trials were not anaesthetized and
largely free from stress.

In our investigations 33 minipigs were prepared
in halothane-nitrous oxide anaesthesia and 3 animals
were prepared in local anaesthesia with 3 - 5 ml of
a 2 % Procaine solution. In the trials with local
anaesthesia the animals were connected to a recording
device immediately upon completion of the preparation.
In the trials with anaesthesia they were allowed a rest
of 24 hours, during this period they could freely move
and received the usual feedstuff.

The arterial blood pressure in the A.saphena and
the ECG were recorded. The antibiotics were infused
into the V.saphena at doses of 16, 24, and 32 mg/kg
over 4, 6, and 8 min resp., each dose group comprising
6 animals. The doses used are about lo - 2o times
higher than the therapeutical single dose of doxycycline,
and about 4 - 8 times higher than the therapeutical
single dose of rolitetracycline.

At a dose of 16 mg/kg, both drugs led to a moderate
yet significant increase of blood pressure in the 1st -
2nd min after the injections. The effect of doxycycline
was only of short duration and not dose-related because
of an adequate extension of the injection period. Thus,
the maximum effect was already over when the injection
of 32 mg/kg was finished. On the other hand, the effect
of rolitetracycline continued for a prolonged period,
being significant until the 6th min after the injection
of 32 mg/kg.

When assessing the ECG results, we found that both
tetracyclines lead to an extension of the P-Q interval.
Here, the difference between the effects of doxycycline
and rolitetracycline was even more pronounced than with
regard to the blood pressure. Again, the effect of
doxycycline reached its peak value in the first min
after the administration of 16 mg/kg. A dose increase
did not result in an increase of effect, whereas the
effect of 32 mg rolitetracycline/kg remained significant
until the 6th min.

A P-Q interval of 16o msec which is positively
pathological for minipigs was reached in none of the
trials using doxycycline, whereas rolitetracycline

given in a dose of 16 mg/kg caused a positively
pathological P-Q extension in 2 out of 6 tests, and
2:1 or 3:1 AV blocks in 4 out of 6 tests.

With regard to the problem of how far the above
results are transferrable to human conditions minipigs
resemble man in several factors of circulatory relevance more than other species do (they are more
suitable for continuous circulatory investigations
in waking conditions).

In our animals, whose age ranged from 146 to 175
days, the systolic blood pressure averaged 155 ± 8.o4
(x ± 2 s$\bar{x}$), while the mean blood pressure was 123 mm
± 3.92.

The mean heart rate amounted to 1o8 ± 5.75 beats
per min and the diastolic-systolic quotient was
assessed to be 1.31 ± o.56. References state a diastolic-systolic quotient of 1.28 in man (Hegglin and
Holzmann 1937), whilst this parameter was found to be
2.o6 in dogs (Spörri 1954).

The mean cardiac output of waking minipigs is
almost the same as that of man, whilst in waking dogs
it is only half that value: 5.34 l/min for minipigs
(Stone and Sawyer 1966), 5.52 l/min for man (Cournand
et al. 1964) and 2.29 l/min for dogs (Bishop et al.
1964).

Also the relative blood volumes of man and pig
largely coincide, whereas the dog has a considerably
higher volume (Grauwiler 1965).

In our trial the relative heart weight was
o.48 ± o.o1 % of the body weight, thus ranging only
slightly below human values. In dogs, however, being
running animals, the percentage is much higher with
o.7 - 1 % (Clark 1927, Howe et al. 1968). A certain
resemblance is claimed between the distribution
patterns of the coronary vessels in man and pig, whereas fundamental differences exist between man and dog
(Lumb and Singletary 1962).

It is obvious from the above findings that the
circulatory system of minipigs is less efficient than
that of man, unlike the dog, whose circulatory
efficiency exceeds that of man by far. This means that
results obtained in minipigs ensure a safety margin
to man, which is indispensable when toxic side effects

of heart and circulatory system are investigated in
animals.

Our trials suggest that with regard to the circulatory* tolerance there are no objections to increasing
the usual dose of intravenous doxycycline, if the injection period is adequately extended.

---

* parameter examined

REFERENCES:

Bishop,V.S.,Stone,H.L., Guyton, A.C.(1964)
Amer.J.Physiol. 2o7, 677

Clark,A.S. (1927)
Comparative physiology of the heart.
McMillan, N.Y., 77

Cournand,R.L., Riley,R.L., Breed,E.S.,
Baldwin,E., Richards,D.W.jr. (1945)
J. clin. Invest. 24, 1o6

Grauwiler, J. (1965)
Experientia, Suppl. 1o

Hegglin,R. and Holzmann, M. (1937)
Z.f.klin.Med. 132, 1

Hergott, I. and Ther,L., (1958)
Münch.med.Wschr. 1oo, 663

Howe,B.B., Fehn,P.A., Pensinger,R.R. (1968)
Acta anat. 71, 23

Lumb, G. and Singletary,H.P. (1962)
Amer.J.Path. 41, 65

Tauberger,G., Schoog,M., Roetzel,V., Kullmann,R.,
Winkler,E. (1971)
Arzneimittelforschung (Drug Res.) 21, 1

Schölkens,B., Gerhards,H., Lindner,E. (1974)
Arzneimittelforschung (Drug Res.) 24, 312

Spörri,H. (1954)
Tierheilkunde 96, 593

Stone, H.D., Sawyer,D.C. (1966)
Swine in Biochemical Research,
Frayn Print.Co. Seattle, USA, 411

AN IN VITRO COMPARISON OF SISOMICIN WITH GENTAMICIN AND TOBRAMYCIN

Smith Shadomy and Christopher Utz

Division of Infectious Diseases, Department of Medicine,
Medical College of Virginia, Virginia Commonwealth University,
Richmond, Virginia, U.S.A.

SUMMARY

The in vitro activity of sisomicin was compared with those of gentamicin and tobramycin against 25 isolates each of Klebsiella, Enterobacter, Pseudomonas and Serratia. Kinetics of bactericidal rates were measured for 3 isolates each of the 4 genera.

Sisomicin was shown to be significantly more active than both of the other drugs against Enterobacter, Klebsiella and Serratia. Tobramycin was the most active against Pseudomonas. In terms of mean bactericidal concen. trations, sisomicin was the most active against Enterobacter and Klebsiella while tobramycin and gentamicin were the most active, respectively, against Pseudomonas and Serratia. Kinetics of bactericidal rates for the 3 drugs were similar for Enterobacter and Klebsiella; tobramycin killed Pseudomonas more rapidly than either of the other drugs. Gentamicin and tobramycin killed Serratia more rapidly than sisomicin. Significant lag periods before onset of death was observed for all three drugs with Serratia and one isolate of Pseudomonas. Evidence of populations partially resistant to sisomicin but not to the other drugs also was observed with Serratia.

INTRODUCTION

Previous in vitro investigations of the aminoglycoside antibiotics gentamicin, sisomicin and tobramycin are in general agreement regarding their comparative activities. Waitz and co-workers ranked them in terms of their decreasing

335

order of activity against gram-negative bacteria other than Pseudomonas and
Serratia as follows: sisomicin, gentamicin and tobramycin (Waitz, et al.,
1972). Tobramycin generally is regarded as being the most active against
Pseudomonas while gentamicin and sisomicin are the most active against
Serratia (Crowe and Sanders, 1973).

However, other workers such as Hyams and associates (Hyams, et al.,
1973) and Jedlickova (Jedlickova and Rye, 1974) do not agree with these
rankings. Thus, this study was undertaken to obtain additional in vitro data
regarding these compounds.

MATERIALS AND METHODS

Three aminoglycoside antibiotics were studied. These included sisomicin,
gentamicin and tobramycin. Twenty five clinical isolates each of four
genera of gram-negative bacteria were tested. These included Enterobacter,
Klebsiella, Pseudomonas and Serratia. All identifications were based on
results obtained with the "API-20 Enteric" test system.

Minimal inhibitory concentration (MIC) were measured using a tube
dilution procedure employing Meuller-Hinton broth. Drug concentrations
ranged from 0.063 to 128 µg/ml. Inocula were prepared from overnight broth
cultures and contained approximately 1×10^5 cells per ml. Incubation was
overnight at 37ºC. The MIC was defined as the lowest concentration of drug
which completely inhibited growth as determined visually. Minimal bactericidal concentrations (MBC) were determined following the first incubation
period by subculturing "negative" tubes to plates of Mueller-Hinton agar which
were then incubated overnight at 37ºC. The MBC was defined as the lowest
concentration from which viable organisms were not recovered on subculture.

In comparing and ranking the three drugs the following criteria were used:
i) per cent of organisms inhibited at concentrations of 0.5, 1.0, 2.0 and 4.0
µg/ml; ii) per cent of organisms killed at these same concentrations; iii) per
cent of organisms resistant to more than 4 µg ml; iv) geometric mean MIC and
MBC values. A concentration of 4 µg/ml, selected on the basis of measured
serum levels and therapeutic responses obtained with gentamicin and tobramycin
was felt to represent the upper limit of probable clinical susceptibility for all
three drugs.

Kinetics of the bactericidal activities of the three drugs were studied in a
limited number of "killing curve" experiments. In these experiments,
logarithmic phase cells were incubated in the presence of 10 µg/ml each of
the three drugs. Quantitative plate counts were made throughout 2 hours of

incubation at 37°C.   Three isolates each of the four genera were tested.
Results of these experiments were depicted as regression lines obtained using
the least squares method.   Times for total kill were calculated from regression
statistics using the estimating equation.

RESULTS

At concentrations of 0.5 and 1.0 μg/ml, all 3 drugs were equally inhibitory for 22 of 25 isolates of Enterobacter or 88 per cent (Table 1).   However
only sisomicin was inhibitory for all 25 at 4 μg/ml.   One isolate was resistant
to less than 16 μg/ml of tobramycin.   On the basis of geometric mean MIC
values, the drugs can be ranked in the order of sisomicin, gentamicin and
tobramycin.   Differences in susceptibilities of individual isolates to the three
drugs, as measured by the student "t" test, were of borderline significance.
Similar results were obtained when MBC concentrations were determined for
Enterobacter (Table 2).   Again, 22 of 25 isolates were killed by 1 μg/ml of
each of the 3 drugs but only sisomicin was bactericidal for all 25 isolates.

Sisomicin was slightly more active than either gentamicin or tobramycin
against Klebsiella with complete inhibition of all 25 isolates at 2 μg/ml
(Table 1).   Gentamicin and tobramycin were essentially identical in activity.
Differences between responses to sisomicin and to gentamicin or tobramycin
were significant.   Greater differences were seen in terms of bactericidal
activities of the three drugs for Klebsiella (Table 2).   Again, sisomicin was
found to be the most active drug.   Two isolates were killed only at concentrations of 8 μg/ml of tobramycin and 16 μg/ml of sisomicin.

Serratia were somewhat more resistant to all three drugs   While 24 of 25
isolates were inhibited by 4 μg/ml of sisomicin, only 20 were inhibited by
similar concentrations of the other two drugs in spite of the fact that the
geometric mean MIC values of sisomicin and gentamicin were similar (Table
1).   Differences in responses to sisomicin and tobramycin were significant.
Again, sisomicin was ranked as the most active drug.   Gentamicin was the
most active drug against Serratia in terms of bactericidal activity (Table 2).
Although both sisomicin and gentamicin were bactericidal for a similar number
of organisms at 4 μg/ml, gentamicin was clearly the more active drug in
having a lower mean MBC value; tobramycin ranked third.

Results for Pseudomonas can be interpreted several ways.   Tobramycin
clearly was the more active drug at lower concentrations with 72 per cent
inhibition at 0.5 μg/ml as compared to 20 and 64 per cent for the other two
drugs (Table 1).   However, in terms of per cent inhibited at 4 μg/ml sisomicin was the more active of the three.   The higher percentage of inhibition

Table 1. Comparison of in vitro inhibitory activities of sisomicin, tobramycin and gentamicin against selected gram-negative bacteria*

Genus antibiotic	Cumulative per cent inhibited, concn. µg/ml						Mean, st.dev.**	geometric mean**
	0.50	1.0	2.0	4.0	8.0	>16.0		
Enterobacter								
Sisomicin	88	88	96	100	-	-	0.49 ± 0.89	0.24
Tobramycin	84	88	88	96	96	100	1.24 ± 3.25	0.41
Gentamicin	88	88	88	92	100	-	1.03 ± 2.23	0.34
Klebsiella								
Sisomicin	92	96	100	-	-	-	0.27 ± 0.41	0.16
Tobramycin	92	92	96	100	-	-	0.46 ± 0.83	0.25
Gentamicin	72	92	100	100	-	-	0.43 ± 0.84	0.24
Serratia								
Sisomicin	64	80	80	96	100	-	1.34 ± 1.93	0.64
Tobramycin	40	56	72	80	92	100	3.22 ± 4.56	1.43
Gentamicin	72	80	80	80	92	100	2.56 ± 4.77	0.68
Pseudomonas								
Sisomicin	64	72	80	92	92	100	8.64 ± 27.9	0.90
Tobramycin	72	72	76	80	92	100	7.20 ± 25.5	0.78
Gentamicin	20	52	76	84	92	100	6.97 ± 17.3	1.79

* Minimal inhibitory concentrations as determined in Mueller–Hinton broth following incubation at 37°C for 18–24 hrs.

** Arithmetic and geometric mean MIC values, µg/ml

Table 2. Comparison of in vitro bactericidal activities of sisomicin, tobramycin and gentamicin against gram-negative bacteria*

Genus antibiotic	Cumulative per cent killed, concn. µg/ml							
	0.50	1.0	2.0	4.0	8.0	>16.0	Mean,st.dev.**	geometric mean**
Enterobacter								
Sisomicin	80	88	92	100	-	-	0.76 ± 1.05	0.46
Tobramycin	68	88	88	92	92	100	3.84 ± 12.92	0.74
Gentamicin	84	88	88	88	92	100	2.59 ± 7.02	0.54
Klebsiella								
Sisomicin	84	88	96	96	96	100	1.66 ± 6.34	0.29
Tobramycin	68	80	88	92	96	100	1.62 ± 3.44	0.57
Gentamicin	76	88	88	92	92	100	2.39 ± 6.95	0.41
Serratia								
Sisomicin	24	44	60	76	84	100	12.78 ± 29.6	2.50
Tobramycin	4	16	28	56	80	100	16.22 ± 29.3	5.74
Gentamicin	52	68	76	76	80	100	14.32 ± 31.5	1.69
Pseudomonas								
Sisomicin	20	48	68	84	92	100	12.29 ± 34.9	2.05
Tobramycin	12	64	72	80	92	100	8.41 ± 25.7	1.84
Gentamicin	8	16	48	68	88	100	14.02 ± 34.5	3.58

* Minimal bactericidal concentration as determined following incubation with subsequent subculture to Mueller–Hinton agar and incubation at 37°C for 48 hrs.

** Arithmetic and geometric mean MBC values, µg/ml

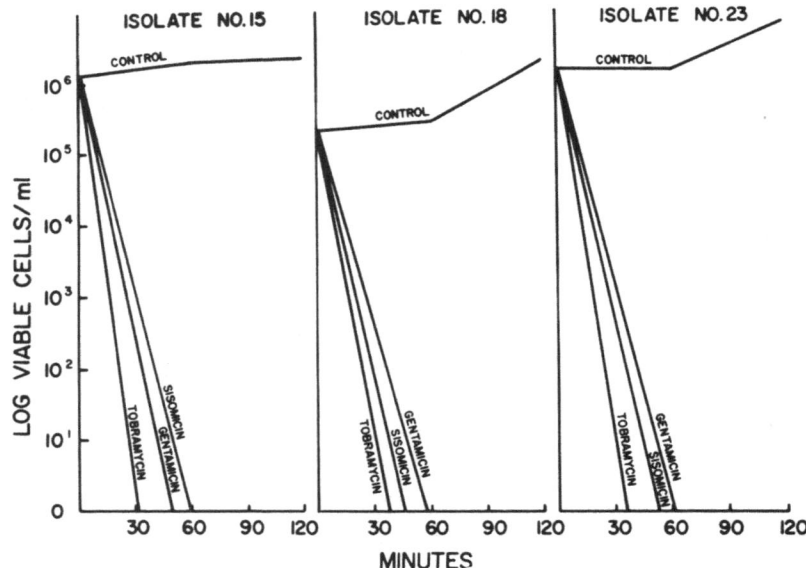

Figure 1.   Bactericidal rates of 10µg/ml of sisomicin, gentamicin and tobramycin against 3 isolates of Enterobacter.

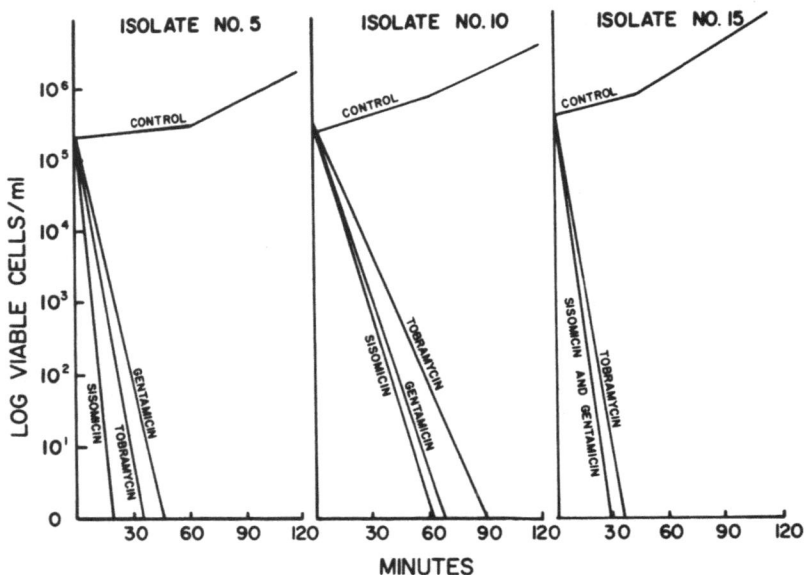

Figure 2.   Bactericidal rates of 10µg/ml of sisomicin, gentamicin and tobramycin against 3 isolates of Klebsiella.

obtained at 2 and 4 µg/ml together with the smaller number of resistant organisms for sisomicin outweigh the somewhat lower mean MBC values of tobramycin and establish sisomicin as the more active drug against Pseudomonas in terms of inhibitory activity.   Tobramycin was ranked as the most active compound against Pseudomonas when MBC values were compared (Table 2) . Again, it was the most active of the three compounds at lower concentrations with 64 per cent being killed by 1 µg/ml as compared with 16 and 48 per cent for gentamicin and sisomicin.   Differences between individual responses to sisomicin and gentamicin as well as to tobramycin and gentamicin were highly significant.

In the kinetics experiments tobramycin killed cells of Enterobacter more rapidly than did either sisomicin or gentamicin (figure 1) .   With all three isolates, complete killing of 10^6 cells occurred within 35 to 45 minutes. Sisomicin was the second most active compound.   Gentamicin required about 1 hour to achieve a total kill.   Sisomicin was the most rapid in terms of time to achieve a 100 per cent kill when tested against Klebsiella while gentamicin was the second most active and tobramycin the least active against 2 of 3 isolates (figure 2) .   With both Enterobacter and Klebsiella, differences in the rates of occurrence of the bactericidal even were not significant.

Significant differences in bactericidal rates were seen with Serratia (figure 3) .   With two of three isolates, tobramycin and gentamicin behaved in essentially identical fashions.   With one isolate they produced complete kills in approximately 80 minutes while with a second isolate, they affected 2 log reductions in numbers only after 2 hours exposure.   The most important finding with Serratia was a delay observed following exposure to drug and on- set of the exponential death phase.   This was observed with all three drugs and all three isolates.   These delays varied in time from 15 to 30 minutes and were essentially identical for each drug.   Another finding, not shown by the regression lines, was the apparent escape of two isolates from the bactericidal action of sisomicin.   With isolate No.5, actual plate counts remained unchanged at approximately 1×10^2 cells for the last hour of the experiment.   A similar escape also was observed in isolate No.7 with both sisomicin and gentamicin.

Tobramycin was the most active drug in killing of Pseudomonas (figure 4) . All three isolates were completely killed within 40 minutes.   Sisomicin was the second most active producing 100 per cent kills with 2 of 3 isolates within 90 to 100 minutes.   Gentamicin ranked third in this experiment.   In the case of isolate No.9, onset of the exponential death phase for gentamicin did not begin until after 60 minutes of exposure to the drug.

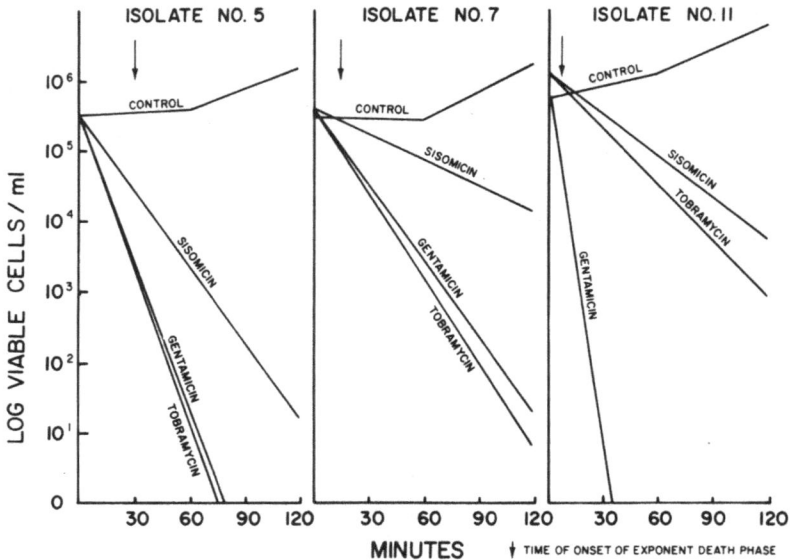

Figure 3.   Bactericidal rates of 10 μg/ml of sisomicin, gentamicin and
             tobramycin against 3 isolates of Serratia.

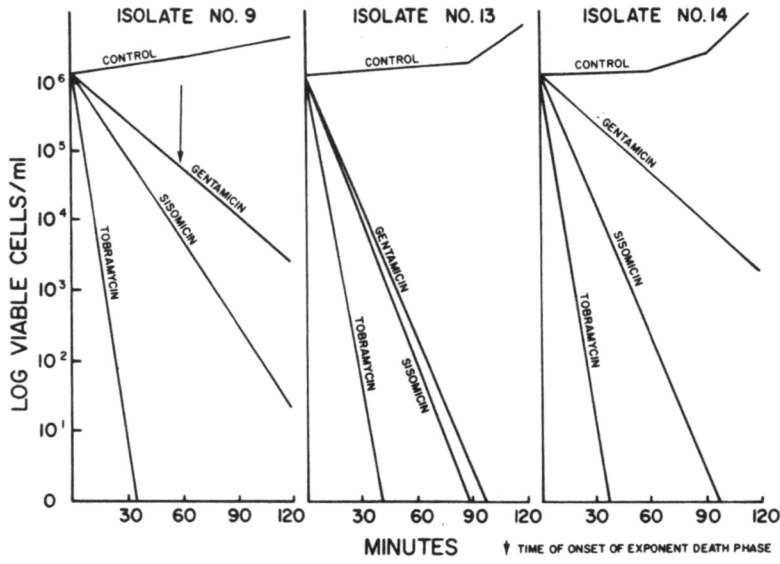

Figure 4.   Bactericidal rates of 10 μg/ml of sisomicin, gentamicin and
             tobramycin against 3 isolates of Pseudomonas.

Table 3.   Comparison of 3 aminiglycoside antibiotics in terms of 3 in vitro parameters

Genus	Inhibitory activity	Bactericidal activity	Rate of bactericidal event
Enterobacter	S > G > T	T > G > T	T > S > G
Klebsiella	S > T = G	S > G > T	S ≏ G > T
Serratia	S > G > T	G > S >> T	T = G >> S
Pseudomonas	S > T > G	T > S >> G	T > S >> G

S = Sisomicin   G = Gentamicin   T = Tobramycin

DISCUSSION

Two conventional as well as a third new parameter were used in this study to compare in vitro activities of sisomicin, gentamicin and tobramycin (Table 3). These included assessments of inhibitory activity, of bactericidal activity and, third, a comparison of rates or kinetics of the bactericidal events of the three drugs. The first two parameters clearly show that sisomicin may be ranked as the most active of the three antibiotics. If we were to conclude the discussion at this point, it would be a fair assessment to say that sisomicin is the most active drug against most gram-negative organisms exclusive of Serratia and Pseudomonas. In contrast, a new assessment would be required if we are to include the third parameter. In the case of Enterobacter, the slight edge that tobramycin had over sisomicin in terms of the rate of killing probably does not outweigh the other parameters and sisomicin remains the most active drug. The rating also remains unchanged with Klebsiella and Pseudomonas. However, in the case of Serratia, the question of both the rate and timing of the bactericidal event may be of major significance in an appraisal of the potential usefulness of the drugs against infections caused by this organism.

REFERENCES

1. Crowe, C.C. and Sanders, E. (1973). Antimicrob. Ag. Chemother., 3, 24.
2. Hyams, P.J., Simberkoff, M.S., and Rahal, J.J., Jr. (1973). Antimicrob. Ag. Chemother., 3, 87.
3. Waitz, J.A., Moss, E.L., Jr., Drube, C.G. and Weinstein, M.J. (1972). Antimicrob. Ag. Chemother., 2, 431.
4. Jedlickova, Z. and Rye, M. (1974). Chemotherapy, 20, 303.

BACTERIOLOGICAL AND CLINICAL EVALUATION OF SISOMICIN, A NEW AMINOGLYCOSIDE ANTIBIOTIC

G.F. Abbate, I. Alagia, V. Leonessa, P. Altucci

Medical Clinic of 1st Faculty of Medicine

Naples University

SUMMARY

Sisomicin exerts a high antibacterial (bactericidal) activity against Pseudomonas, most Coliform Bacilli and Staphylococcus aureus strains.

Rate of killing studies demonstrate the greater activity of Sisomicin within the first 4 hours, depending also on concentration and MBC; the effect of inoculum size on MIC of the drug is almost always very moderate.

Comparison of Sisomicin with other antibiotics show a good correlation of it with other aminoglycosides (Tobra- and Gentamicin) and some distinct advantage of Sisomicin toward other unrelated antibiotics over all for Salmonella B Wien strains.

The few resistant (or less susceptible) strains not infrequently show the lack of cross-resistance within the group.

Clinical preliminary data suggest the usefulness of Sisomicin in the treatment of gram-negative bacilli infections, over all respiratory and/or systemic also if severe or re-exacerbated.

INTRODUCTION

The present study was undertaken to assess the in vitro antibacterial activity of the new aminoglycoside antibiotic Sisomicin, and to compare it with other drugs chemically related or unrelated.

Preliminary data about clinical trial with Sisomicin will also be reported.

EXPERIMENTS AND RESULTS

1. Antibacterial Activity of Sisomicin

It was determined by the antibiotic dilution method in Brain Heart Infusion, using a 10^{-4} dilution of an 18 hour culture (10^{-3} for the more slowly growing gram-positive cocci), against 188 bacterial strains recently isolated from humans. The results are summarized in Figure 1.

It can be seen that a MIC of 3.12 mcg/ml is effective against all Pseudomonas and Staphylococcus strains and most strains of E.coli, Citrobacter, Klebsiella-Enterobacter and Salmonella B (both Paratyphi and Wien). Proteus species were also susceptible, indole-positive more than indole-negative (70% and 58% respectively).

The relative resistance of Streptococcus faecalis (7 strains) must be stressed; already known not to be intensely susceptible to Sisomicin, and also of 6 Serratia strains, only two of which were inhibited by 6.25 mcg/ml of the drug. This does not agree with our previous observations (Abbate et al., 1974) about the high susceptibility of Serratia to aminoglycosides.

The MBC determinations (see Fig. 1) confirm the good bactericidal activity of Sisomicin. The mean increase of MBC toward MIC is also shown for each species: the most susceptible is nearer 1 than the relatively resistant.

2. Rate of Killing by Sisomicin

It has been studied over all for Pseudomonas and indole-positive Proteus, calculating, at different times, the bacterial titre of fluid cultures incubated with different concentrations of the drug.

The bacterial titre was obtained through successive subcultures in Brain Heart Infusion.

Figure 2 reports in detail the behaviour of two strains belonging to the above species. Sisomicin displays an early bactericidal activity (highest within 4 hours). However, it is definitive only if the drug has a concentration

Microrganisms	N. of strains tested	minimal inhibitory concentrations (MIC, µg/ml)										% strains inhibited by 3.12 µg/ml	minimal bactericidal concentrations (MBC, µg/ml)										mean increase of MBC toward MIC
		0.19	0.39	0.78	1.56	3.12	6.25	12.5	25	50	>50		0.19	0.39	0.78	1.56	3.12	6.25	12.5	25	50	>50	
Pseudomonas	28	2	10	10	2	4	-	-	-	-	-	100%	-	2	8	10	8	-	-	-	-	-	2.1
E. Coli	15	-	-	2	6	6	-	-	1	-	-	93.4%	-	-	-	2	8	4	-	-	-	1	1.1
Kebsiella	8	-	2	-	-	4	2	-	-	-	-	75%	-	2	8	4	-	-	-	-	-	1	1.1
Enterobacter	16	-	2	6	6	-	2	-	-	-	-	87.5%	-	-	2	8	2	2	2	-	-	-	2
Serratia	6	-	-	-	-	-	2	1	3	-	-	0%	-	-	-	-	-	1	1	1	1	3	≥3.1
Salmonella Group B	39	-	-	2	13	18	6	-	-	-	-	87.3%	-	-	-	5	9	19	6	-	-	-	1.8
Citrobacter	10	-	-	1	2	6	1	-	-	-	-	90%	-	-	1	1	5	3	-	-	-	-	1.5
Proteus indole⁻	19	-	-	2	2	7	5	2	1	-	-	57.9%	-	-	-	-	2	4	2	6	-	6	≥4.5
Proteus indole⁺	10	-	-	1	4	2	3	-	-	-	-	70%	-	-	-	-	2	-	8	-	-	-	3.6
Staphylococcus aureus	30	7	12	9	1	1	-	-	-	-	-	100%	2	8	13	5	1	1	-	-	-	-	1.8
Streptococcus faecalis	7	-	-	-	-	-	1	3	2	1	-	0%	-	-	-	-	-	-	-	2	3	2	≥3.1
T o t a l	188																						

Fig. 1. Susceptibility to Sisomicin of various bacterial species.

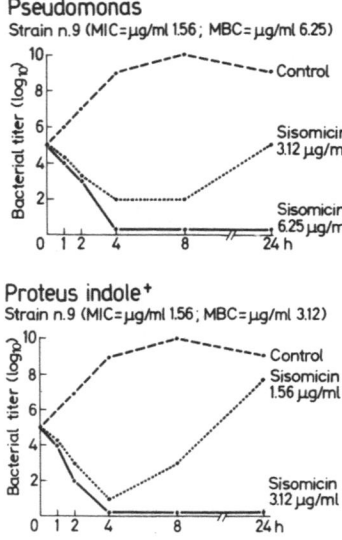

Fig. 2.   Rate of killing by Sisomicin.

corresponding to MBC for the strains under study.

3. Effect of Inoculum Size on MIC of Sisomicin

This aspect has been evaluated by challenging various doses of Sisomicin against different concentrations of bacterial inoculum (10^3, 10^6 and 10^9 cells per ml respectively) and calculating the increase of MIC with more concentrated inocula.

The results are shown in Figure 3: the inoculum effect is much less marked for Pseudomonas than for Proteus strains, especially the indole-positive, for which the MIC increase reaches 32-fold.

Microrganisms	Strains	Inoculum 10^3	Inoculum 10^6		Inoculum 10^9	
		MIC µg/ml	MIC µg/ml	Increase (Fold)	MIC µg/ml	Increase (Fold)
Pseudomonas	1	0.39	0.39	–	0.78	2
	2	0.39	0.78	2	1.56	4
Proteus	1 (indole⁻)	1.56	6.25	4	12.5	8
	2 (indole⁺)	0.78	6.25	8	25.0	32

Fig. 3.   Effect of inoculum size on MIC of Sisomicin.

4. Comparison of Sisomicin with other Antibiotics

Comparison was made, through MIC calculation for each strain of the various bacterial species examined, not only with regard to other amino-glycoside antibiotics (Gentamicin, Tobramycin) but alos to chemically unrelated antibiotics (Colimycin, Carbenicillin, Cefazolin, Ampicillin and Chloramphenicol).

Figure 4 shows that all aminoglycosides are inhibitory at 3.12 mcg/ml for Pseudomonas strains, but Sisomicin is a little more active than Tobramycin at lower concentrations and both are more active than Gentamicin (at concentrations of 0.78 mcg/ml Gentamicin does inhibit only 25% of the strains, Tombramycin 70% and Sisomicin 80%).

The results are also good, but less impressive, for Colimycin and Carbenicillin considering the serum levels obtainable with these drugs.

For Klebsiella-Enterobacter strains all aminoglycosides are inhibitory at

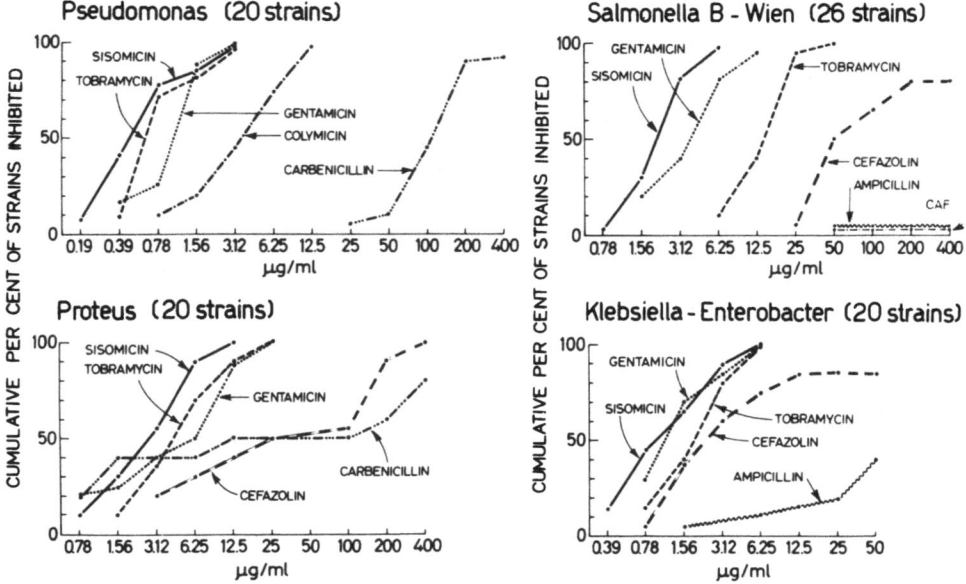

Fig. 4. Minimal inhibitory concentrations of various antibiotics for various strains of four bacterial species.

6.25 mcg/ml but the above phenomenon is repeated (i.e. Sisomicin is more active also at lowere concentrations).

The good behaviour of Cefazolin must be emphasized on strains which are probably producers of beta-lactamase and resistant to Ampicillin.

For Proteus strains Sisomicin shows the best activity (over all on indole-positive strains), while there are no significant differences between Tobramycin and Gentamicin. The susceptibility of the strains to Cefazolin and Carbeni-cillin is moderate but not high.

For Salmonella B Wien (important in our country because it is very frequently isolated, Altucci et al., unpublished), the higher activity of Sisomicin stands out in comparison with the resistance to Ampicillin and Chloramphenicol and the very moderate susceptibility to Cefazonlin.

We have not found in the present researches, strains resistant to amino-

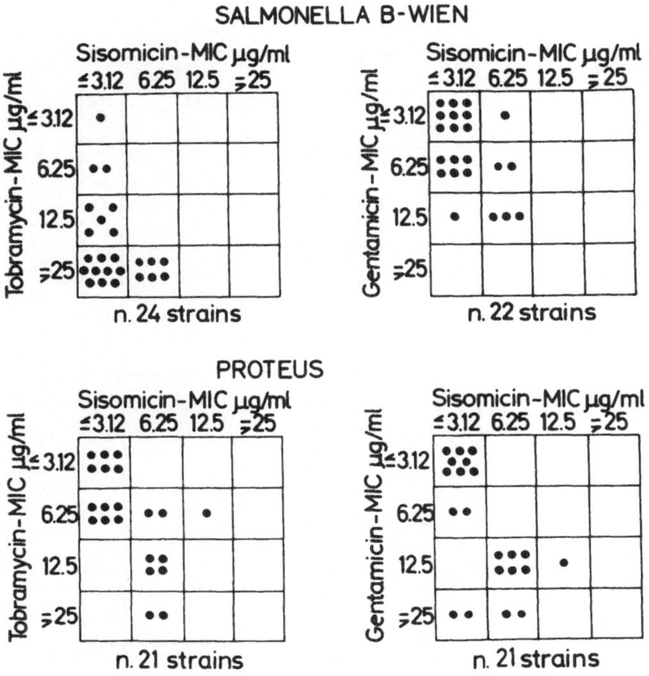

Fig. 5. Comparison of resistance between Sisomicin and other aminoglycosides: very sensitive, <3.12 - 3.12; less sensitive, 6.25; moderately resistant, 12.5; very resistant 25 - >25.

glycoside within Pseudomonas, E. coli, Klebsiella-Enterobacter. Some resistant (or less susceptible) strain appears within Salmonella B and Proteus less frequently for Sisomicin than for the others: it is interesting that in some cases there is no cross resistance between aminoglycosides (figure 5).

5. Preliminary Clinical Data

At present Sisomicin has been given i.m. (70-100 mg three times daily, every 8 hours, i.e. 2.8-3.8 mg/kg) for 7-13 days, to seven patients, all suffering from bronchopneumonia (acute or chronic or exacerbated) by Pseudomonas or Coliform Bacilli.

Figure 6 shows infecting agents; clinical diagnosis, sensitivity to Sisomicin, and clinical and bacteriological results.

Infecting agent	Diagnosis (and underlying diseases)	N.	Sensitivity to Sisomicin μg/ml	Dosage mg/kg p d	Duration of treatment (days)	Results			
						Clin. resolution (or marked improvement)	Eradication of pathogen	Bact. improved	Clinical or bacteriol. failure
Pseudomonas	Chronic bronchopneumonia (exacerbation)	3	0.39÷0.78	2.0÷3.0	7÷13	3	1	2	0
	Acute bronchopneumonia (after cardiac surgery)	1	0.39	2.5	8	1	1	0	0
Coliforms(*)	Chronic obstructive bronchopneumonia (one with bronchiectasias)	2	1.56	2.2÷3.0	8÷10	2	0	2	0
Proteus indole-	Chronic obstructive bronchopneumonia	1	1.56	2	7	1	0	1	0
Total		7				7/7	2/7	5/7	0/7

(*) {Klebsiella, E. Coli}

Fig. 6.   Preliminary results obtained with Sisomicin.

We have constantly observed clinical cure or marked improvement. In two acute and exacerbated cases respectively it was associated with respiratory eradication of pathogens, in the other five with its clear reduction.

No adverse reaction was registered through haematology, liver, renal and 8th cranial nerve function tests.

DISCUSSION AND CONCLUSIONS

Our results confirm the high antibacterial (bactericidal) activity of Sisomicin against Pseudomonas, Coliform Bacilli (with some exception for indole-negative Proteus and over all Serratia), Staphylococcus aureus, and agree with previous data of others with only some minor differences (Crowe and Sanders, 1973; Hyams et al., 1973; Ries et al., 1973; Waitz et al., 1973; Young and Hewitt, 1973; and Levison and Kaye, 1974).

Levison and Kaye, (1974) have reported higher MIC of Pseudomonas in agar than broth and have related this observation to the higher magnesium and calcium contents found in most agar as compared with broths.

Rate of killing and inoculum effect are also, in our actual experiments, very favourable evaluation parameters for Sisomicin.

Although there was some trend for bacteria that were resistant to one of the aminoglycosides to be relatively resistant to others, the phenomenon is not absolute at all and examples exist, in the present researches also, of non-corssed resistance, over all within Proteus and Salmonella B Wien species. However, we know how complex the situation of bacterial resistance to amino-glycoside antibiotics actually is, related to some R Factors and various inactivating enzymes, and depending also on the specificity of these for aminoglyco-side substrates (Holmes et al., 1974; Bryan et al., 1974; Kabins et al., 1974; Minshew et al., 1974).

As far as Salmonella B Wien is concerned (so diffuse in our country) the high in vitro activity of Sisomicin and other aminoglycosides is important considering the resistance to CAF, Ampicillin and in part to Cephalosporins, and could deserve some clinical development and implication.

Finally, the preliminary therapeutical results obtained by us with Sisomicin in humans bring us to consider it very promising in the treatment of gram-negative bacilli infections, over all respiratory and/or systemic, also if severe or exacerbated.

REFERENCES

Abbate, C.F., Leonessa, V. and Algia, I. (1972). Attivita antibatterica in citro della Tobramicina. 1st Congr. Naz.Tobramicina, Roma.

Bryan, L.E., Sharabadi, M.S., Van Der Elzen, H.M. (1974). Gentamicin resistance in Pseudomonas: R.Factor mediated resistance. Antim. Agents a. Chemoth., 191-199.

Crowe, C.C., and Sanders, E. (1973). Sisomicin: evaluation in vitro and comparison with Gent- and Tobramycin. Antim.Agents a. Chemoth., 3, 24-38

Holmes, R.K., Minshew, B.H., Gould, K. and Sanford, J.P. (1974). Resistance of Pseudomonas A. to Gentamicin and related aminoglycosides antibiotics. Antim.Agents a.Chemoth., 253-262

Hyams, P.J., Simberkoff, H.S. and Rahal, J.J. Jr. (1973). In vitro bactericidal effectiveness of four aminoglycoside antibiotics. Antim. Agents. a.Chemoth. 3, 87-94.

Kabins, S., Nathan, C. and Cohen, S. (1974). Gentamicin adenyl-transferase activity as a cause of Gentamicin resistance in clinical isolates of Pseudomonas aeruginosa. Antim.Agents.a.Chem., 565-570.

Levison, M.E. and Kaye, D. (1974). In vitro comparison of four amino-glycoside antibiotics: Siso-, Genta-, Tobramycin and BB-K8. Antim. Agents a.Chemoth., 667-669.

Minshew, B.H., Holmes, R.K., Sanford, J.P. and Baxter, C.R. (1974). Transferable resistance to Tobramycin in Klebsiella-Enterobacter asso-ciated with enzymatic acetylation of Tobramycin. Antim. Agents a. Chemoth. 492-497.

Ries, K., Levison, M.E. and Kaye, D. (1973). In vitro evaluation of a new aminoglycoside derivative of Kanamycin - a comparison with Tobra-mycin and Gentamicin. Antim. Agents a. Chemoth., 3, 532-533.

Waitz, J.A., Moss, E.L., Jr., Drube, C.G. and Weinstein, M.J. (1972). Comparative activity of Siso-, Genta-, Kana- and Tobramycin. Antim. Agents a.Chemoth., 2, 431-437.

Young, L.S. and Hewitt, W.L. (1973). Activity of four aminoglycoside antibiotics in vitro against gram-negative bacilli and Staphylococcus aureus. Antim. Agents a. Chemoth., 4, 617-626.

PHARMACOKINETICS OF SISOMICIN IN PATIENTS WITH RENAL IMPAIRMENT

G. Heinecke, K. Finke, E. Renner

Medical Clinic I, City Hospital Köln-Merheim

Ostmerheimerstr. 200, D-5 Cologne 91, GFR

SUMMARY

Serum levels and urinary excretion rates of sisomicin were measured after a single i.v. injection of 1 mg/kg body wt. in 24 patients with various degrees of impaired renal function. A good correlation was found between the elimination constants and the half-lives on the one hand and creatinine clearances, serum creatinine and blood urea levels on the other hand. The retention of sisomicin increases with decreasing renal function. On the basis of these results a dosage regimen for the sisomicin therapy in patients with renal insufficiency is suggested.

INTRODUCTION

Sisomicin is a new aminoglycosid antibiotic similar to gentamicin (Crowe and Sanders 1973, Hyams et al. 1973, Waitz et al. 1972, Waitz et al. 1970). As a gentamicin derivate sisomicin is eliminated nearly completely by glomerular filtration (Gingell and Waterworth 1968, Lockwood and Bower 1973). In patients with impaired renal function this antibiotic will cumulate.

The present study tries to correlate the decrease of sisomicin serum levels after a single i.v. injection with the degree of renal insufficiency in order to develop guidelines for an appropriate dosage regimen for patients with renal impairment.

Table I: Age, sex, and diagnosis of the patients

C_{cr} groups	Case No.	Age	Sex	Diagnosis
I >85	1	24	F	Normal
	2	25	M	Renal artery embolism
	3	22	F	Normal
II 85 - 65	4	38	F	Chronic P.N.
	5	46	F	Chronic P.N.
	6	25	F	Normal
	7	78	F	Nephrosclerosis
III 65 - 45	8	47	F	Accel. Hypertension
	9	38	M	Accel. Hypertension
	10	48	F	Renal artery stenosis
	11	30	F	Renal artery stenosis
IV 45 - 25	12	59	M	Nephrosclerosis
	13	56	F	Chronic P.N.
	14	68	M	Nephrosclerosis
V 25 - 10	15	59	F	Diabetic Nephrosclerosis
	16	55	F	Chronic P.N.
	17	63	F	Plasmocytoma
	18	61	F	Chronic P.N.
VI <10	19	37	F	Acute renal failure
	20	61	M	Chronic G.N.
	21	67	F	Chronic P.N.
VII I.H.D.	22	56	F	Chronic P.N.
	23	54	F	Chronic G.N.
	24	55	F	Chronic P.N.

I.H.D. = Intermittent haemodialysis

MATERIAL AND METHODS

24 patients, 19 women and 5 men, 22 to 78 years old, were included in the study. Renal function was normal in 3 patients. The remaining 21 individuals had various degrees of impaired renal function due to diseases such as chronic pyelonephritis, glomerulonephritis, nephrosclerosis, renal artery stenosis, renal artery embolism, acute renal failure, accelerated hypertension and plasmocytoma. Age, sex and diagnosis of the patients are shown in table I. Patients were assigned to one of seven groups, depending on their renal function as measured by

creatinine clearance. Each group consisted of 3 to 4 patients.

Sisomicin was provided as sisomicin sulfate injection in 2-ml ampoules (50 mg/ml; batch No. 213017). Each patient received a single i.v. injection of the drug at a dosage of 1,0 mg/kg body wt. dissolved in 20 ml of physiological saline slowly administered exactly within five minutes.

Serum concentrations of sisomicin were measured in blood samples drawn from the contralateral arm at standardised time intervals after the end of the injection depending on the degree of impaired renal function.

The urine for the sisomicin assay was collected before and during periods of 0 - 6, 6 - 12 and 12 - 24 hours p.i. All assays were performed by Dr. Scheer at the Microbiological Institute of Bayer, Wuppertal, GFR. The serum and urine levels were determined microbiologically.

Clinical tests to evaluate vestibular and auditory functions were carried out before and regularly after the injection. Endogenous creatinine clearances, serum creatinine and blood urea levels were determined before and after the examination period.

The biological half-live of sisomicin in serum was derived for each patient from the semilogarithmic plot of serum concentration versus time p.i., using the one hour level and the time, when a serum level of 1 mcg/ml was reached (Dost 1968). The half-live determinations were performed by Prof. Dr. Pütter, Bayer, Wuppertal.

Sisomicin serum levels were plotted as a function of time after the i.v. injection following the method of S.D. Foss (1970). We used the Wang computer 600 with the "plot decay 2" program. It determines all parameters of a model expressible as a sum of two exponential equations. The data are fitted following the function:

$$y = A_1 \cdot e^{-B_1 \cdot x} + A_2 \cdot e^{-B_2 \cdot x}$$

Correlation coefficient (r), coefficients A_1, A_2, B_1, B_2, F-value, t-value and the graph of the function were printed automatically. The coefficient B_2 represents

Table II: Serum levels (M ± SD) of Sisomicin at various times after single i.v. injection of 1 mg/kg body wt. in patients with different degrees of renal insufficiency

time p.i.	C_{cr} groups I	II	III	IV	V	VI	VII
5 min	7,4 ± 0,9	7,9 ± 0,3	8,5 ± 0,6	8,0 ± 0,2	7,5 ± 1,2	7,1 ± 0,9	7,9 ± 0,4
30 min	5,4 ± 1,0	5,5 ± 0,5	6,8 ± 1,1	5,8 ± 0,8	5,8 ± 0,3	-	-
1 h	4,4 ± 0,3	3,9 ± 0,3	5,5 ± 1,6	4,5 ± 0,4	4,5 ± 0,6	4,1 ± 0,2	4,5 ± 0,6
2 h	2,6 ± 0,2	3,0 ± 0,3	-	-	-	-	-
4 h	1,3 ± 0,5	1,5 ± 0,5	2,2 ± 0,8	-	-	-	-
6 h	-	-	-	2,1 ± 0,15	1,8 ± 0,6	2,1 ± 0,5	2,7 ± 0,8
8 h	0,3 ± 0,1	0,7 ± 0,2	1,3 ± 0,3	-	-	-	-
12 h	0,1 ± 0,06	0,4 ± 0,3	0,8 ± 0,2	1,0 ± 0,1	1,3 ± 0,3	1,3 ± 0,06	1,7 ± 0,36
16 h	-	-	0,8 ± 0,4	0,8 ± 0,15	-	-	-
24 h	-	-	0,3 ± 0,22	0,6 ± 0,1	1,2 ± 0,18	1,2 ± 0,1	1,3 ± 0,23
30 h	-	-	-	0,4 ± 0,15	1,0 ± 0,1	-	-
36 h	-	-	-	-	1,1 ± 0,15	1,0 ± 0,1	-
48 h	-	-	-	-	-	0,8 ± 0,15	1,1 ± 0,2

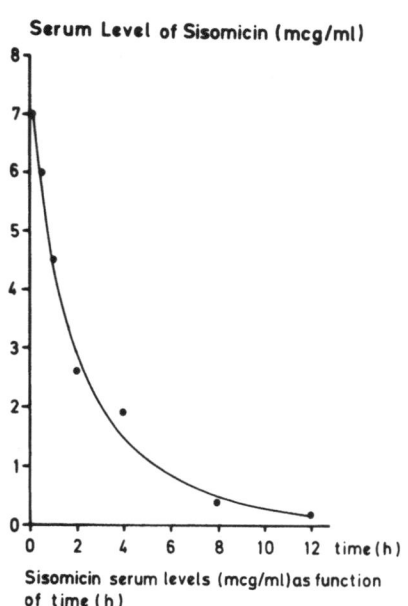

Sisomicin serum levels (mcg/ml) as function of time (h)
Patient with normal kidney function
(Case No. 2 | C_{cr} 145 ml/min | r = 0,994)

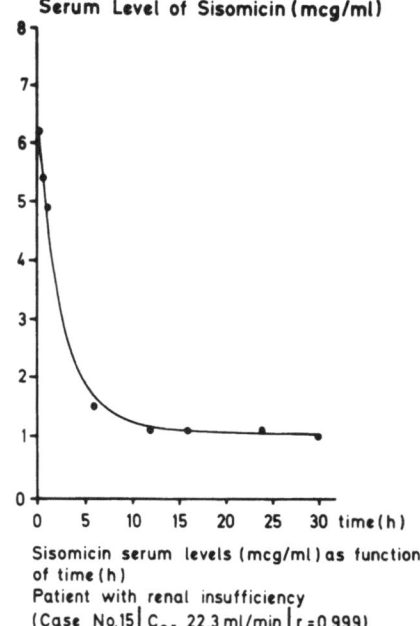

Sisomicin serum levels (mcg/ml) as function of time (h)
Patient with renal insufficiency
(Case No.15 | C_{cr} 22,3 ml/min | r = 0,999)

Figure 1

Table III: Sisomicin half-lives and elimination constants after single i.v. injection in patients with various degrees of renal impairment

Case No.	C_{cr} (ml/min)	half-life t 1/2 (h)	elimination constant
1	162,0	1.43	0.329
2	145,0	2,40	0.255
3	94,0	1,42	0,301
4	83,5	3.70	0.148
5	83,0	1 65	0.239
6	83,0	1,54	0,237
7	76,0	3,05	0,194
8	66,5	3,00	0.083
9	61,0	5,04	*
10	61,0	2,96	0,126
11	58,0	3,43	0,152
12	41,4	4,78	0,079
13	27,5	6,88	0,054
14	26,3	4,93	0,077
15	22,3	12,60	0,003
16	17,9	11,15	0,007
17	16,0	18,40	0,015
18	12,7	21,10	0,012
19	9,5	16,80	0,015
20	5,0	16,50	0,020
21	4,2	18,90	0,010
22	I.H.D.	28,90	0,006
23	I.H.D.	9.74	0,055 [x]
24	I.H.D.	23,00	0,058

I.H.D. = Intermittent haemodialysis
* = not determined
x = one haemodialysis included

Table III: Sisomicin half-lives and elimination constants
after single i.v. injection in patients with
various degrees of renal impairment.

the elimination constant k.

The rate constants of elimination were determined
for all patients. Elimination constants and creatinine
clearances were compared using linear regression models.
In addition the correlation of the elimination constant
with the serum creatinine or blood urea concentration
respectively were analysed with the same already mentioned two compartment model (Foss 1970). This was done
because of the hyperbolic relationship of the serum creatinine and the blood urea to the creatinine clearance
(Siegenthaler 1973).

RESULTS

The single i.v. injection of sisomicin was well
tolerated. No local side effects, no auditory or vestibular alterations were observed. No decrease of renal
function was seen following a single application.

Table II shows the mean values and standard deviations of sisomicin serum levels in the seven groups of
renal insufficiency after a single i.v. injection of the
drug. One can see how the time chosen for blood sampling
depends on the degree of impaired renal function.

The sisomicin serum levels as a function of the
time p.i. is shown in Fig.I. For an example the graph
shows a patient with normal kidney function and another
patient with renal insufficiency. In all patients correlation coefficients r were above 0,97.

Table III summarises creatinine clearances, biological half-lives and elimination constants of all cases.

Fig.II shows the correlation between the elimination
constants and the creatinine clearances calculated by linear regression analysis. The correlation coefficient
r = 0,928.

Fig.III shows the results when the elimination constants are plotted versus the serum creatinine levels.
The correlation coefficient r = 0,916.

Fig.IV shows the corresponding analysis of the elimination constants as a function of the blood urea. The
correlation coefficient r = 0,878.

Fig.V shows the plot of the sisomicin half-live versus the creatinine clearance. Correlation coefficient

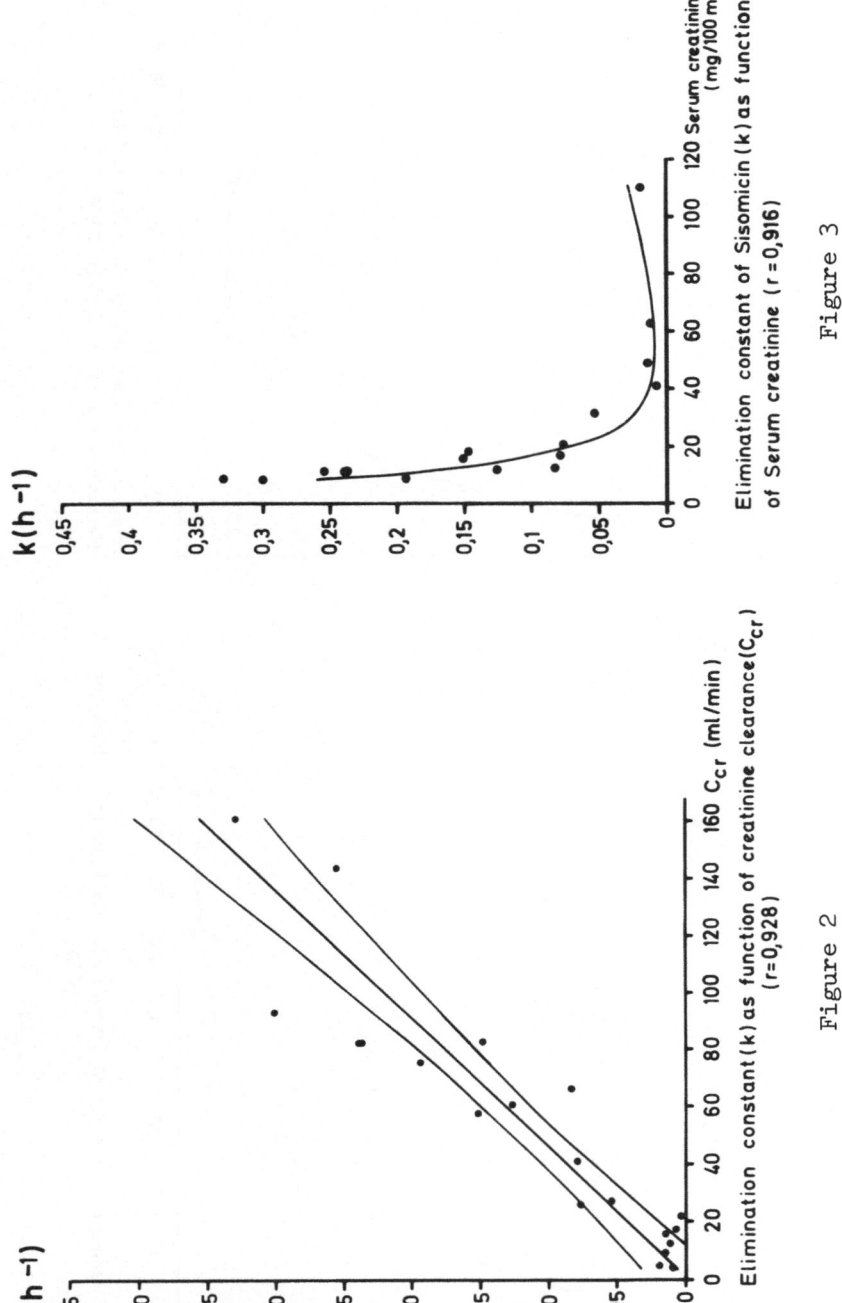

Elimination constant of Sisomicin (k) as function
of Serum creatinine (r=0,916)

Figure 3

Elimination constant (k) as function of creatinine clearance(C$_{cr}$)
(r=0,928)

Figure 2

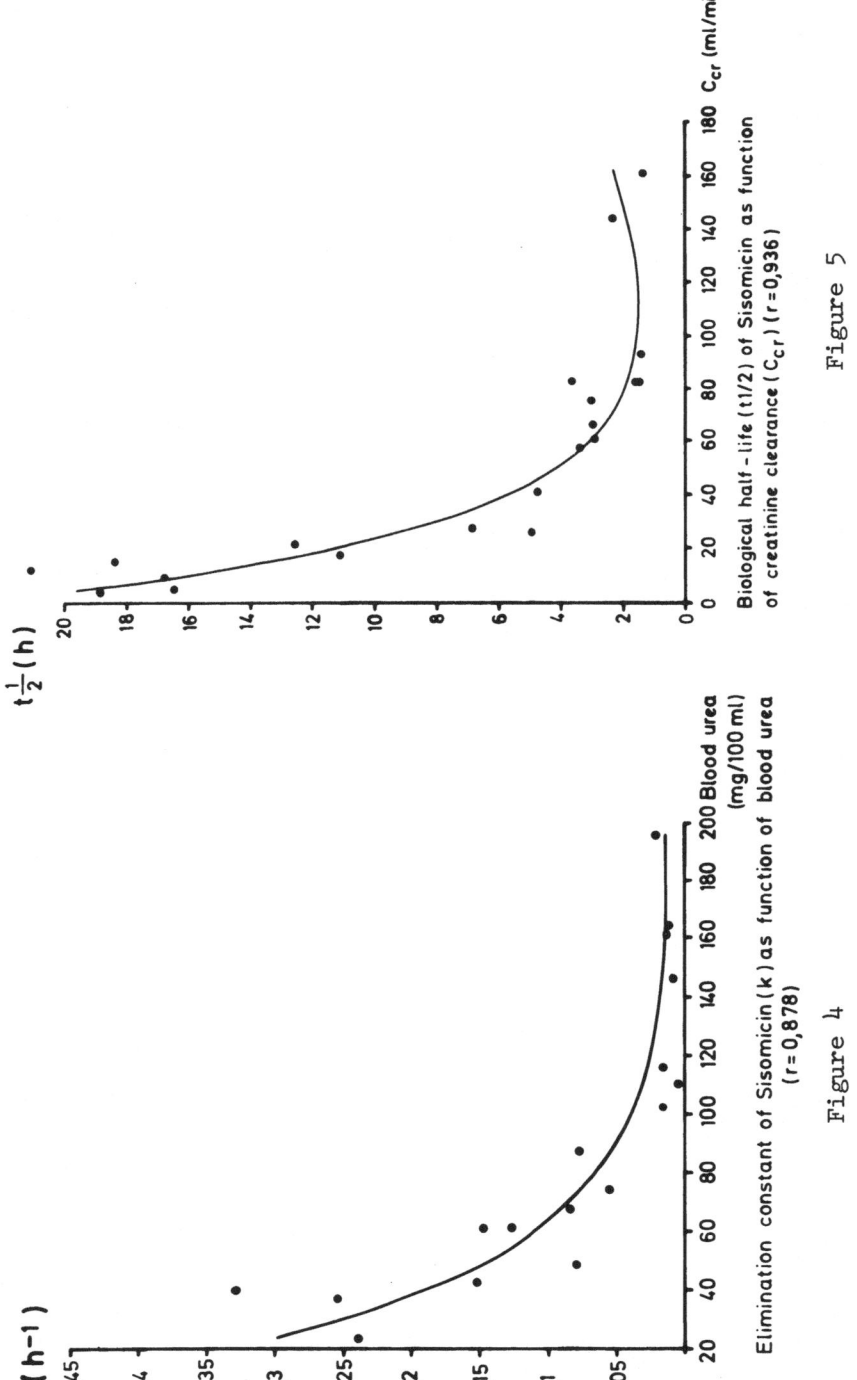

Biological half-life (t1/2) of Sisomicin as function
of creatinine clearance (C_{cr}) (r=0,936)

Figure 5

Elimination constant of Sisomicin (k) as function of blood urea
(r=0,878)

Figure 4

Table IV: Sisomicin excretion rates (%) after single i.v. injection of 1 mg/kg body wt. in patients with various degrees of renal impairment (M ± SD)

C_{cr} groups	0-6 h p.i.	6-12 h p.i.	12-24 h p.i.	0-24 h p.i.
I n = 3	55,5 ± 11,4	13,3 ± 10,2	5,4 ± 4,3	74,2 ± 25,6
II n = 4	26,7 ± 11,8	9,7 ± 5,4	7,5 ± 3,0	43,9 ± 5,9
III n = 4	35,0 ± 22,0	15,8 ± 5,2	12,0 ± 5,8	62,8 ± 16,5
IV n = 3	15,1 ± 2,2	15,6 ± 7,3	15,8 ± 4,4	46,5 ± 9,1
V n = 4	10,6 ± 3,6	7,6 ± 1,3	11,5 ± 0,8	29,7 ± 5,0
VI n = 3	5,2 ± 1,8	5,0 ± 1,6	7,3 ± 3,6	17,5 ± 6,7
VII n = 3	-	-	-	6,6 ± 7,6

Table V: Preliminary dosage regimen of Sisomicin in patients with impaired renal function

Initial and repeated dosage:		1,0 mg/kg body wt.
Creatinine clearance (ml/min)	serum (mg/100 ml)	Dose interval (h)
>35	<1,2	12
65 - 85'	1,3 - 1,5	12
45 - 65	1,6 - 2.5	16
25 - 45	2,6 - 4,0	24
10 - 25	4,1 - 7,5	36
<10	>7,5	48
Dialysis		after each dialysis

was r = 0,936.

Table IV shows the sisomicin excretion rates in %
of the given dose now subdevided into different collection periods. There is a significant decrease of the
sisomicin excretion rate between the groups I to III
and the groups IV to VI in the collection period 0-6
hours (p ‹ 0,001). The difference of the total excretion rate per day is significant between the groups I
to III and the groups V to VII (p ‹ 0,001).

We determined the serum levels of sisomicin before
and after a haemodialysis with a Kiil dialyser. Sisomicin is dialysable. Similar to gentamicin (Stratford et
al. 1974) a single 8 hours haemodialysis leads to a decrease of the sisomicin serum level of about 50 %.

                            DISCUSSION

The evaluation of the biological half-life of renally
eliminated drugs is equivocal. The conditions for a calculation cannot be standardised because of the various
interferences of the drug distribution into the extra-
vasal compartment and the renal elimination. Many ex-
perts prefere therefore the calculation of the elimination constant (Dettli et al. 1971, Dost 1968, Stratford
et al. 1974).

We calculated the elimination constant of sisomicin
in our 24 patients using a two compartment model (Foss
1970). The linear regression analysis of elimination
costants as a function creatinine clearances with a correlation coefficient r = 0,928 proves that this model
describes very well the correlation of the parameters.

Similar to gentamicin (Gingell and Waterworth 1968,
Stratford et al. 1974) the retention of sisomicin increases with decreasing renal function.

On the basis of our results we suggest the following
dosage regimen for the sisomicin therapy in patients with
impaired renal function (Table V). In order to test this
suggestion this dosage regimen was used under the control
of repeated sisomicin serum level determinations in patients with renal insufficiency. in now 4 cases we saw
that the chosen dose intervals led to satisfactory serum
levels and a good antibacterial efficiency.

REFERENCES

Crowe,C.C. and Sanders,E. (1973), Antimicrob.Ag. and Chemother. 3,1,24.

Dettli,L., Spring,P., and Ryter,S. (1971), Acta Pharmacologica 29,3,211.

Dost,F.H. (1968), Georg Thieme Verlag Stuttgart.

Foss,S.D. (1970), Biometrics 26,4,815.

Gingell,J.C. and Waterworth,P.M. (1968), British Medical Journal, 2,19.

Humair,L. (1973), Münchener Medizinische Wochenschrift 115,39,1657.

Hyams,P.J., Simberkoff,M.S. and Rahal,J.J. (1973), Antimicrob.Ag. and Chemother. 3,1,87.

Lockwood,W.R. and Bower,J.D. (1973), Antimicrob.Ag. and Chemother. 3,1,125.

Stratford,B.C., Dixson,S. and Gobkoff,A.J. (1974), The Lancet 378.

Siegenthaler,W. (1973), Georg Thieme Verlag Stuttgart.

Waitz,J.A., Moss,E.L., Drude,C.G. and Weinstein,M.J. (1972), Antimicrob.Ag. and Chemother. 2,6,431.

Waitz,J.A., Moss,E.L., Oden,E.M. and Weinstein,M.J. (1970), Journal of Antibiotics 23,11,559.

SERUM AND TISSUE LEVELS OF SISOMICIN IN DOGS

SCHEER, M.

BAYER AG, Institute for Medical Microbiology

D-56 Wuppertal-1 / West Germany, Box 130105

Studies were performed on 32 beagles after a single or after seven daily intramuscular injections of 5 and 10 mg/kg sisomicin. Two dogs were used for each dose and sacrifice time. At 1 - 2 - 4 and 24 hours after the last injection the animals were sacrificed and the following fluids and tissues were taken for sisomicin determination: Serum, bile, spinal fluid, heart, lung, liver, kidney, spleen, musculature, brain, ovaries/testicles, uterus/prostate, bones, ribs, fatty tissue, adrenal glands and eyes. Antibacterial activity in varying amounts and dependent on the dose level and time was found in all the organs examined except the eyes. No difference was noted between the single or the seven dose administration at each dose level except the kidney.

For successful antibacterial therapy it is important to achieve adequate concentrations of the antibiotic in various organs.

Not only the amount but also the duration of activity is important.

To date publications on the results of studies with sisomicin deal only with serum- and urine concentrations in animals (Waitz et al. 1970) and humans (Lode et al. 1974, Rodriguez et al. 1975, Klastersky et al. 1975).

It was the aim of the present investigations to determine the concentrations of sisomicin in various
organs of dogs.

MATERIALS AND METHODS

Studies were performed on 32 beagles after a single
or after seven daily intramuscular injections at
5 mg/kg and 10 mg/kg sisomicin. Two dogs, one male
and one female were used for each dose and sacrifice
time. The dogs were eight months old and had an
average weight of 8 to 10 kg. Sisomicinsulfate was
dissolved in saline buffer and administered in an
amount of 0.03 ml per mg sisomicin.

At 1 - 2 - 4 and 24 hours after the last injection the animals were sacrificed in ether anesthesia
and the following fluids and tissues were taken for
sisomicin determination: Serum, bile, spinal fluid,
heart, lung, liver, kidney (renal cortex and medulla),
spleen, musculature, brain, ovaries/testicles, uterus/
prostate, bones, ribs, fatty tissue, adrenal glands
and eyes. For technical reasons urine could not be
taken. The fluids and most organs were worked up
immediately after their removal, only fatty tissue,
long bones, ribs, eyes and adrenal glands were deep-
frozen at - 20° C. Special attention was given to
organs extracted from blood.

The organs were triturated in an Ultra-Turrax
in a ratio of 1 : 1 or more with phosphate buffer at
pH 8.0. After one hour at + 4° C, the samples were
centrifuged and the supernatant fluid was worked up.

The serum assays were done against a standard
curve (dog serum), the other fluids and the tissues
were assayed against a phosphate buffer standard
(pH 8.0). The determination of the sisomicin-concen-
trations in the samples was carried out with the
disc diffusion test with Staphylococcus aureus ATCC
6538 on antibiotic agar No. 11 (Difco).

RESULTS AND DISCUSSION

Antibacterial activity in varying amounts and dependent on the dose level and time was found in all the
organs examined, except the eyes. Tables 1 and 2
show the mean values after a single and after seven

daily intramuscular injections of 5 mg/kg sisomicin.
The concentrations in tissues are given in descending
order.

Table 1
Tissue Levels* of Sisomicin in Dogs After
a Single Injection of 5 mg/kg

	Hours	1	2	4	24
Renal Cortex		29,0	44,0	51,0	54,0
Renal Medulla		17,5	12,0	3,6	1,0
Serum		6,2	2,4	0,7	-
Ovary		3,5	1,3	+	+
Uterus		3,3	1,2	0,1	+
Prostate		2,0	2,8	0,4	0,1
Lung		1,7	0,8	0,3	-
Testicles		1,6	0,8	0,2	-
Long Bones		1,5	1,1	0,3	-
Ribs		0,9	1,5	0,4	0,1
Bile		0,2	0,9	0,4	-
Heart		0,6	0,3	+	-
Spinal Fluid		0,3	0,6	-	-
Spleen		0,5	0,3	+	-
Adrenal Glands		0,3	0,2	0,1	-
Fatty Tissue		0,2	0,2	-	-
Muscle		0,2	-	-	-
Liver		+	+	-	-
Brain		-	-	-	-
Eyes		-	-	-	-

-: No activity   * in mcg/ml or mcg/g

Tables 3 and 4 show results after a single and after
seven daily injections of 10 mg/kg sisomicin. The
injections were well tolerated in all dogs.

In all cases the largest quantities were measured
in the renal cortex and in the renal medulla, while
the smallest quantities were found in the brain. No
activity could be found in the eyes.

The serum concentrations were on the order of
magnitude to be expected. Surprisingly good tissue
concentrations were found in the reproductive organs
(ovary/testicles, uterus/prostate). They rank in
value directly behind the serum concentrations.

Table 2
Tissue Levels* of Sisomicin in Dogs After
Seven Daily Injections of 5 mg/kg

Hours	1	2	4	24
Renal Cortex	249,5	168,0	266,5	175,5
Renal Medulla	26,0	27,5	5,9	5,9
Serum	5,4	3,2	0,6	–
Uterus	2,8	1,1	1,0	0,1
Ovary	2,3	1,2	0,6	0,1
Prostate	1,8	1,5	0,1	0,5
Ribs	1,3	1,7	1,1	0,5
Long Bones	1,4	0,8	0,3	0,2
Lung	1,3	1,2	0,6	0,3
Testicles	1,3	0,8	0,1	+
Spleen	0,5	0,4	0,3	+
Adrenal Glands	0,5	0,3	0,2	0,1
Heart	0,5	0,5	–	–
Bile	0,3	0,5	0,1	–
Spinal Fluid	0,2	0,2	0,3	–
Fatty Tissue	0,2	0,2	–	–
Muscle	0,2	+	–	–
Brain	+	+	–	–
Liver	+	–	–	–
Eyes	–	–	–	–

–: No activity   * in mcg/ml or mcg/g

Significant levels were also detected in the lungs,
long bones and ribs. Levels in other tissues or
fluids, like heart, spleen, adrenal glands, fatty
tissue or bile and spinal fluid, were generally
lower. The concentrations in the muscle and in the
liver proved to be low and furthermore could be detected for only a brief period of time.

In general, a continuous decrease in the values
of the concentrations from one to 24 hours áfter
treatment was noted. This occurs also for the renal
medulla. The renal cortex however behaves completely
different. After single application in dosages of
5 mg/kg and up to 10 mg/kg the concentrations in
tissue rise in the following 24 hours. After multiple
applications however, various concentrations are
found at different times. After 4 hours all four
regimes of administration do not show residues in

liver (one exception) muscle and brain. After 24 hours
the same occurs for serum, heart and fatty tissue.
After a single application with 10 mg/kg sisomicin,
adrenal glands, spleen and spinal fluid are free of
antibacterial activity at the same time. This occurs
after a single application with 5 mg/kg also for
lung, testicles, long bones and bile.

In some cases, the concentrations detected after
the administration of seven doses are higher and in
many cases longer lasting than those after a single
dose.

Table 3
Tissue Levels* of Sisomicin in Dogs After
a Single Injection of 10 mg/kg

Hours	1	2	4	24
Renal Cortex	41,5	59,5	40,0	100,0
Renal Medulla	53,0	28,5	5,8	1,4
Serum	11,5	8,7	1,3	–
Uterus	5,4	4,4	0,4	0,7
Prostate	3,4	3,4	5,0	+
Ovary	4,4	2,2	0,4	+
Testicles	3,6	1,0	0,3	+
Ribs	2,7	1,7	0,6	0,2
Lung	2,3	2,2	0,4	+
Long Bones	1,6	1,4	0,6	0,2
Adrenal Glands	1,4	1,0	0,1	–
Heart	1,3	0,8	+	–
Bile	0,7	0,7	0,3	1,0
Spleen	0,8	0,6	+	–
Spinal Fluid	0,4	0,3	0,1	–
Muscle	0,4	0,2	–	–
Fatty Tissue	0,3	0,2	0,1	–
Liver	0,3	0,2	–	–
Brain	+	–	–	–
Eyes	–	–	–	–

–: No activity   * in mcg/ml or mcg/g

Table 4
Tissue Levels* of Sisomicin in Dogs After
Seven Daily Injections of 10 mg/kg

	Hours	1	2	4	24
Renal Cortex		235,0	313,0	337,5	234,0
Renal Medulla		95,0	52,0	14,4	7,2
Serum		13,9	7,7	1,2	–
Uterus		6,2	4,0	1,0	0,3
Prostate		6,2	2,0	1,2	0,1
Ovary		4,0	1,9	0,6	0,3
Lung		3,8	2,6	1,4	0,6
Testicles		3,2	1,9	0,7	0,3
Ribs		2,6	2,3	1,2	0,8
Long Bones		1,7	1,2	0,5	0,5
Heart		1,7	1,1	0,1	–
Adrenal Glands		1,6	0,8	0,4	0,2
Spleen		1,4	1,0	0,7	0,4
Spinal Fluid		1,3	0,3	0,2	0,2
Bile		0,3	0,7	0,2	–
Fatty Tissue		0,5	0,2	0,1	–
Liver		0,5	0,3	+	–
Muscle		0,5	0,2	–	–
Brain		+	+	–	–
Eyes		–	–	–	–

–: No activity   * in mcg/ml or mcg/g

In table 5 peak levels of sisomicin are summarized in direct comparison.

As expected, higher tissue levels were found after doses of 1 x 10 or 7 x 10 mg/kg than after the administration of 1 x 5 or 7 x 5 mg/kg. The activity detected is not twice as high in every case, but higher values, especially in the renal cortex are noted. No cummulation of sisomicin takes place.

The most interesting finding is the high tissue concentration in the kidneys. These concentrations are extremely higher than concentrations in serum at the same time; this is distinctly marked after multiple application.

Table 5
Peak Levels* of Sisomicin in Various Dog
Tissues Following Single or Seven Daily Injections

	1x 5 mg/kg	7x 5 mg/kg	1x 10 mg/kg	7x 10 mg/kg
Serum	6,2	5,4	11,5	13,9
Bile	0,9	0,5	0,7	0,7
Spinal Fluid	0,6	0,3	0,4	1,3
Lung	1,7	1,3	2,3	3,8
Heart	0,6	0,5	1,3	1,7
Spleen	0,5	0,5	0,8	1,4
Liver	+	+	0,3	0,5
Renal Cortex	54,0	266,5	100,0	337,5
Renal Medulla	17,5	27,5	53,0	95,0
Adrenal Glands	0,3	0,5	1,4	1,6
Muscle	0,2	0,2	0,4	0,5
Brain	−	+	+	+
Eyes	−	−	−	−
Fatty Tissue	0,2	0,2	0,3	0,5
Ribs	1,5	1,7	2,7	2,6
Long Bones	1,5	1,4	1,6	1,7
Ovary	3,5	2,3	4,4	4,0
Uterus	3,3	2,8	5,4	6,2
Testicles	1,6	1,3	3,6	3,2
Prostate	2,8	1,8	5,0	6,2

* in mcg/ml or mcg/g

Wahlig et al. (1974) made similar observations in his studies of gentamicin in dogs. Furthermore activity data which were found by our investigations in other organs are comparable with results of Wahlig.

Weinstein/Waitz (1974) carried out pharmacokinetic investigations with sisomicin in rats. They also detected very high concentrations of the drug in kidneys.

If it is assumed, that observations carried out in tests with animals can be transferred to humans, sisomicin is expected a therapeutic agent with good efficiency against bacterial infections. This was proved by investigations in humans against infections

of kidneys and urinary tract, against bronchopneumoniae
affects, septicemia and soft tissue infections.

The results of these trials are not yet
published.

References:

Klastersky, J., Hensgens, C., Geraro, M. and Daneau,
D. (1975)
J. Clin. Pharm., 252

Lode, H., Kemmerich, B. and Langmaack (1974)
14th ICAAC, San Francisco
11 - 13 September, 1974

Rodriguez, V., Bodey, G.P., Valdevieso, M. and
Feld, R. (1975)
Antimicrob. Ag. Chemother. 7, 38

Wahlig, H., Metallinos, A., Hameister, W. and
Bergmann, R. (1974)
Inst. J. Clin. Pharmacol. 10, 212

Waitz, J.A., Moss, E.L., Oden, E.M. and Weinstein,
M.J. (1970)
J. Antibiotics 23, 559

Weinstein, M.J. and Waitz, J.A. (1974)
personal information

Sisomicin Treatment of Urinary Tract Infections

Gilbert A. Dale and Clair E. Cox

University of Tennessee Center for the Health Sciences
Department of Urology
Memphis, Tennessee 38163

Sisomicin is a new aminoglycoside antibiotic produced by the
growth of a species of Micromonospora, M. inyoensis. The
antibiotic is produced substantially as a single component and
most closely resembles gentamicin C_{1a}, a component of the
gentamicin complex (C_1, C_{1a}, C_2). Minimal inhibitory concentrations (MIC) of sisomicin appear less than of the other aminoglycosides. This new antibiotic has a spectrum of in vitro
antimicrobial activity similar to that of gentamicin, however, it
is more active particularly against strains of Pseudomonas
aeruginosa and indole positive proteus. Bacterial strains
resistant to gentamicin are usually resistant to sisomicin. In
the presence of serum, sisomicin appears to be more bactericidal
than gentamicin, and in in vivo mouse protection studies, it has been
shown to be two to four times more effective. In mice, rats, and
guinea pigs, the acute LD_{50}'s for sisomicin are between one-half
and three-fourths of those for gentamicin. In the cat, sisomicin
appears to be slightly more vestibular toxic than gentamicin.
Auditory toxicity studies in the guinea pig show that it is
slightly less toxic than gentamicin, and based on the projective
therapeutic dose, probably less toxic than kanamycin. Comparative
studies of nephrotoxicity in the dog indicate that the
nephrotoxic potential of sisomicin is similar to that of gentamicin.
However, in the rat and cat, it appears to be slightly more
nephrotoxic.

In man, single intramuscular doses of sisomicin ranging from
0.5 to 3.0 mg/kg have been well-tolerated. One of seven subjects
receiving a single injection of 3.0 mg/kg described transient
paresthesias of the face and hands two hours after injection. More
than 60 individuals with normal renal function have received
between 1.5 and 3.0 mg/kg/day for up to seven days. Ten healthy

young males have been given 3.75 mg/kg/day for seven days. The
total daily dose was usually administered in divided doses every
eight hours. Serum concentrations were dose-related, usually
peaking one hour after injection. Peak serum concentrations were
approximately four times the single dose; i.e., a dose of 1.0 mg/kg
resulted in a peak serum concentration of approximately 4 mcg/ml.
Sisomicin is mainly excreted by the kidneys resulting in high
concentrations in the urine. Careful monitoring of auditory,
vestibular, and renal function failed to reveal any serious drug-
related toxicity. Local tolerance to intramuscular injection has
been excellent. Because of its increased antimicrobial activity
against Enterobacteriaceae and Pseudomonas aeruginosa and because
of the comparatively lower MIC's we initiated studies with
sisomicin.

Materials and Methods

Three studies involving sisomicin have been completed. The
first study was an open study using sisomicin in a dose of 2 mg/kg
per day intramuscularly, given in two equally divided doses every
12 hours. Twenty patients were evaluated in this study. These
were hospital in-patients ranging in age from 26-84 years. The
average age was 62 years. Their weights ranged from 50 to 102
kilograms, the median being 72 kilograms. There were 14 males and
6 females. Most of the patients had underlying urologic disease.
Pre-therapy urine cultures were obtained, following which the
patients were treated for from 5-10 days. All patients had urinary
infection as evidenced by a urine culture revealing greater than
100,000 bacteria per ml of urine. All organisms were sensitive to
sisomicin , as evidenced by a zone of at least 16 mm utilizing
standard disc sensitivity methods. Cultures were also taken at
the completion of therapy and at followup 2-4 weeks later. Pre
and post therapy hematologic studies and measurements of renal
and hepatic function were made. Additionally, all patients
underwent pre and post therapy audiograms to monitor VIII cranial
nerve function.

The second study group consisted of twenty-five patients
ranging in age from 15-99 years, mean age 59 years. Their weights
ranged from 46-91 kilograms, with a mean weight of 64 kilograms.
There were 21 males and 4 females. All patients had a urinary
tract infection as evidenced by a urinary bacterial count of
100,000 bacteria per ml of urine. This study was performed in a
similar manner to the first, except that sisomicin given intramuscularly every 12 hours was compared by random allocation to
sisomicin administered once daily. Patients receiving twice daily
therapy were given 50 mg every 12 hours if they weighed less than
60 kilograms and 75 mg every 12 hours if they weighed greater than
60 kilograms. Those receiving once daily therapy were given 75 mg
every 24 hours if they weighed less than 60 kilograms and 100 mg
every 24 hours if they weighed greater than 60 kilograms. Thirteen

patients received sisomicin twice daily and twelve received
sisomicin once daily. Similar pre and post therapy studies were
performed on the 25 patients in this study.

The third study compared gentamicin and sisomicin. Again all
patients had a urinary tract infection as evidenced by a urinary
bacterial count of 100,000 bacteria per ml of urine. Patients
were monitored in the same fashion as in the previous two studies.
There were 43 patients, 32 males and 11 females. Their ages
ranged from 17 to 87 years, mean 62 years. Their weights ranged
from 39 to 96 kilograms, mean 63 kilograms. The 20 patients
randomly chosen to receive gentamicin received 60 mg every 8 hours
if they weighed less than 60 kilograms and 80 mg every 8 hours if
they weighed more than 80 kilograms. The 23 patients receiving
sisomicin were given 50 mg every 12 hours if they weighed less than
60 kilograms and 75 mg every 12 hours if they weighed greater
than 60 kilograms. All were treated from 6-12 days.

Results and Discussion

Study one: As can be seen in Table I, sisomicin, 1 mg/kg every
12 hours was effective in treating urinary infection. The post
treatment urine culture revealed no growth on 19 of 20 occasions.
This is a 95% cure rate. On the other occasion the original
organism was eradicated, but superinfection with Proteus rettgeri,
resistant to sisomicin, developed. Followup cultures, obtained
two to four weeks after completion of treatment revealed reinfection in two of the nineteen patients whose cultures had revealed
no growth at the completion of treatment. These reinfections were
considered "patient failures" rather than antibiotic failures and
therefore did not detract from the 95% cure rate.

Study two: In the second study, 12 patients received sisomicin
once daily and 13 received the drug twice daily. As evidenced
by post treatment urine cultures, (Table II) there were three
treatment failures in the group receiving one dose daily and four
failures in those receiving two doses daily. This reveals a cure
rate of 9/12 or 75% in the group treated once daily and a cure
rate of 9/13, or 69% in the group treated twice daily. One patient,
treated twice daily, developed superinfection. No patients who
were cured developed reinfection at followup. These cure rates
are statistically not significantly different. The failure rate
in the second study (comparing one and two daily doses) was 7 of
25 patients. This higher failure rate may be accounted for by
the observation that, in general, underlying urologic disease was
more prominent in the second study than in the first.

Study three: In the third study (Table III) all 43 post therapy
urine cultures revealed no growth. There were three followup

Table I. Sisomicin Q 12 H

Pt.	Age	Sex	Treatment Days	Total dose (mg)	Urine Cultures Pre	Post	Follow up	Serum Creatinine Pre Rx	Post Rx	Diagnosis	Surgery
E.E.	49	M	7	1008	E.Coli	NG	NG	1.3	1.0	Epididymitis	Rt. Orchiectomy
J.H.	84	M	8	832	E.Coli	NG	NG	1.4	1.5	Suspected Bladder Tumor	None
R.T.	26	M	7	1204	P.Mirabilis	NG	NG	.7	1.0	Epididymitis	None
D.C.	60	F	7	924	Serratia	NG	E.Coli Serratia	.8	.9	Renal Calculus	None
I.T.	78	M	7	896	Enterobacter	NG	NG	1.3	1.3	B.P.H.	None
J.M.	46	M	8	1168	E.Coli	NG	NG	1.2	1.2	Epididymitis	Epididymectomy Orchiectomy
H.C.	76	M	5	580	P.Mirabilis	NG	NG	1.1	.9	Ca. of Prostate	None
E.H.	76	M	5	640	Pseudomonas	NG	NG	.9	.9	Urethral Stricture	None
C.G.	67	M	7	952	Pseudomonas	NG	NG	1.4	1.4	B.P.H.	TURP
F.A.	66	M	10	1200	Pseudomonas Klebsiella	NG	NG	.9	1.2	B.P.H.	TURP

Table I. Sisomicin Q 12 H

Pt.	Age	Sex	Treatment		Urine Cultures			Serum Creatinine		Diagnosis	Surgery
			Days	Total dose (mg)	Pre	Post	Follow up	Pre Rx	Post Rx		
K.H.	59	F	8	864	P.Mirabilis	NG	NG	.9	1.0	Neurogenic Bladder	Cystoscopy
L.J.	59	M	8	1200	Klebsiella	NG	NG	1.3	1.1	B.P.H.	Prostatectomy
J.G.	78	M	7	1120	Pseudomonas	NG	NG	1.2	1.3	B.P.H.	TURP
F.K.	47	F	7	980	E.Coli	NG	NG	1.0	1.0	Neurogenic Bladder	Cervical biopsy with D & C
W.B.	68	M	7	784	Pseudomonas	NG	NG	1.1	1.0	B.P.H.	TURP
J.B.	54	F	8	1440	Klebsiella	NG	NG	1.1	1.3	Bladder tumor	None
G.L.	50	F	8	1488	Klebsiella	NG	NG	.9	1.0	Bladder tumor	Bladder Biopsy
E.C.	76	M	9	1476	Klebsiella	NG	NG	1.5	1.5	Urethral Stricture	Internal Urethrotomy
V.S.	53	F	7	1400	Klebsiella	NG	NG	.8	.8	Urethral Stricture	Cystoscopy Internal Urethrotomy
R.A.	60	M	8	1200	Klebsiella	P. Rettgeri	P. Retteri	1.2	1.2	B.P.H.	TURP

Table II. Sisomicin Q 24 H vs. Sisomicin Q 12 H (Q 24 H)

Pt.	Age	Sex	Treatment			Urine Cultures			Serum Creatinine		Diagnosis	Surgery
			Days	mg/day	mg	Pre	Post	Follow up	Pre Rx	Post Rx		
B.J.	63	F	6	75	450	Pseud. E.Coli	NG	NG	1.3	2.5	Ureteral Stricture	None
W.P.	99	M	7	75	525	P.Mirabl.	NG	NG	.9	1.1	Vesical Calculus	Cysto: extraction of bladder stone
B.F.	18	F	7	75	525	E.Coli	E.Coli	E.Coli	.9	1.0	Vesicoureteral Reflux	None
J.W.	15	M	7	75	525	P.Mirabl.	P.Mirabl.	P.Mirabl.	1.5	1.1	Renal Calculus	(R) Nephrolithotomy (R) Heminephrotomy
L.P.	59	M	6	75	450	Klebsiella	NG	NG	1.2	1.1	Renal Pelvic Calculus	(L) Pyelolithotomy
R.T.	26	M	7	100	700	P.Mirabl.	P.Mirabl.	P.Mirabl.	.8	.8	Neurogenic bladder	None
W.N.	77	M	8	100	800	P.vulgaris	NG	NG	1.3	1.0	B.P.H.	TURP
L.H.	59	M	8	100	800	E.Coli	NG	NG	1.4	1.0	B.P.H.	TURP
J.N.	73	M	9	100	900	Klebsiella	NG	NG	1.3	1.1	B.P.H.	TURP
J.B.	71	M	10	100	1000	Klebsiella	NG	NG	1.6	1.6	Ca.Prostate	None
W.R.	74	M	7	100	700	E.Coli	NG	NG	1.4	1.4	B.P.H.	TURP
R.K.	74	M	8	100	800	Pseud.	NG	NG	1.2	1.1	B.P.H.	TURP

Table II. Sisomicin Q 24 H vs. Sisomicin Q 12 H (Q 12 H)

Pt.	Age	Sex	Days	Treatment mg/day	mg	Urine Cultures Pre	Post	Follow up	Serum Creatinine Pre Rx	Post Rx	Diagnosis	Surgery
J.J.	51	M	7	100	700	P.Rettgeri	P.Rettgeri	P.Rettgeri	.9	1.0	Vesical Calculi	Vesicolithotomy
E.B.	74	M	8	100	800	Klebsiella	NG	NG	.8	1.0	Ca.Prostate	TURP
L.H.	66	M	8	100	800	P.Rettgeri	P.Rettgeri	P.Rettgeri	1.7	1.7	Neurogenic Bladder	Cysto; bil. Cath. Explor. Lap
V.H.	67	M	12	100	1200	Klebsiella	Pseud.	Pseud.	.8	.9	Neurogenic Bladder	None
M.D.	78	M	7	100	700	Klebsiella	NG	NG	1.2	1.1	B.P.H.	TURP
E.D.	74	M	7	150	1150	Klebsiella	NG	NG	1.1	1.2	B.P.H.	TURP
W.J.	73	M	7	150	1050	Klebsiella	NG	NG	1.1	1.1	B.P.H.	TURP
A.F.	70	M	7	150	1050	Klebsiella P.vulgaris	mina Polymorpha	mina Polymorpha	.7	1.0	Ureteral Stricture	None
A.P.	72	M	6	150	900	Pseud.	NG	NG	.9	.9	B.P.H.	TURP
L.R.	28	F	7	150	950	E.Coli	NG	NG	1.0	.9	Pyelonephritis	None
A.M.	64	M	8	150	1200	P.Mirabi. Pseud.	NG	NG	1.1	1.4	Urethral Stricture	1st Stage Urethroplasty
O.J.	50	F	13	150	1950	Klebsiella	NG	NG	.6	.6	Neurogenic Bladder	ileal conduit
H.R.	83	M	7	150	1050	E.Coli	NG	NG	1.6	1.4	B.P.H.	TURP

Table III. Sisomicin vs. Gentamicin (Sisomicin)

Pt.	Age	Sex	Treatment Days	mg/day	mg	Urine Cultures Pre	Post	Follow up	Serum Creatinine Pre Rx	Post Rx	Diagnosis	Surgery
K.W.	52	F	8	100	800	E.Coli	NG	Pseud.	1.4	1.0	Neurogenic Bladder	None
W.W.	33	M	12	100	1200	P.vulgaris	NG	NG	1.0	.8	Neurogenic Bladder Vesical Calculi	Lithopaxy
W.R.	70	M	7	100	700	E.Coli	NG	NG	1.1	1.2	B.P.H.	TURP
M.C.	76	M	7½	100	750	Klebsiella	NG	Klebsiella	1.2	1.5	B.P.H.	Retropubic Prostatectomy
S.P.	17	F	7½	100	750	E.Coli	NG	NG	1.1	1.0	Pyelonephritis	None
S.P.	78	M	8	100	700	E.Coli	NG	NG	1.7	2.0	B.P.H.	TURP
A.G.	66	M	6	50	300	P.Mirabi.	NG	NG	2.8	1.4	B.P.H. Urethral Stricture	TURP and Cysto; internal urethrotomy
J.G.	51	M	7½	100	750	Klebsiella	NG	NG	3.4	2.8	B.P.H.	TURP
B.D.	18	F	7	100	700	Klebsiella	NG	NG	1.6	1.5	Ureteral Calculus	1/3 lower Ureterolithotomy
A.O.	71	M	8½	150	1275	E.Coli	NG	NG	1.1	1.2	B.P.H.	TURP and internal urethrotomy
A.L.	62	M	8½	150	1275	E.Coli	NG	NG	1.3	1.4	B.P.H.	TURP
G.W.	70	M	7	*75	525	E.Coli	NG	NG	2.4	2.7	Urethral Stricture	2nd Stage Urethroplasty
E.P.	38	F	8½	150	1275	E.Coli	NG	NG	1.3	1.4	Renal Calculus	(R) Nephrolithotomy
A.W.	68	M	8	*75	600	Klebsiella	NG	Pseud.	2.1	2.8	B.P.H.	None

Table III. Sisomicin vs. Gentamicin (Sisomicin)

Pt.	Age	Sex	Treatment			Urine Cultures			Serum Creatinine		Diagnosis	Surgery
			Days	mg/day	mg	Pre	Post	Follow up	Pre Rx	Post Rx		
R.R.	63	M	7	150	1050	E.Coli	NG	NG	1.2	1.2	Urethral Stricture	Urethroplasty
T.C.	74	M	7	150	1050	P.Morgarii	NG	NG	1.1	1.2	Urethral Stricture	Urethroplasty
O.B.	75	M	7	150	1050	Enterbact.	NG	NG	2.4	3.1	B.P.H.	TURP
E.T.	76	M	5½	150	825	P.rettgeri	NG	NG	1.3	1.5	B.P.H.	TURP
J.B.	79	M	8	*75	600	Klebsiella	NG	NG	1.4	1.8	Urethral Stricture	Cystoscopy
T.F.	54	F	7	150	1050	Klebsiella	NG	NG	1.0	1.0	Neurogenic bladder	None
H.B.	65	M	8½	150	1275	Pseud.	NG	NG	1.2	1.2	Periurethral Abscess	Debridement of Scrotum and perineum
A.P.	82	M	10	*75	750	Klebsiella	NG	NG	1.8	1.9	B.P.H.	Open Prostatectomy
J.B.	54	F	8	240	1920	Pseud. P.rettgeri	NG	NG	1.0	1.2	Vesical Calculus	Lithopaxy and bladder biopsy

*Dosage reduced because of creatinine elevation.

Table IV. Sisomicin vs. Gentamicin (Gentamicin)

Pt.	Age	Sex	Days	mg/day	mg	Urine Cultures Pre	Post	Follow up	Serum Creatinine Pre Rx	Post Rx	Diagnosis	Surgery
D.G.	20	F	8	100	800	E.Coli	NG	NG	.8	1.0	Bladder Contusion	None
N.J.	66	M	8	180	1260	Pseud.	NG	NG	.8	1.0	Hydrocele	Hydrocelectomy
C.H.	87	M	6	180	1080	E.Coli	NG	NG	1.7	1.3	Ca.prostate	None
E.B.	65	M	6	180	1080	P.rettgeri Pseud.	NG	NG	1.9	2.5	B.P.H.	TURP
C.L.	76	M	7	120	840	Enterobact.	NG	E.Coli	1.6	1.8	Ca.prostate	None
R.W.	81	M	8	180	1440	Klebsiella	NG	NG	1.3	1.5	B.P.H.	TURP
T.R.	70	M	6	180	1080	P.Mirabl.	NG	NG	1.1	1.4	Ca.prostate	None
M.C.	33	M	7	180	1260	P.Mirabl.	NG	P.Mirabl	.8	.7	Urethral Stricture	None
I.H.	74	M	9	180	1620	P.Mirabl.	NG	NG	1.1	1.2	Renal Calculus	None
M.W.	56	F	7	240	1680	Pseud.	NG	NG	1.0	1.0	Renal Cyst	Exploration of (R) kidney
E.C.	69	M	9	240	2160	E.Coli	NG	NG	1.2	1.2	B.P.H.	TURP
R.E.	69	M	9	240	2160	Klebsiella	NG	NG	1.6	1.7	Ca.prostate	Radical perineal Prostatectomy
M.F.	67	M	7	240	1680	Pseud.	NG	NG	1.2	1.5	Urethral Stricture	Urethroplasty
A.E.	71	M	6	240	1440	Enterobact.	NG	NG	1.0	1.0	Ca.prostate	None
R.G.	78	M	7	80	560	E.Coli	NG	NG	2.6	1.7	B.P.H.	Retropubic Prostatectomy

Table IV. Sisomicin vs. Gentamicin (Gentamicin)

Pt.	Age	Sex	Days	Treatment mg/day	mg	Urine Cultures Pre	Post	Follow up	Serum Creatinine Pre Rx	Post Rx	Diagnosis	Surgery
R.T.	68	M	7	80	560	Klesiella	NG	NG	2.0	2.3	B.P.H. Urethral Stricture	TURP Internal Urethrotomy
E.W.	70	F	8	240	1920	E.Coli P.Mirabl.	NG	NG	1.5	2.5	CA. kidney	Radical nephrectomy
J.M.	51	M	8	240	1920	Klebsiella	NG	NG	2.3	2.2	Periurethral Abscess	Incision & Drainage of Periurethral Abscess
L.S.	69	F	8	240	1920	P.Mirabi.	NG	NG	.8	.8	Bladder Tumor	None
L.O.	42	F	7	240	1680	Klebsiella	NG	P.rettgeri	1.5	1.2	Interstitial Cystitis	Uretero-ileo-ceco cystoscopy

reinfections in the 20 patients treated with gentamicin and two
followup reinfections in the 23 receiving sisomicin. This
difference is not statistically significant.

No apparent side effects developed in any of the studies.
Sixty-eight patients in the three studies received sisomicin.
Intramuscular injection was tolerated well in all cases. There
was no evidence of allergic manifestations, hepatic or hematopoetic
toxicity. There were five instances of transient rise in BUN or
creatinine during therapy. All these were mild and returned to
pre-treatment values following discontinuation of therapy.
Clinical tests of vestibular function and audiograms were
performed before, during and after treatment in all cases. In no
instance was a significant change in auditory function noted. The
20 patients treated with gentamicin were monitored for toxicity
in a similar fashion. In this group there were no cases of auditory
impairment and one instance of transient elevation in creatinine.

Sisomicin serum and urine levels were performed on most of
these patients and will be discussed in a future communication.
In general, serum concentrations one hour following sisomicin
injection, range between three and six mcg/ml. These concentrations were significantly above the MIC of sensitive infecting
organisms. Urinary concentrations, during the first eight hours
following injection, ranged between 12 and 120 mcg/ml. Again,
this is well above the MIC of sensitive organisms.

Sisomicin, a new aminoglycoside antibiotic, was utilized in
three studies. Sixty-eight patients with urinary tract infection
received sisomicin. Clinical efficacy was demonstrated for a
variety of organisms, including Enterobacteriaceae and Pseudomonas.
Toxicity was limited to 5 transient elevations in serum BUN or
creatinine. In our opinion sisomicin is as effective as gentamicin
in the treatment of urinary infections. Additionally, sisomicin
MIC's for sensitive infection organisms are often lower than for
gentamicin and in vitro studies indicate a greater effectiveness
against some Enterobacteriaceae and Pseudomonas.

From these studies, it appears that the potential VIII nerve
toxicity of sisomicin is no greater than gentamicin.

Bibliography

1. Hyams, P.J. et al. In vitro bactericidal effectiveness of four aminoglycoside antibiotics. Antimicrob. Ag. Chemother. 3: 87-94, 1973.

2. Levinson, M.E. and Kaye,D. In vitro comparison of four aminoglycoside antibiotics: sisomicin, gentamicin, tobramycin, and BB-K8. Antimicrob. Ag. Chemother. 5: 667-669, 1974.

3. O'Hara, K. et al. Enzymatic inactivation of a new aminoglycoside antibiotic, sisomicin, by resistant straws of Pseudomonas aeruginosa. Antimicrob. Ag. Chemother. 5:558-561, 1974.

4. Waite, J.A. et al. Comparative Activity of sisomicin, gentamicin, kanamycin, and tobramycin. Antimicrob. Ag. Chemother. 2:431-437, 1972.

PARENTERAL SISOMICIN FOR SURGICAL INFECTIONS

H.H. Stone, L.D. Kolb, and C.E. Geheber

Department of Surgery
Emory University School of Medicine
69 Butler St., SE, Atlanta, Georgia 30303, U.S.A.

Sisomicin, a newly developed aminoglycoside with properties similar to those of gentamicin and tobramycin, recently became available for clinical investigation (3). Initial studies demonstrated it to be highly effective in the treatment of urinary, pulmonary, and selective bacteremic infections due to gram-negative bacilli; yet in few patients with peritonitis, burn infection, or other types of wound sepsis has the antibiotic been evaluated (3). Accordingly, a clinical study of sisomicin in the management of gram-negative surgical infections was undertaken.

PROCEDURES

From 1 January 1974 through 31 July 1974, all patients admitted with or developing gram-negative sepsis on the Trauma, Burn and Pediatric Surgical Services of Grady Memorial Hospital were given sisomicin as the sole therapeutic antimicrobial agent. Clinical findings, course, response to therapy, and complications were carefully recorded. Special note was made of type of infection and establishment of drainage in relationship to success of treatment.

Generally, sisomicin dosage was 1 mg/kg body weight given every 8 hours either intravenously or intramuscularly. Antibiotic concentrations in the blood were determined at 0, 2, and 6 hours twice weekly by well diffusion techniques (5). Similar biologic methods were used to measure urinary excretion.

Both aerobic and anaerobic cultures were taken of the focus responsible for the infection. In particular, aerobes were isolated and speciated by routine laboratory procedures, while antibiotic

389

sensitivities of such isolates were tested to sisomicin and comparable antimicrobial drugs according to disc (1) and tube dilution
(2) methods.

Patient hospital course was closely monitored, not only to
document the antimicrobial benefit of sisomicin, but also to detect
any adverse response — ototoxicity by audiograms (cochlear division)
and electronystagmograms (vestibular division) prior to, during, and
after therapy (4); nephrotoxicity by frequent urine analysis, blood
urea nitrogen, serum creatinine, and creatinine clearance; hepato-
toxicity by means of repeated liver function tests; and bone marrow
injury by initial and then weekly blood counts and smears.

RESULTS

During the seven month period of study, 110 hospitalized
patients received parenteral sisomicin for the treatment of established surgical infection. Average age was 35.7 years, with a range
of 1 to 89. There were 87 blacks and 23 whites, 71 males and 39
females. The majority were cases with some component of peritonitis — generalized, localized into an intra-abdominal abscess, or
primarily of the biliary tract (Table 1). Another large group had
wound sepsis, not evolving as a postoperative complication, but
developing because of a significant injury or thermal burn.

Seriousness of the infection was characterized by the fact that
half of the patients had temperatures in excess of $39^{\circ}C$, a third had
leukocytosis greater than $15,000/mm^3$, and a sixth were hypotensive.
Indeed, three patients were hypothermic, five had white blood counts
less than $5,000/mm^3$, and two were in frank septic shock. Based on
these three parameters — temperature, leukocytosis, and blood
pressure — the patient's condition was critical in 42, serious in
47, and fair in 21.

Dose, Distribution, and Excretion

Although the goal of antibiotic therapy had been set at 1 mg/
kg/8 hours, doses ranged from 0.6 mg to 1.7 mg/kg/8 hours on account
of severity of infection, errors in calculation, and variations required by impairment in renal function. Intravenous administration
over a 5 to 30 minute period gave serum levels that averaged 6 mcg/
ml at 15 minutes, fell to 4 mcg/ml by 1 hour, and equalled the 3
mcg/ml average from intramuscular injection at 3 hours. By the
sixth to eighth hour, serum concentrations of antibiotic were 1 mcg/
ml or less, irrespective as to mode of administration. The urinary
excretion of sisomicin was reflected in its serum half-life of 2
hours and its almost total excretion by glomerular filtration. By

6 hours, 68% of administered sisomicin had been excreted in the urine; 87% by 12 hours.

Bacteriology

In 11 of the patients, no growth was noted from what appeared to be the responsible site of infection. Nevertheless, 197 pathogenic bacteria were isolated from the remaining 99 cultures. There were 146 gram-negative rods, 23 gram-positive cocci, and 28 other species with known resistance to aminoglycoside antibiotics.

Disc and tube dilution testing for antibiotic sensitivities of the 169 pathogens potentially susceptible to sisomicin revealed a superior response to sisomicin over all other comparable antimicrobial agents. Such was true for both likelihood of susceptibility, i.e., disc testing (Table 2), as well as degree of sensitivity, i.e., tube dilution (Table 3).

Clinical Results

The overall clinical response to sisomicin was excellent in that 92 patients had their infection eradicated and another 11 demonstrated significant improvement (Table 1). The 7 deaths produced a mortality of 6%, quite low considering the seriousness of the infections treated. Of these deaths, 3 were due to antibiotic failure — mixed flora pneumonia, Pseudomonas burn sepsis, and gas gangrene. Uncontrolled hemorrhage caused another 2 deaths when poorly drained abscesses suddenly eroded into adjacent major vessels. The final 2 deaths were the result of massive pulmonary embolism and pre-existant anuric renal failure complicating prior hemorrhagic shock.

TABLE 1

DISEASE CATEGORIES AND RESPONSE TO SISOMICIN THERAPY

	Well	Improved	Died	Total
Gen. Peritonitis	56	3	4	63
Abd. Abscess	16	4	1	21
Biliary	5	–	1	6
Burns	1	2	1	4
Wounds	4	1	–	5
Pneumonia	2	–	–	2
Miscellaneous	8	1	–	9
TOTAL	92	11	7	110

TABLE 2

DISC SENSITIVITIES OF BACTERIAL ISOLATES

| | ISOLATES | PERCENT SENSITIVE (mcg) | | | | | |
		SIS 10	TOB 10	GEN 10	CAR 50	KEF 30	KAN 30
E. coli	88	100	99	99	90	43	82
Kleb-Entero	24	100	100	100	33	38	88
Ps. aerug.	19	100	95	95	79	0	0
Proteus sp.	15	93	93	93	60	60	80
Staph. aureus	8	100	88	100	88	100	-
Enterococcus	15	27	13	80	100	0	-

Patient response was obviously dependent upon seriousness of the infection. However, equally critical was the establishment of drainage of the septic focus. The mortality was only 4% if the infection drained as a result of wound disruption, operation, or spontaneous erosion. Without such drainage, the mortality rate was more than double, i.e., 10%.

Complications

There were no instances of ototoxicity, nor did any new pathogens evolve. Nevertheless, 2 patients did develop mild and eventually reversible nephrotoxicity. In both, an episode of hypovolemia preceded the renal injury and may well alone have accounted for subsequent impairment in renal function.

COMMENT

The present study has demonstrated a significant benefit from parenteral sisomicin in the control of surgical infections due to gram-negative bacteria. However, complete eradication of sepsis in such patients is usually dependent upon eventual debridement and/or drainage of the infectious process (4). Irrespective of the antibiotic regimen chosen and the dosage give, the definitive therapy provided by establishment or improvement in surgical drainage is of utmost importance.

Aminoglycosides are ideal antimicrobial agents for the treatment of peritonitis and burn wound sepsis (4). Properly administered according to existing renal function, risks of ototoxicity (both cochlear and vestibular) are minimal. Likewise, delay in

TABLE 3

TUBE DILUTION SENSITIVITIES OF BACTERIAL ISOLATES

	ISOLATES	AV. MIN. INHIB. CONC. (mcg/ml)				
		SIS	TOB	GEN	KEF	KAN
E. coli	88	3.4	7.3	6.6	19.8	19.1
Kleb-Entero	24	1.2	3.1	3.0	16.6	10.6
Ps. aerug.	19	0.2	0.4	0.8	48.0	41.5
Proteus sp.	15	6.9	11.2	8.5	15.6	22.2
Staph Aureus	8	0.0	2.1	0.0	1.1	4.8
Enterococcus	15	37.5	39.4	27.0	18.1	46.4

aminoglycoside therapy until hypovolemia has been corrected and the patient is out of shock is another consideration that, when feasible, consistently reduces the incidence of nephrotoxicity.

Overall, sisomicin has appeared to be the most reliably effective aminoglycoside yet tested. Safety with its use, as for similar antibiotics, is dependent more on the knowledge and skill of the prescribing physician, rather than any inherent toxicity of the drug alone.

SUMMARY

Sisomicin, a new aminoglycoside, was administered parenterally to 110 surgical patients, primarily with peritoneal and various wound infections. The usual dose was 1 mg/kg body weight/8 hours, adjusted to serum creatinine levels. Patients were also monitored for toxicity to inner ear, kidneys, bone marrow, and liver.

Success of antibiotic therapy was dependent upon eventual establishment of surgical drainage. Bacteriologic analysis revealed a predominance of gram-negative rods, with greatest susceptibility to sisomicin on comparison to other antibiotics by disc and tube dilution methods. No drug toxicity was noted, that is except for possible contribution to already developing ischemic renal damage in 2 patients.

REFERENCES

1. Bauer, A.W., Kirby, W.M.M., Sherris, J.D., and Tuck, M.: Antibiotic Susceptibility Testing by a Standardized Single Disc Method. Amer. J. Clin. Path. 45:493, 1966.

2. Gavin, T.L., and Town, M.A.: A Microdilution Method for Anti-
         biotic Susceptibility Testing: An Evaluation. Amer. J.
         Clin. Path.,53:880, 1970.

3. Schering Corporation: Investigators Manual, Bloomfield, 1974.

4. Stone, H.H., Kolb, L.D., Geheber, C.E., and Currie, C.A.:
         Treatment of Surgical Infections with Tobramycin. Amer.
         Surg.,41:301, 1974.

5. Winters, R.E., Litwack, K.D., and Hewitt, W.L.: Relation
         Between Dose and Levels of Gentamicin in Blood. J.
         Infect. Dis., 124:590, 1971.

CLINICAL TRIAL OF SISOMYCIN: EVALUATION OF TWO DIFFERENT DOSAGES

M. Jonsson, E. Bengtsson, S. Jonsson, I. Julander and
G. Tunevall

Roslagstull Hospital; Karolinska Institute; University of Lund
Roslagstull; Stockholm; Lund., Sweden

INTRODUCTION

Sisomicin is a new aminoglycoside antibiotic structurally related to gentamicin. From data in the literature it is known that the antimicrobial activity of sisomicin is similar to that of gentamicin. However, sisomicin has been reported to have advantageous characteristics, e.g. higher activity against certain bacterial species, effectivity against strains resistant to gentamicin and also a higher bactericidal effect in the presence of serum. These data qualified the drug for a clinical trial. The main purpose of the study was to investigate the pharmacokinetics at two different dose regimens in patients with normal and impaired renal function.

MATERIALS AND METHODS

The material studied comprised 25 in-patients, aged between 26 and 90 years. They had no history of renal or otological diseases, and they had not taken any nephro- or ototoxic drugs during 3 months prior to therapy. Thorough laboratory investigations were performed before the start of therapy and then repeated during and at the end of therapy and in addition 2 weeks later. The investigations comprised complete blood cell counts, ESR, routine liver and uring analysis. Renal function was estimated by measuring serum creatinine and creatinine clearance. Audiograms were carried out and the vestibular function was evauluated at the beginning, during, at the end of treatment and also 2-3 weeks later. Similarly, blood and specimens from nose, throat, urine and other suspect infectious foci were repeatedly taken

and bacteria isolated were identified by standard bacteriological methods.
The MICs of the bacterial strains were determined by the paper disc method,
oridinarily used for routine test. A series of disc tests in parallel with serial
agar dilution tests was also performed on gram-negative strains in order to
obtain a provisional regression line.

Sisomicin concentrations were measured in two ways in two laboratories
600 km apart: at the Department of Bacteriology of Serafimerlasarettet in
Stockholm a microbiological method was applied, mainly a modification of
that one described by Sabath and co-workers using B.subtilis. Sera reported
to contain penicillin were treated with penicillinase. At the Department of
Medical Microbiology in Lund the sisomicin levels were measured with a
newly developed radioimmuno-assay technique. It is based upon an immunological dross-reactivity between sisomicin and gentamicin and upon the use
of a conjugate of gentamicin and human serum albumin labelled with 125
iodine as a tracer and also based upon the use of a suspension of killed protein
A-containing staphylococci as a separation reagent.

It happens that we have examined a rather heterogenous group of patients.
There is a great variation as to age, severity and type of infection and also
concerning renal function, although serum creatinine was below 1.5 mg/ml
in all patients.

Sisomicin was given at two different dosage levels in two consecutive
patient groups. The first patient group was treated at a level of 1.5 mg/kg
a day. This relatively low dosage was chosen because of indications of
sisomicin being more effective but also slightly more toxic than gentamicin.
After having gained experience from 11 patients we had a basis for doubling
the dosage to 3 mg/kg a day.

Figure 1 : 14 patients were   given 1.5 mg/kg of the drug.
6 patients had septicemia, but the causative agent could only be found in
four. Three patients suffered from pulmonary infections. Pyelonephritis
and skin infection was the diagnosis in the other cases. The causative agents
found are listed to the right. In patients no. 5,6,8,10 and 11, creatinine
clearance was decreased to about half the normal level.

Fig.2:11 patients were given 3 mg/kg. Also in this group the most
frequent diagnosis was septicemia (6 patients). Three patients suffered from
urinary tract infection, 3 patients had skin infections, one had oseitis, and
one bronchopneumonia. Out of these patients all except the first five had
impaired renal function.

The total patient material was divided into 5 groups. 2 groups,

Figure 1.   Data on 11 patients given sisomicin 1.5 mg/kg body weight

Pat. No.	Age years	Sex	Diagnosis	Microorganism
1	26	F	Septichaemia suspecta	-
2	26	F	Septicaemia with subphrenic liver abscesses	S.aureus, Str.faecalis, Clostridia, coliforms
3	27	F	Empyema pulm. bilat.	S.aureus
4	35	M	Septichaemia with septic liver metastases	Peptostreptococcus micros, Streptococcus intermedius
5	63	F	Pyelonephritis acuta	E.coli
6	64	M	Bronchopneumonia	-
7	65	M	Septichaemia	β-haemolytic streptococci, not group A, Bacteroides fragalis
8	67	F	Septichaemia	P.mirabilis
9	69	F	Furunculosis	S.aureus
10	74	M	Bronchopneumonia	-
11	79	M	Septichaemia suspecta	-

Figure 2.   Data on 14 patients, given sisomicin 3.0 mg/kg body weight

Pat. No.	Age years	Sex	Diagnosis	Microorganism
1	30	M	Osteitis	S.aureus
2	31	F	Septichaemia, c.arthritis	-
3	45	M	Erysipelas	β-haemolytic streptococci, Group A
4	45	M	Erysipelas	β-haemolytic streptococci, Group A
5	50	M	Pyelonephritis acuta	-
6	63	M	Septichaemia Bronchopneumonia	α-haemolytic streptococci H. influenzae
7	67	M	Septichaemia suspecta	-
8	73	M	Septichaemia	Fusibacterium aquatilis Propriumbacterium acne
9	73	M	Bronchopneumonia	-
10	79	M	Abscessus regio colli	Peptostreptococcus products
11	82	M	Urinary tract infection	-
12	84	F	Septichaemia suspecta	-
13	86	M	Urinary Tract Infection	Str.faecalis
14	90	F	Septichaemia	E.coli

receiving 1.5 mg/kg of sisomicin a day: one group with normal renal function and the other with impaired. Three groups received 3 mg/kg a day: one with normal renal function, one with creatinine clearance 61-74 and the last one with clearance 31-38 ml/min.

All patients received sisomicin by intramuscular injection every 8 hours for between 2 and 11 days, on the average for 7 days. Twenty patients were concomitantly treated with benzylpenicillin or ampicillin intravenously. Serum samples for sisomicin determination were obtained immediately before and at 0.5, 1, 1.5, 2,4,6, and 8 hours after the first weekday's morning injection, then on two occasions during therapy further samples were obtained before the morning dose and also 2 and 6 hours later (see figure 3).

Initial data analysis was based on the results of the microbiological assay. All groups gave maximum serum levels half to one hour after injection, indicating rapid absorption from the intramuscular sites. If we consider only the patients with normal renal function: with the lower dose mean peak level of 2.3 µg/ml was obtained at 1 hour. A mean serum concentration greater than 1 µg/ml was maintained for about 2.5 hours, mean serum concentration at 2 and 4 hours being 1.3 and less than 0.5 µg/ml, respectively. The serum half-life was 120 min.

After administration of 3 mg/kg the mean peak level of 2.9 µg/ml occurred at half hour. Mean serum concentrations at 2,4 and 5 hours were 2, 0.65, and less than 0.5 µg/ml respectively.

In patients with moderately impaired renal function, i.e. creatinine clearance ranging between 41 and 74, serum half-life was about 3 hours and in patients with highly impaired renal function, i.e. clearance about 30 ml/min half-life was 5 hours. Measurable levels of the drug 8 hours after administration was found in this group only.

On the bases of radio-immunoassay data it can be seen there is good agreement in the overall results between the two assay techniques. The correlation coefficient was calculated to 0.8, may be acceptable when two laboratories are each setting up a new technique.

Which dose regimen is to be preferred? We performed in vitro tests of sensitivity of 398 clinical isolates obtained at the Department of Infectious Diseases in Stockholm 1975 (figure 4). It includes the strains isolated from the patients we are discussing. We compared sisomicin, gentamicin, kanamycin, and streptomycin. All strains of E.coli were sensitive to 2 µg/ml or less of sisomicin. There was no significant difference in the activity of

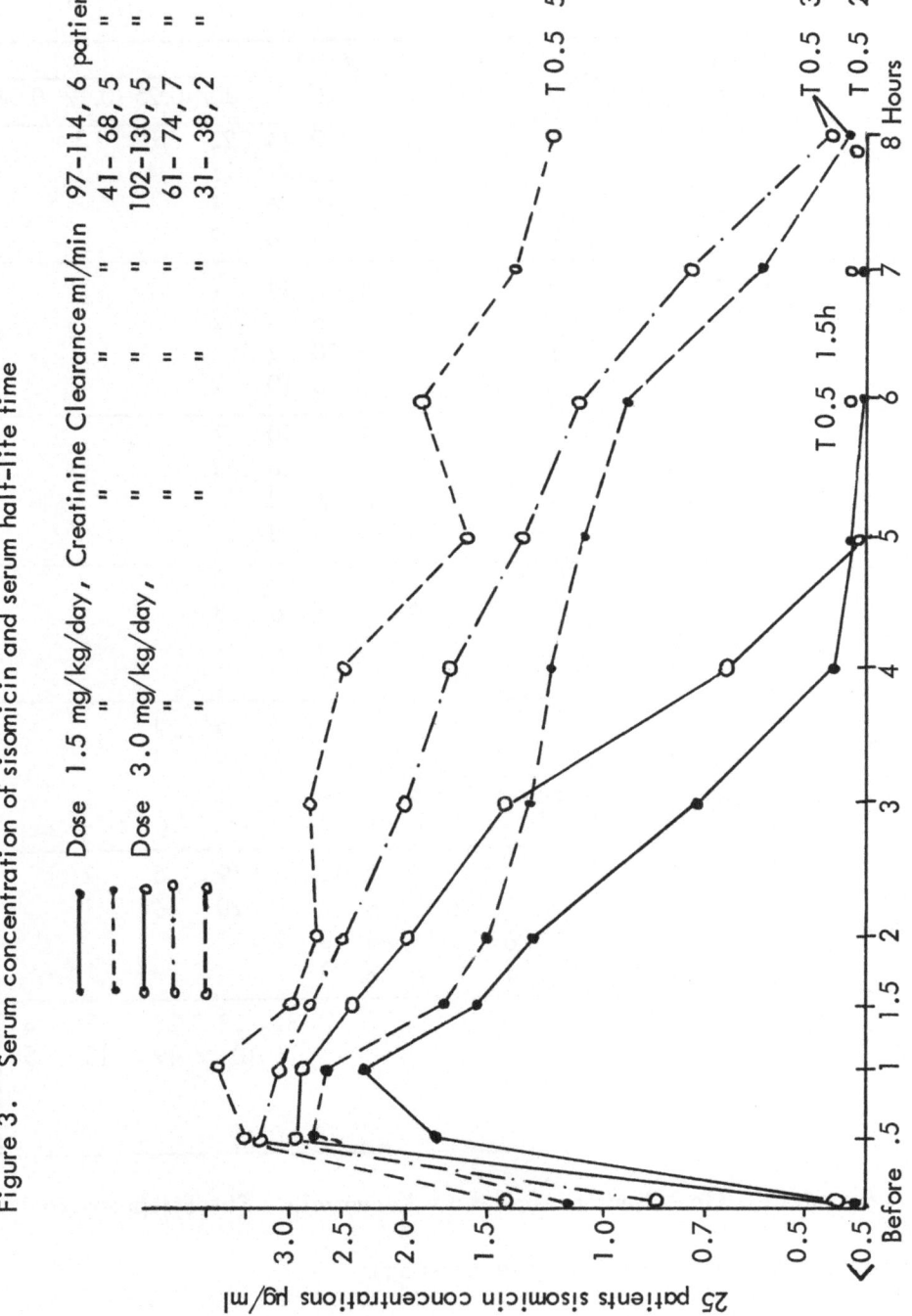

Figure 3.   Serum concentration of sisomicin and serum half-life time

Figure 4.   398 clinical isolates from Roslagstull Hospital 1975*

Strains	Anti-biotic	µg/ml											
		>125	64	32	16	8	4	2	1	0.5	0.25	0.12	0.06
E. coli 60	Si							10	14	23	10	3	
	Ge						2	11	27	16	4		
	Ka	2	3	3	5	7	17	16	6	1			
	St			1	1	4	21	25	6	2			
Enterobacter 28	Si					1	4	7	14	1	1		
	Ge					1	2	8	15	2			
	Ka	4	1	1			10	10	2				
	St		1			1	6	8	10	2			
Klebsiella 24	Si							2	5	10	7		
	Ge					1	3	9	8	3			
	Ka			1	1	8	6	6	2				
	St					5	10	6	3				
Proteus mirabillis 26	Si					2	5	9	6	3	1		
	Ge					2	7	8	6	3			
	Ka	3	1		1	8	5	5	3				
	St				1	4	11	7	2	1			
Proteus (indole +) 20	Si						1	6	7	5	1		
	Ge					2	2	5	6	4	1		
	Ka		2				3	8	4	2	1		
	St				1	4	8	4	3				
Pseudomonas aeruginosa 54	Si					1	2	11	14	19	5	2	
	Ge			1	2	3	6	6	9	20	6	1	
	Ka	8	3	6	11	11	4	8	2	1			
	St	26	10	4	5	4	3	2					
St. aureus 186	Si							7	82	69	23	2	3
	Ge								16	101	49	15	5
	Ka												
	St												

Si = Sisomicin   Ge = Gentamicin   Ka = Kanamycin   St = Streptomycin

* Disc tests on petone-free 5% horse blood agar

siso- and gentamicin against E.coli.   In the Enterobacter/Klebsiella group
almost all 52 isolates were sensitive to 4 μg/ml or less of sisomicin and gentamicin.   Among strains of P.mirabilis there was no significant difference in
the effectiveness of the different aminoglycosides except for kanamycin.
Against indole-positive proteus strains sisomicin was the most active drug with
MIC 2 μg/ml or less.   Also P.aeruginosa strains isolated were more sensitive
to sisomicin than to the other aminoglycosides.   We could not find any
difference between siso- and gentamicin in effectiveness against strains of
S.aureus; almost all strains were sensitive to 1 μg/ml or less.

So, on the basis of our serum concentration analyses, the sensitivity testings
and also information as to how long serum concentration should exceed MIC
to obtain cure we have taken the opinion that a dosage of 3 mg/kg is safe in
patients with normal renal function.

What about the side-effects seen at the different doses?   Sisomicin, like
other aminoglycosides, is potentially oto- and nephrotoxic; it is not possible
to predict the occurrence of these side-effects.   During therapy we noticed
transient increase of serum creatinine beyond the upper normal limit in 3 out
of 25 patients.   However, already initially all 3 had creatinine clearance
values lower than 67.   Two of these 3 patients were given 1.5 and the third
patient, 3 mg sisomicin per kg.   Ototoxic side-effects were seen in 3 out of
25 patients.   All 3 received 3 mg/kg body weight.   Only one patient had
impaired renal function.   Very slightly impaired hearing was noticed after
therapy in two of them and in the third the vestibular function was damaged.
Other side-effects as measured by the other laboratory parameters were not
noticed.

CONCLUSION

1. Sisomicin is a drug more efficient in vitro against indole-positive
proteus and P.aeruginosa strains than gentamicin;
2. A dosage regimen of 3 mg/kg body weight is to be recommended in
patients with normal renal function;
3. In patients with impaired renal function the dose must be based upon
creatinine clearance and serum concentrations of the drug.

IN VIVO ACTIVITY OF SISOMICIN IN MICE

SCHEER, M.

BAYER AG, Institute for Medical Microbiology

D-56 Wuppertal-1 / West Germany, Box 130105

The in vivo antibacterial activity of sisomicin was
demonstrated by its ability to protect mice from death
following an intraperitoneal infection by a lethal
dose of pathogenic bacteria (Klebsiella pneumoniae,
Pseudomonas aeruginosa, Proteus spp., E. coli,
Serratia marcescens, Staphylococcus aureus. The
therapeutic activity was compared to that of gentamicin.
The results indicate, that sisomicin is on average
2 - 3 times more effective in vivo than gentamicin.

In 1970 Weinstein et al. described a new broad-
spectrum aminoglycoside antibiotic which was later
named sisomicin. In comparison to gentamicin, sisomicin has better in vitro activity against a number
of bacterial strains and a higher potency in infected
animals (Weinstein et al. 1970; Waitz et al. 1970).

The purpose of this study was to compare, under
identical conditions, the in vivo effectiveness of
sisomicin and gentamicin against bacterial infections
in mice.

MATERIALS AND METHODS

For protection tests in mice, we used sisomicin- and
gentamicin-sulfate. Drug solutions were prepared in
sterile saline buffer. Comparisons were made in terms
of base of activity.

The animals used were female white CF-1 mice weighing
from 20 to 22 g. Before treatment the test animals
had been infected with the appropriate bacterial
strains. Per strain 8 different dosages were tested
in 10 animals each. Each trial was repeated 6 times
at least, so that each bacterial strain was tested
in 480 mice. Every trial was carried out with 10
control-animals each which were infected but not
treated.

The infection was induced intraperitoneally in
a volume of 0,25 ml with approximately 10^7 organisms/
mouse. The infections were carried out with 3 strains
each of E. coli, Proteus spp., Klebsiella pneumoniae,
Serratia marcescens, Pseudomonas aeruginosa and
Staphylococcus aureus. The treatment was administered
as a single subcutaneous dose at the time of infection.
Drug was administered in a volume of 0,5 ml per animal.
Untreated infected controls generally died within
24 hours after infection.

The survival rates on the first and the third
days after infection/treatment were used for the
statistical evaluation of the PD_{50} and the PD_{95}
(protective dose in 50 % and 95 % of mice). Minimal
inhibitory concentrations (MIC) were determined by
serial twofold dilution technique in Mueller-Hinton
broth.

RESULTS AND DISCUSSION

Table 1 shows the PD_{50}- and PD_{95}-values in terms of
mg/kg of the two antibiotics in direct comparison
against 18 bacterial infections, based on surviving
mice 24 hours after infection/treatment. In all cases
sisomicin had a better therapeutic effect than gentamicin. This was most significant against Pseudomonas
aeruginosa and less significant against Serratia marcescens. In addition MIC-values of the infecting
organisms are listed in this table. Against 13 of 18
strains sisomicin and gentamicin have the same in
vitro activity; in 3 cases the MIC-value of sisomicin
is lower, in 2 cases it is lower for gentamicin.

It is clear that a correlation between sensitivity in vitro and efficacy in vivo does not always
exist.

Table 1
Comparative in vivo Activity of Sisomicin
and Gentamicin

(protection test in mice)
(statistical evaluation on day 1)

Infecting organism	Sisomicin MIC mcg/ml	Sisomicin PD$_{50}$ mg/kg	Sisomicin PD$_{95}$ mg/kg	Gentamicin MIC mcg/ml	Gentamicin PD$_{50}$ mg/kg	Gentamicin PD$_{95}$ mg/kg
E. coli 774	0,25	0,12	0,33	0,25	0,24	0,74
E. coli 6922	0,25	0,15	0,34	0,25	0,27	0,87
E. coli C165	0,5	0,22	0,58	0,5	0,42	1,06
Prot.mir. 4	2,0	0,57	1,47	2,0	0,97	3,07
Prot.mir. 8	2,0	0,43	1,74	2,0	1,02	3,69
Prot.morg.932	0,25	0,42	0,98	0,25	0,90	2,05
Klebs. 70	0,06	0,11	0,21	0,12	0,24	0,61
Klebs. 63	0,06	0,15	0,27	0,12	0,32	0,58
Klebs. 8085	0,06	0,13	0,40	0,06	0,26	1,31
Serratia 6	0,5	0,50	1,93	0,5	0,65	1,95
Serratia 4	1,0	0,60	1,69	0,25	0,92	4,17
Serratia 2	0,5	0,45	1,68	0,25	0,53	1,89
Psdm. 08	0,5	1,92	5,00	0,5	7,85	19,05
Psdm. 87	0,12	4,86	14,41	0,25	20,93	42,67
Psdm. W	0,25	2,57	6,20	0,25	5,96	21,55
Staph. 133	0,06	0,42	1,03	0,06	0,98	3,10
Staph. 860	0,06	0,48	1,18	0,06	1,04	3,90
Staph. 873	0,06	0,41	1,26	0,06	0,99	3,52

In table 2 dosages are given which are necessary to protect 50 or 95 % of the animals, based on survivors 3 days after infection/treatment. With 3 exceptions, it is obvious that sisomicin has a better efficacy also on the third day.

A comparison between the PD$_{50}$- and the PD$_{95}$-values of the first and the third day shows, that the protective dosages on the third day are slightly higher than those of the first day. In some cases however this dose has to be doubled or tripled.

Table 2
Comparative in vivo Activity of Sisomicin
and Gentamicin

(protection test in mice)
(statistical evaluation on day 3)

Infecting organism	Sisomicin		Gentamicin	
	PD_{50} mg/kg	PD_{95} mg/kg	PD_{50} mg/kg	PD_{95} mg/kg
E. coli 774	0,16	0,45	0,29	0,77
E. coli 6922	0,18	0,38	0,33	0,93
E. coli C165	0,26	0,61	0,45	1,16
Prot.mir. 4	0,83	1,79	1,53	3,97
Prot.mir. 8	1,38	5,83	1,59	3,38
Prot.morg.932	0,55	1,44	1,15	3,10
Klebs. 70	0,20	0,42	0,46	0,82
Klebs. 63	0,18	0,34	0,40	0,74
Klebs. 8085	0,21	0,53	0,56	1,77
Serratia 6	0,78	2,14	1,01	2,97
Serratia 4	1,51	5,65	2,06	6,93
Serratia 2	1,20	3,18	1,27	2,54
Psdm. 08	3,10	7,23	14,08	25,98
Psdm. 87	9,02	51,06	28,33	56,95
Psdm. W	5,16	20,38	12,11	44,61
Staph. 133	0,51	1,24	1,08	3,62
Staph. 860	0,56	1,37	1,21	4,51
Staph. 873	0,65	1,93	1,13	3,99

Table 3 shows the relative potency of sisomicin and gentamicin. In most cases it is obvious that sisomicin is superior to gentamicin. The larger the relative activity value, the greater the activity of sisomicin. The PD_{50}-values of Serratia marcescens show, that the efficacy of sisomicin is only one and a half times better. Against E. coli, Proteus spp., Klebsiella pneumoniae and Staphylococcus aureus the dose of gentamicin has to be doubled to reach the same effect as with sisomicin. Against Pseudomonas aeruginosa sisomicin is up to four and a half times more active than gentamicin.

With the PD_{95}-values the same trend is demonstrated. In 2 cases, against Serratia marcescens 2 and Proteus mirabilis 8, gentamicin is more efficient. Against most of the strains however sisomicin is 2 - 3 times more effective than gentamicin. The calculation of the mean of all PD_{50}- and PD_{95}-values shows that sisomicin is superior to gentamicin by a factor 2.1 to 2.7.

Table 3
In vivo Activity Relative to Gentamicin

| | Gentamicin PD_{50} | | Gentamicin PD_{95} | |
| | Sisomicin PD_{50} | | Sisomicin PD_{95} | |
	Day 1	Day 3	Day 1	Day 3
E. coli 774	2,0	1,8	2,2	1,7
E. coli 6922	1,8	1,8	2,6	2,4
E. coli C165	1,9	1,7	1,8	1,9
Proteus mir. 4	1,7	1,8	2,1	2,2
Proteus mir. 8	2,4	1,2	2,1	0,6
Proteus morg. 932	2,1	2,1	4,9	2,2
Klebsiella 70	2,2	2,3	2,9	2,0
Klebsiella 63	2,1	2,2	2,1	2,2
Klebsiella 8085	2,0	2,7	3,3	3,3
Serratia 6	1,3	1,3	1,0	1,4
Serratia 4	1,5	1,4	2,5	1,2
Serratia 2	1,2	1,1	1,1	0,8
Psdm. aerug. 08	4,1	4,5	3,8	3,6
Psdm. aerug. 87	4,3	3,1	3,0	1,1
Psdm. aerug. W	2,3	2,3	3,5	2,2
Staph. aureus 133	2,3	2,1	3,0	2,9
Staph. aureus 860	2,2	2,2	3,3	3,3
Staph. aureus 873	2,4	1,7	2,8	2,1
$\bar{x}$	2,2	2,1	2,7	2,1

The reason that sisomicin is more effective in the protection tests in mice is not yet known. Generally strains were used for infections which had the same MIC-values for sisomicin and gentamicin (see table 1). Therefore greater in vitro activity does not explain the better in vivo activity of sisomicin.

It is possible that the better activity of sisomicin in vivo may be related to some difference in the
pharmacokinetics of two substances.

It is evident from these studies that sisomicin
is clearly superior to gentamicin against bacterial
infections in mice.

How well these results correlate with the results
of the treatments to human infections one has to await
the completion of clinical studies in man.

References:

Waitz, J.A., Moss, E.L., Oden, E.M. and Weinstein,
M.J. (1970)
J. Antibiotics 23, 559

Weinstein, M.J., Marquez, J.A., Testa, R.T., Wagman,
G.H., Oden, E.M. and Waitz, J.A. (1970)
J. Antibiotics 23, 551

NEW DATA ON PHARMACOLOGY OF GENTAMYCIN

Zhelyazkov, D., Ivanova, K., Gueorguiev, N., Marinova, R., Beltcheva, A., Mangurova, M. and Temnyalov, N.

Department of Pharmacology, Medical Faculty
Varna, Bulgaria

During the last eight years we have carried out a detailed study of the pharmacology and toxicology of gentamycin, produced in Bulgaria. It included investigations of the acute, subacute and chronic toxicity of the antibiotic; observations on the sex and species differences in its toxicology; comparison of its acute toxicity with those of the other aminoglycoside antibiotics (8, 9); study of its influence on the normal microbial flora of the macro-organism (6), of its relation to the mineral metabolism (5); elucidation of its action on the blood pressure (2), intestinal smooth musculature (2), myoneural synapses of the skeletal muscles (3), as well as its direct effect on the striated musculature and muscle fatigue (7) and many others.

As a result of this work much new data has been accumulated on the pharmacology and toxicology of gentamycin, some of which are summarised in the present paper.

Using the method of potentiometric titration (4) we have studied the pKa - ionisation constants of the antibiotic, that are, as is well known, one of the most important parameters, determining its kynetics. In connection with that it is necessary to remember that gentamycin belongs to the group of aminoglycoside antibiotics and represents a complex of three components - C_1, C_2 and C_{1a}. As can be seen in figure 1, its basic structure can be looked at as 1,3- disubstituted with amino sugar residues deoxystreptamin (14). The three antibiotic components differ from each other in the presence of one methyl group (C_2), two methyl groups (C_1) and by the lack of any methyl group (C_{1a}) in the structure of one of the aminosugar substituents (14, 18, 19). The gentamycin structure described determine its behaviour of poly-

Figure 1.   Gentamycin components (C_1, C_2 and C_{1a})

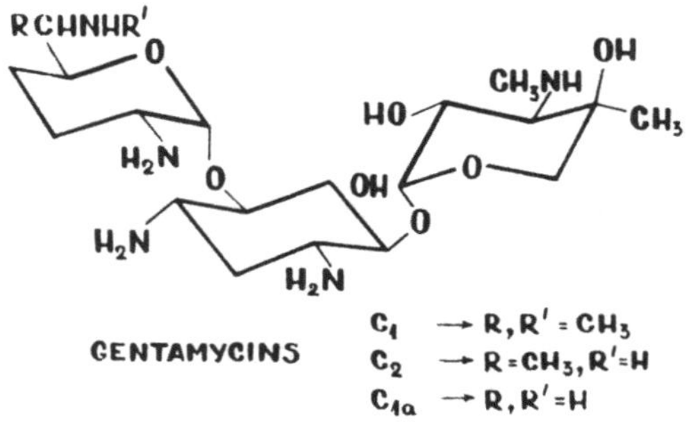

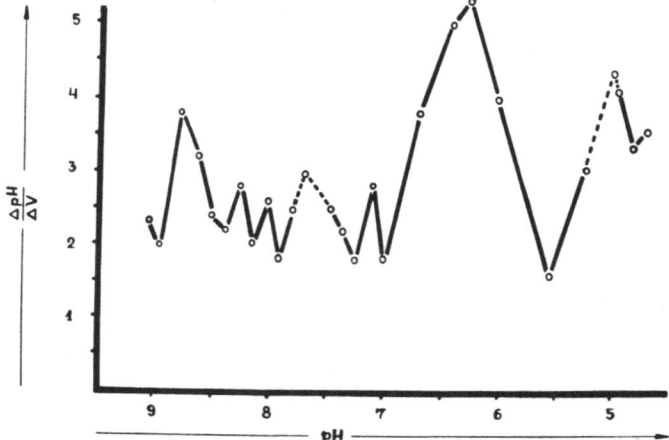

GENTAMYCINS $C_1 \rightarrow R, R' = CH_3$
               $C_2 \rightarrow R = CH_3, R' = H$
               $C_{1a} \rightarrow R, R' = H$

ion with a relatively high molecular weight.   This fact creates considerable difficulties in determination of the values of the antibiotic.

With a view to avoiding the deformation of the antibiotic molecular form the titration has been carried out in a medium with constant ionic force - potassium chloride saturated solution.   To determine the inflex points of the curve so obtained, a differential titration curve has been constructed (fig. 2). As it is seen it has two maximums, to which two pH values correspond, equal to 8.77 and 6.24 each.   Conforming with the gentamycin structure, the two pKa values - pKa_1 and pKa_2, found can be addressed respectively to the primary and secondary antibiotical amino groups (10).

The values established for the pKa_1 and pKa_2 of gentamycin give the possibility of explaining some essential aspects of its pharmacological

Figure 2. Potentiometric titration of gentamycin-base with 1 N hydrochloric acid

Table 1

MINIMUM INHIBITORY CONCENTRATIONS /MIC/ OF GENTAMYCIN /G/ AT DIFFERENT CONTENTS OF CALCIUM IONS IN NUTRIENT MEDIUM

№	BACTERIAL STRAIN	MEAT-PEPTONIC BROTH /LIQUID MEDIUM/		MEAT-PEPTONIC AGAR /SOLID MEDIUM/	
		WITHOUT ADDITION OF CALCIUM IONS	ADDITION OF CALCIUM IONS TO MIC OF G 100:1 μM	WITHOUT ADDITION OF CALCIUM IONS	ADDITION OF CALCIUM IONS TO MIC OF G 100:1 μM
1	2	3	4	5	6
1	PS.AERUG.24	3,6	10,2	17,2	28,6
2	PS.AERUG.III	4,8	10,0	15,4	29,8
3	PS.AERUG.355	1,8	9,3	12,0	19,2
4	B.COLI 231	2,8	3,0	12,0	12,2
5	B.COLI 256	3,0	3,4	12,0	12,0
6	B.PROTEUS 431	3,0	3,2	10,2	10,6
7	B.PROTEUS 261	25,0	26,2	30,2	30,4
8	SALM.ENTERIT.10	6,0	6,0	11,0	11,4
9	SCHIG.FLEX.1310	5,4	5,6	9,0	9,2
10	STAPH.AUREUS 21	0,8	0,8	0,8	0,8

characterisation such as very low resorbtion in gastro-intestinal tract and higher antimicrobial activity in the basic medium (11). It seems quite reasonable that the primary amino groups are responsible for the antimicrobial activity, which at that must be maximally ionized. The hypothesis discussed is supported by the data showing that the acetylation of the primary anti-biotic groups results in its activation (13, 16).

Our further investigations show that the nutrient medium, in which the micro-organisms are cultivated, is a factor that determines the Minimum Inhibitory Concentrations (MIC) of the antibiotic. As can be seen in Table 1. the MIC are always higher in solid nutrient medium (meat-peptonic agar) in comparison with those for the liquid nutrient medium (meat peptonic broth). The only exception observed concerns Staphylococcus aureus (strain 21).

On the other hand, the addition of calcium ions in the nutrient medium increases several times the gentamycin MIC only towards Pseudomonas strains, cultivated both in liquid and solid medium (see table 1). The MIC towards the other micro-organisms do not change significantly.

To the well known myoneural blocking action of gentamycin (12, 17) confirmed by us (4) our studies add new data, showing that the antibiotic also exerts a direct depressing influence on the skeletal musculature (fig. 3). Together with inhibition of myoneural synapses, this direct action of genta-mycin on the striated muscles explains its fatiguenic effect established by us is experiments with rats by the test "swimming till refuse", even in the cases when the antibiotic is administered in considerably small doses (7).

The finding (see fig. 3) that calcium ions successfully antagonise not only myoneural inhibition of gentamycin, but also its direct depressing effect

Figure 3. Direct effect of gentamycin on the muscle contraction and antagonistic action of calcium ions. From above: respiration;
contraction of m.gastrocnemius upon direct electrical stimulation

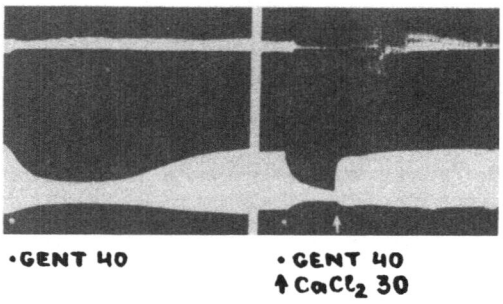

·GENT 40   · GENT 40
                        ↑CaCl₂ 30

on the skeletal muscles and fatiguenic action may be of importance for the use of the antibiotic in the therapeutic practice.

Further, our experiments on the histamine liberating properties of genta-mycin show (fig. 4) that the antibiotic provokes the strongest statistically significant release of histamine from the proximal parts of the small intestine, where this amine is stored in non-mast cell depots. At the same time its effect on the mast-cell stored histamine is insignificant. These data in the light of the concept for lack of connection between non-mast cell histamine liberation and allergic phenomena (15) lead to the conclusion that gentamycin has or has not slight allergogenic properties. On one hand, this conclusion has been confirmed by the administration of the antibiotic to patients with a marked polyallergy without any allergic manifestations and, on the other, on the strength of this conclusion gentamycin has been introduced by inhalation to many patients with chronic bronchitis, without any complications.

Finally, our experiments confirmed that gentamycin is deprived of epi-leptogenic and other exciting effects on the central nervous system. Based on the results just described, the antibiotic has been introduced directly into the brain of pateints with Escherichia coli encephalomyelitis, without any side effects.

In conclusion it can be said that the new data, discussed in this paper and concerning the pharmacological characterisation of gentamycin, enlarge the indications, augment the routes of administration and make more rational the utilisation of this unique antimicrobial agent.

Figure 4.   Liberation by gentamycin of mast-cell (ears) and non-mast cell (small intestine) stored histamine

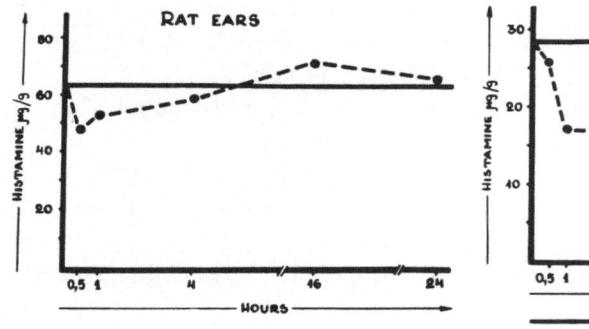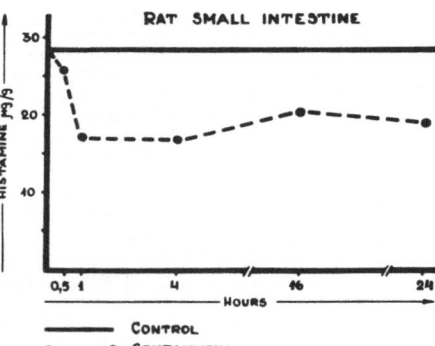

REFERENCES

1. Albert, A., Serjent, E. (1964). Konstanti ionizacii i kislot o snovanii (in Russian), Moscow.

2. Gueorguiev, N.M., Zhelyazkov, D.K., Beltcheva, A., Temnyalov, N., Mangurova, M. (1972). Symposium po Oleandomycin, Tetraolean i Gentamycin, Sofia. 5, 25-57.

3. Gueorguiev, N.M., Zhelyazkov, D.K., Temnyalov, N., Mangurova, M., Beltcheva, A. (1972). In: Gentamycin, p. 55. Ed. D.K. Zhelyazkov, Sofia.

4. Ivanova, K. (1973). V Nautchna sessia na Med. fac. - Varna, 12, 14-15.

5. Mangurova, M., Gueorguiev, N.M., Beltcheva, A., Temnyalov, N., Zhelyazkov, D.K., Yakimov, G. (1972). In: Gentamycin, p. 65, Ed. D.K. Zhelyazkov, Sofia.

6. Marinova, R., Temnyalov, N., Zhelyazkov, D.K., Gueorguiev, N.M., Beltcheva, A., Mangurova, M., Yakimov, G., Markov, D. (1972). In: Gentamycin, p. 33. Ed. D.K. Zhelyazkov, Sofia.

7. Temnyalov, N., Mangurova, M., Beltcheva, A., Gueorguiev, N.M., Zhelyazkov, D.K. (1972). Symposium po Oleandomycin, Tetraolean i gentamycin, Sofia, 5, 25-27

8. Zhelyazkov, D.K., Gueorguiev, N.M., Belthceva, A., Mangurova, M., Temnyalov, N., Yakimov, G.I., Markov, D (1971). VIIIth International Congress of Chemotherapy, Prague.

9. Zhelyazkov, D.K., Mangurova, M., Beltcheva, A., Gueorguiev, N.M., Temnyalov, N., Markov, D., Yakimov, G., Marinova, R. (1972). In: Gentamycin, p. 13. Ed. D.K. Zhelyazkov, Sofia.

10. Zhelyazkov, D.K., Ivanova, K. (1973). V. Nautchna sessia na Med. Fac. - Varna, 12, 14-15

11. Barber, M., Waterworth, M. (1966). Brit.Med.J., 1, 203.

12. Barnte,A. and Ackerman,E.(1969). Arch.int.Pharmacocyn., 181,109.

13. Brzezinaka, M., Benveniste, R., Davies, J., Daniels, P.J.L. and Weinstein, J. (1972). Biochemistry, 11, 761.

14. Cooper, D.J., Mariglino, H.M., Yudis, M.D., and Traubel, T. (1969). J. Infect. Dis., 342, 1199.

15. Mariani, L. (1968). Bull. Soc. ital. biol. sperum., 37, 1478.

16. Mitsuhashi, S., Kobayashi, F., Tamaguchi, N. (1971). J. Anti-biotics, 24, 400.

17. Vital-Brazil, O. and Prado-Fraceshi, J. (1971). Arch.int. Pharmacodyn., 78, 179.

18. Wagman, G.H., Marquez, J.A. and Weinstein, N.J. (1968). J. Chromatogr. 34, 210.

19.   Weinstein, M.J., Wagman, G.H. and Marquez, J.A. (1976).
        J. Bact., 94, 789.

BACTERIOLOGICAL,CLINICAL AND PHARMACOLOGICAL INVESTIGATIONS

WITH TOBRAMYCIN

Éva Iván,A.E.Nagy and Klára N.Csatáry

Szőnyi T.Hospital,H-2601 Vác,Hungary

Aminoglycoside antibiotics have played a significant role
in combating infections due to gram-negative bacteria.In our
country Tobramycin is a very new antibiotic and never used before in practice.

During our in vitro studies on Tobramycin we observed an
excellent high antibacterial effect against a lot of bacterium
strains,derived from clinical sources belonging mainly to the
genera of Enterobacteriaceae family,Pseudomonas,Staphylococcus
and Acinetobacter.In this group of bacteria Tobramycin was excellent especially against Pseudomonas aeruginosa and polyresistant Staphylococcus aureus strains,against indol-positive Proteus strains and against Acinetobacter anitratus and lwoffii/see
table 1./.

Having compared the sensitivity spectra of the strains to
other aminoglycoside antibiotics it was obvious that Tobramycin
is the most effective antibiotic in this group beside Gentamicin
having a broad antibacterial spectrum similar to that of Gentamicin,with the same low or even less toxicity.

The antibacterial spectrum was determined by the standardized Bauer-Kirby disc sensitivity method on Mueller-Hinton agar.
Susceptibility test discs containing lo µg of Tobramycin were
supplied by Lilly Research Laboratories.Bacteria giving zone diameters 14 mm or more were regarded as susceptible and less than
14 mm were regarded as resistant.

	No of strains	Sm	Km	Pm	Nm	Gm	Tm	Note
E.coli	568	26	6	6	5	0,4	4,2	
Klebsiella	88	34	14	14	5	2,3	4,5	
Enterobacter	94	58	11	9	9	9	15	
Proteus/indol-/	116	35	16	12	2	3,5	1oo	
Proteus/indol±/	2o	12	8	8	6	0	0	No of res
Acinetobacter	3o	3	1	0	0	0	0	strains!
Pseudomonas	118	7o	75	92	9	5	8,5	
S.aureus	228	16	0	0	0	0		
Total	1262							

TABLE 1.Totally resistant strains in % against aminoglycoside
antibiotics/□=not in %,but number of resistant strains/

Clinical studies:a total of 5o hospitalized patients aged
from 17-7o years,suffering from serious urinary tract infection
were treated with Tobramycin.These were mainly chronic infections and received several times antibiotic therapy with more or
less success before Tobramycin.The drug was administered alone.
Patients received 2-2,5 mg/kg per day Tobramycin divided into
2 twelve hourly i.m. injections for a total of 7 days.In the case of Pseudomonas aeruginosa infections the therapy lasted till
1o days.For main parameter of recovery we regarded the total
abolishment of bacteriuria immediatelly,3 months and 6 months
after therapy/figure 1./.

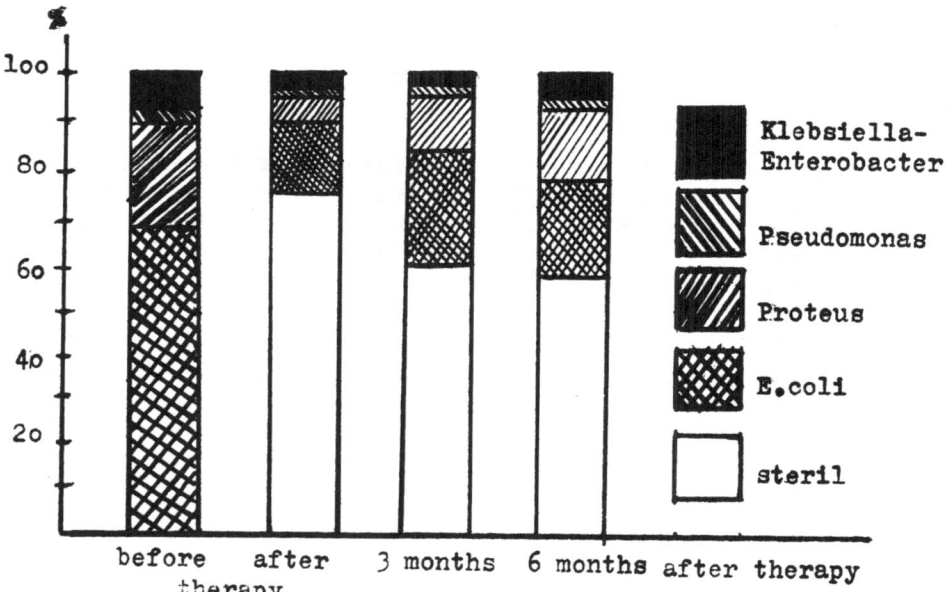

FIGURE 1.Change of bacteriuria following Tobramycin therapy

However we took into account the development of clinical status,renal function and radiology,too.The therapy resulted good clinical effect in the infections of the urinary tract with no or only slight side effects.We never observed oto-,or nephro-toxicity using 2-2,5 mg/kg per day Tobramycin.

Comparing the parameters of recovery to another group of patients suffering from the same disease group treated with Genta-micin we obtained similar good,occasionally better clinical results with Tobramycin,especially in Pseudomonas aeruginosa infections.

Pharmacological studies were performed in patients suffer-ing from end-stage disease/renal/ who have been nephrectomized. They received 15o mg Tobramycin i.m. two hours previous to the operation.From the kidney a fine tissue homogenate was prepaired with Biomix homogenizator by aseptic technic.From renal homoge-nate and from the two hour blood and urin sample serial dilut-ions were performed and bioassays were carried out by agar diff-usion method on Grove-Randall N°5 medium/pH:8/ with S.aureus ATCC 6538P strain as the test organism.Figure 2.shows the average of Tobramycin level of 5 renal tissue homogenate and of serum samples obtained at the time of nephrectomy.

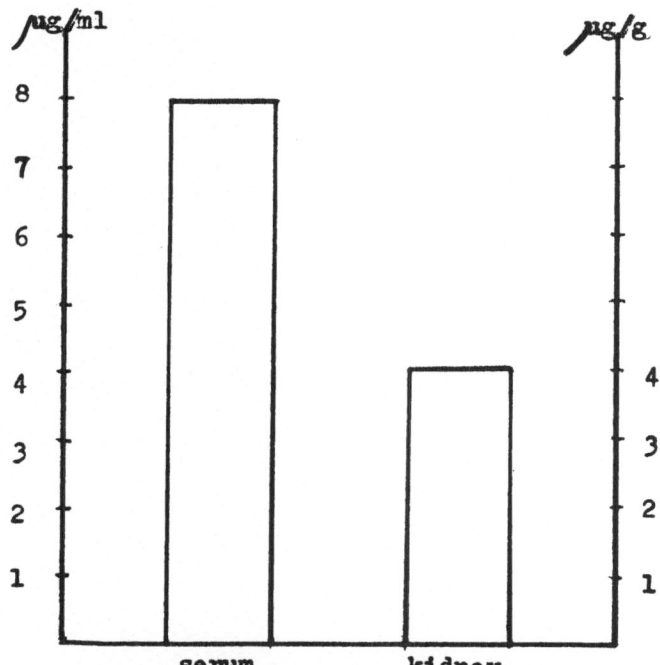

FIGURE 2.Average of Tobramycin concentrations obtained in 5 patients/15o mg i.m. 2 h previous to the operation/

Now we got answer to our question:whether Tobramycin does reach renal parenchyma in sufficient quantity or not.The answer is yes,because the average MIC-s are well below the average renal tissue level of Tobramycin we found.I.e. we can obtain therapeutic concentration in the kidney.

In summary:It is obvious that Tobramycin is the choice of antibiotic when Pseudomonas aeruginosa is present in the urinary tract.When other polyresistant bacterium strain is the infecting agent one has to know that there are two very effective aminoglycoside antibiotics with similar antibacterial spectra and with the same low toxicity.These are:Tobramycin and Gentamicin.

THE URINARY EXCRETION OF TOBRAMYCIN AND GENTAMICIN

M.J. Wood and W. Farrell

The London Hospital Medical College

London E1 2AD

INTRODUCTION

Previous studies of the urinary excretion of the aminoglycoside antibiotics, gentamicin and tobramycin, have employed microbiological assay methods and the results obtained have been very variable. The values obtained for the 24 hour urinary excretion of gentamicin in adults with normal renal function have ranged from 0 to 100% of the administered dose and there has been a similar wide range of values for tobramycin excretion (Black and Griffith, 1971, 1974; Regamey et al, 1973; Geddes et al, 1974). This variability in the results obtained is due chiefly to changes in antibiotic activity with different levels of urinary pH (Lamb et al, 1972) and variation in the electrolyte constituents of urine.

The adenylase method of assaying aminoglycoside antibiotics (Smith et al, 1972) is independent of urinary pH and a study was therefore undertaken of the urinary excretion of gentamicin and tobramycin in normal adults, using such an assay method, in order to assess its suitability for such estimations.

METHOD

Six adult males aged 28 to 35 years and with normal renal function volunteered for the study. Each was given a single intramuscular injection of 1 mg/Kg body weight tobramycin followed one week later by a similar injection of 1 mg/Kg gentamicin. Venous blood was sampled 30 minutes and 1, 2, 4 and 6 hours after each injection. Each subject collected the urine passed in the intervals 0-1 hour, 1-2 hours, 2-4 hours, 4-6 hours, 6-12

hours and 12-24 hours following injection and the serum and urine
samples were stored at -70°C until assayed. Assay of the specimens was performed using the method of ten Krooden and Darrell
(1974) with the modification that the enzyme was prepared by
sonication (Andrews et al, 1974). This involved centrifuging
an overnight culture of Escherichia coli JR66/W677 at 4,000 rpm
for 15 minutes and then washing the cells in 0.01M Tris-HCl-
0.03M NaCl buffer, pH 7.8. The cells were then resuspended in
cold 5 x 10^{-4}M $MgCl_2$ and sonicated for 10 minutes in an ice bath
using an MSE ultrasonic probe. The cellular debris was removed
by centrifuging at 18,000 rpm for 20 minutes at 0°C.

RESULTS

The mean serum levels for the six subjects are shown in
Figure 1. The peak levels ranged from 4.7 to 7.6 µg/ml for
gentamicin and from 3.9 to 5.9 µg/ml for tobramycin.

The cumulative urinary excretion of the drugs expressed as
a percentage of the administered dose is shown in Figure 2.
Within 24 hours between 50 and 71% (mean 63.5%) of the gentamicin

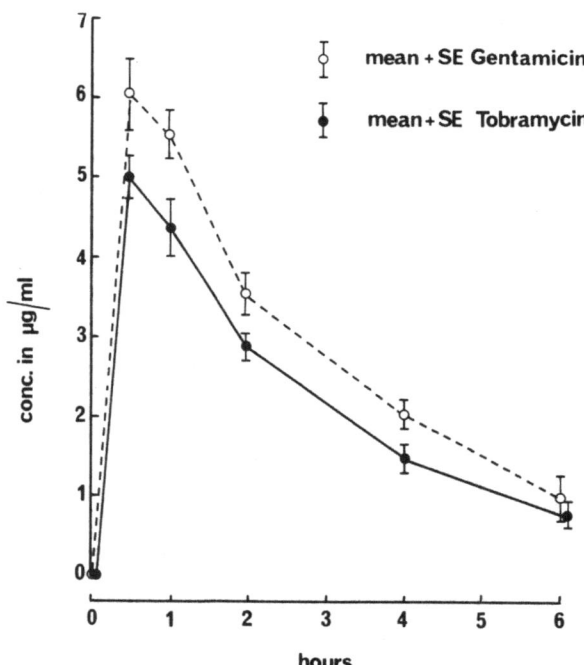

Fig. 1 Serum concentrations following intramuscular administration
        of 1 mg/Kg

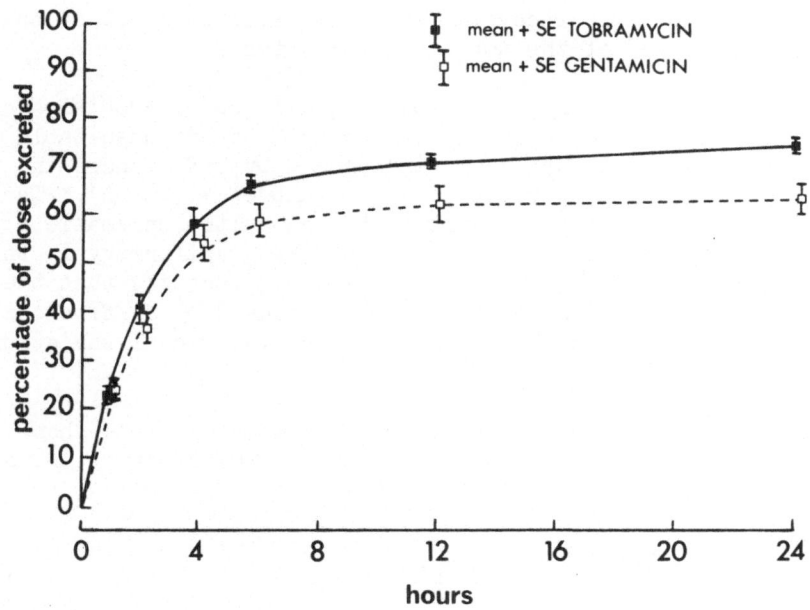

<u>Fig. 2</u> <u>Cumulative urinary excretion of tobramycin and</u>
          <u>gentamicin following intramuscular administration of</u>
          <u>1 mg/Kg</u>

was excreted and the amount of tobramycin recovered ranged from
70 to 77% (mean 74%) of the administered dose. A large proportion of this excretion occurred within four hours of administration and 23% of the gentamicin and 22% of the tobramycin was
recovered in the first hour following injection. There was no
statistical difference between the amounts of the two drugs
excreted during the first six hours but there was significantly
greater urinary excretion of tobramycin (p < 0.05) 12 and 24
hours after administration.

DISCUSSION

There has been marked variation in previous estimates of the
urinary excretion of gentamicin and tobramycin. Black and
Griffith (1971, 1974) found that the proportion of either drug
excreted was dependent on the amount administered. However, the
values obtained at each dosage level varied greatly between
individual subjects. In dosages similar to those used in the
present study both these authors and Geddes et al (1974) noted
lower urinary excretion than that found in our volunteers.
Regamey et al (1973), however, found a greater proportion of the

administered dose was recoverable in the urine with 80% of the
gentamicin and 93% of the tobramycin excreted.

These other studies have, however, all used microbiological
assays and it has been shown that such methods are unsuitable for
urinary assays because they are influenced by differences in
urinary pH as well as certain cations (Lamb et al, 1972). These
factors do not affect the results obtained by the enzymatic
method and the present study shows a striking uniformity in the
results for each of the subjects studied and suggests that the
variability in previous reports has been caused by differences
in the pH of the urine samples rather than individual variation
in urinary excretion.

The adenylylase method appears to be more suitable than
microbiological assays for the accurate determination of urinary
excretion of aminoglycoside antibiotics.

REFERENCES

Andrews, J., Gillette, P., Williams, J.D. and Mitchard, M.
    Analysis of gentamicin in plasma : a comparative study of
    four methods. Postgrad. Med. Journal, 50 (Suppl.7), 17-20
    (1974)

Black, H.R. and Griffith, R.S. Preliminary studies with
    nebramycin, factor 6. Antimicrobial Agents Chemother.,
    1970 p.314-321 (1971)

Black, H.R. and Griffith, R.S. Comparative pharmacology of
    tobramycin and gentamicin in adult volunteers. In Progress
    in Chemotherapy, Vol.1. ed. Daikos, G.K., Hellenic Society
    of Chemotherapy, Athens, p.638-643 (1974)

Geddes, A.M., Goodall, J.A.D., Speirs, C.F., Gillett, A.P.,
    Andrews, J. and Williams, J.D. Clinical and laboratory
    studies with tobramycin. Chemotherapy. 20 : 245-256 (1974)

Laub, J.W., Mann, J.M. and Simmons, R.J. Factors influencing
    the microbiological assay of tobramycin. Antimicrobial
    Agents Chemother., 1 , 323-328 (1972)

Regamey, C., Gordon, R.C. and Kirby, W.M.M. Comparative pharm-
    acokinetics of tobramycin and gentamicin. Clin.Pharmacol.
    Ther., 14, 396-403 (1973)

Smith, D.H., van Otto, B. and Smith, A.L. A rapid chemical assay
     for gentamicin. New Engl. J. Med., 286, 583-586 (1972)

Ten Krooden, E. and Darrell, J.H. Rapid gentamicin assay by
     enzymatic adenylylation. J. clin. Path., 27, 452-456(1974)

PHARMACOKINETICS AND OTOTOXICITY OF GENTAMICIN, TOBRAMYCIN AND AMIKACIN

FEDERSPIL, P. and TIESLER, E.

UNIVERSITY OF THE SAAR

6650 HOMBURG (SAAR) - WEST GERMANY

The aim of this paper is to give a survey of the pharmacokinetical studies on the ototoxicity of the new aminoglycoside antibiotics Gentamicin, Tobramycin and Amikacin. The animal used was the guinea pig and the antibiotic concentrations were determined by the microbiological method (Bac subtilis ATCC 6633).

The pharmacokinetics of Gentamicin, Tobramycin and Amikacin in the serum and inner ear of the guinea pig are almost similar (fig. 1). The perilymph concentrations increase slowly, however, after 5 hours they are as high as the serum concentrations and after 18 hours they are many times higher. There is a distinct retention of these antibiotics in the inner ear fluids. The half-life times of Gentamicin, Tobramycin and Amikacin are 12, 11 and 10 hours respectively.

The Gentamicin concentrations in the perilymph are in linear relation to the doses injected. The Gentamicin, Tobramycin and Amikacin concentrations in the perilymph are similar on both sides and many times higher than the concentrations in the brain. The Gentamicin concentrations in the endolymph are 80 to 90 % of those in the perilymph 2 and 5 hours after the injection.

No retention of Gentamicin, Tobramycin and Amikacin in the cerebrospinal and eye fluids is found.

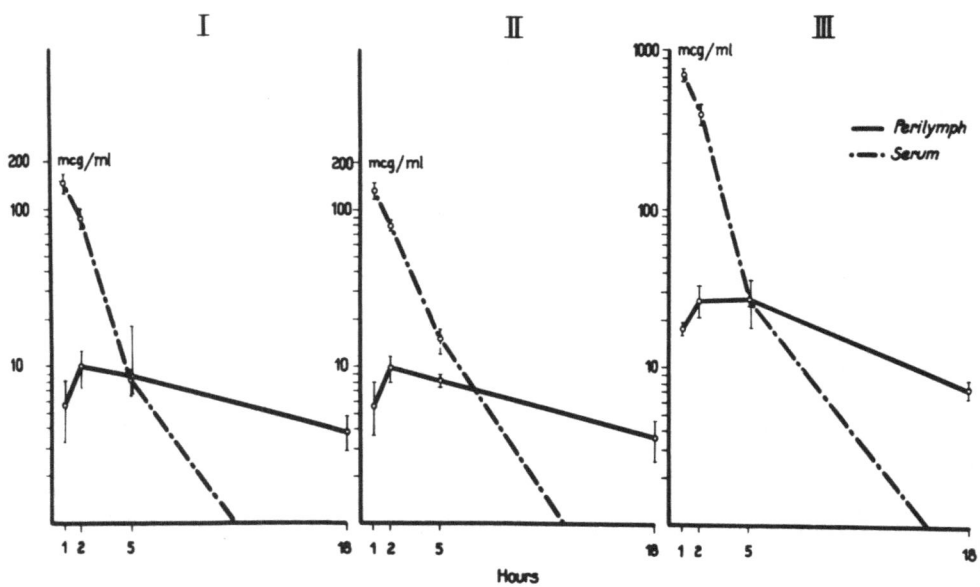

Fig. 1.   Gentamicin (I), Tobramycin (II), and Amikacin (III) levels
in serum and perilymph.

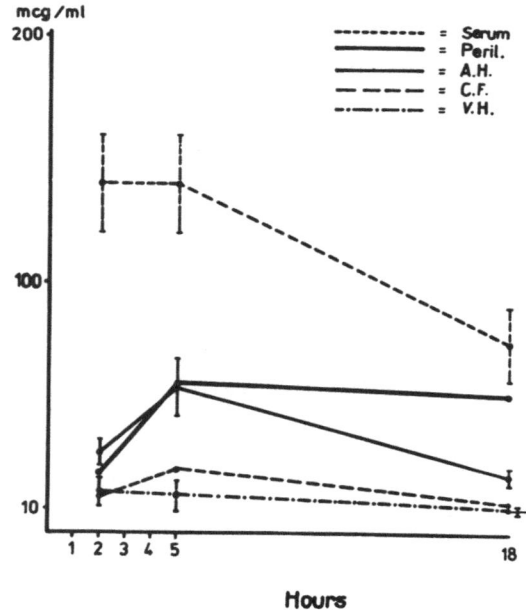

Fig. 2.   Gentamicin concentrations after bilateral nephrectomy and
1 x 50 mg/kg (84 samples).   Peril. = perilymph, A.H. = aqueous
humour, C.F. = cerebrospinal fluid, V.H. = vitreous humour.

The results obtained by using C 14 labelled Gentamicin are strikingly consistent with those obtained by
the microbiological method and confirm the pharmacokinetics in the serum, inner ear, eye and cerebrospinal
fluids as well as in the brain, heart and liver.

Pharmacokinetical studies about long-term treatment
with Gentamicin, Tobramycin and Amikacin showed results
explaining the clinically known additional effect of
long-term treatment with aminoglycoside antibiotics.

The pharmacokinetics of Gentamicin in anuric guinea
pigs give an explanation of the increased ototoxicity
in uremia (fig. 2). This figure with its constant high
blood levels may be considered as an experimental model
to evaluate the ototoxicity of continuous i.v. infusions.
The rather high perilymph concentrations prove that the
continuous i.v. infusion therapy with aminoglycoside
antibiotics does not only increase the effectiveness of
the aminoglycoside antibiotic treatment but also its
ototoxicity.

A certain percentage of the cases of otitis media
treated with Gentamicin, Tobramycin and Amikacin shows
higher perilymph levels and increased ototoxicity.

In order to study the treatment of ototoxic damage,
we started with the working hypothesis that the concentration of aminoglycoside antibiotics in the inner ear
lymph is a graduator for measuring the ototoxicity of
these antibiotics and tested the effectiveness of the
suboccipital puncture and hydro-, osmo- and salidiuresis.
No effect could be found.

Finally, the pharmacokinetics of the aminoglycoside
antibiotics in the inner ear allow an estimation of the
ototoxicity of these antibiotics. Figure 1 shows the
perilymph and serum levels after a subcutaneous injection of 50 mg Gentamicin or Tobramycin per kg body
weight or a 5 times higher Amikacin dose. According to
these studies and taking the general toxicity of these
antibiotics into consideration, the ototoxicity of
Amikacin lies below that of Tobramycin and the Tobramycin ototoxicity below that of Gentamicin on a weight-
for-weight basis.

Further data about the ototoxicity of these new
aminoglycoside antibiotics were found by histological
investigations (in Journal of Infectious Diseases).

CLINICAL EXPERIENCE ON TOBRAMYCIN

S. Ishiyama, I. Nakayama, H. Iwamoto, S. Iwai,
I. Murata, and M. Ohashi

Department of Surgery
Nihon University School of Medicine
8, 1-chome, Kandasurugadai, Chiyodaku, Tokyo, Japan

The results of our clinical experience on Tobramycin in severe surgical infections indicate that the frequency of administration would be more important than increasing a single dose of the drug.

As previously reported by several investigators, Tobramycin is a new aminoglycoside antibiotic, which shows wide activities against both Gram-negative and positive bacteria except for anaerobic ones (Table 1).

The shortcoming of this class of drugs is, as is widely known, a potential side effect such as ototoxicity or nephrotoxicity. This necessitates a serious examination of what dosage regimen will result in clinical efficacy together with minimal side effects.

Table 1. Sensitivity Distribution of Pseudomonas aeruginosa

(49 str.)	MIC (µg/ml)											
	≤0.1	0.2	0.4	0.8	1.56	3.13	6.25	12.5	25	50	100	>100
Tobramycin		2	11	11	18	3	2				1	1
Gentamicin	1	1	10	13	17	5						2
Amikacin			2	1	9	19	11	1	2		1	3
Dibekacin			2	18	22	1	1	1	1		1	2
Lividomycin						2	2	10	25	5	1	4
Kanamycin									2	11	23	13

From this point of view, we clinically tried Tobramycin in serious surgical infections due to Gram-negative bacilli, particularly to Pseudomonas aeruginosa.

Forty mg of Tobramycin, 3 times daily, was successful in some cases which had not responded to previous antibiotic therapy. This case was a patient with a diffuse peritonitis after a cholecysto-duodenostomy for malignancy in the pancreas head. Sulbenicillin and cefazolin and 80 mg daily of Tobramycin were all ineffective, while 120 mg daily of Tobramycin was successful. The isolated microorganisms were klebsiella, citrobacter, and pseudomonas (Fig. 1).

Some cases resisted a BID regimen of Tobramycin, while they responded to a TID regimen. Case 2 was a 63 year old man with pyelonephritis complicated with a recurrent rectal cancer. Forty mg twice a day was not successful, but when the dosage was increased to forty mg three times a day, the treatment succeeded promptly (Fig. 2).

In some cases a decreasing dosage resulted in failure. The patient was a 67 year old man with diffuse peritonitis due to leakage after a gastrectomy for cancer. E. coli and pseudomonas were cultured from the abdominal discharge. Administration of Tobramycin three times a day succeeded at first, but as the frequency of injection was reduced to two times a day the temperature rose again and klebsiella and staphylococcus epidermidis were detected from his urine (Fig. 3).

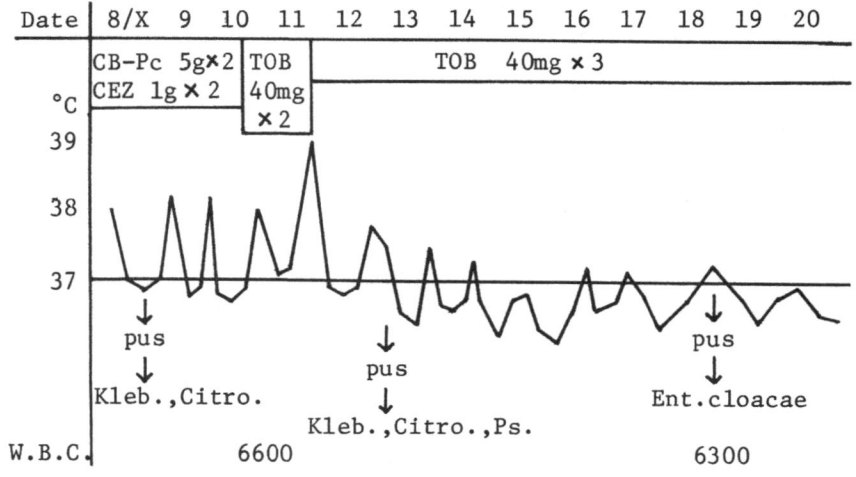

Fig. 1. 58 yr M 60 kg Peritonitis (Pancreas cancer).

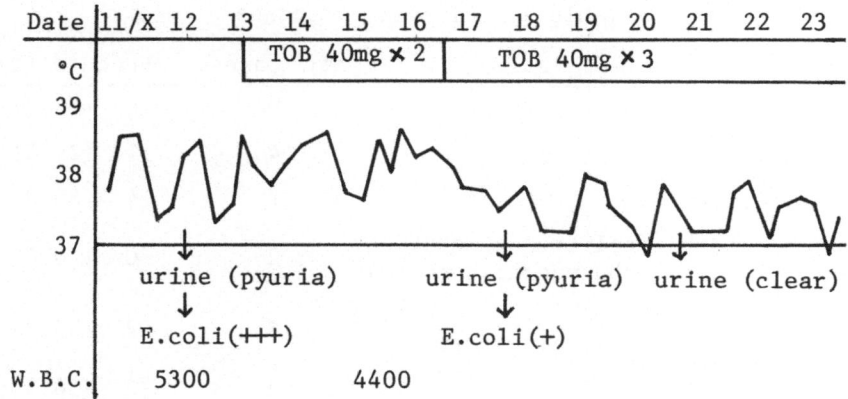

Fig. 2.   63 yr M 36 kg Pyelonephritis
(Cancer of pancreas head).

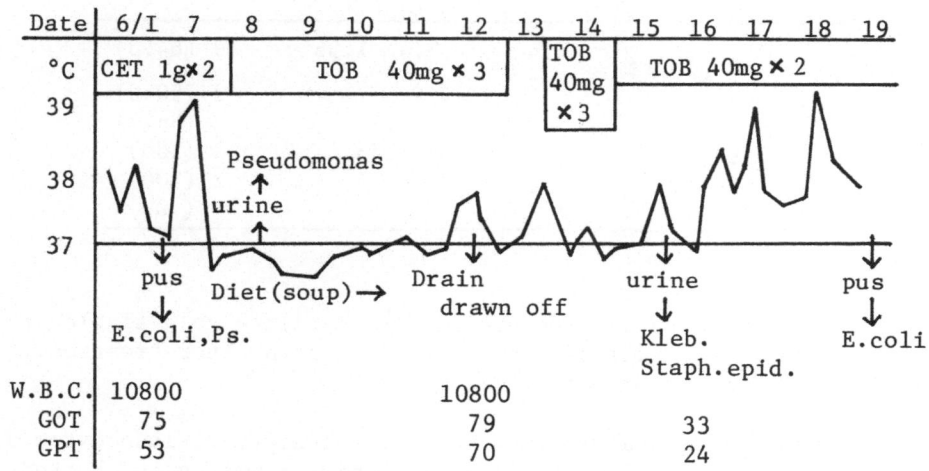

Fig. 3.   67 yr M 52 kg Peritonitis (Gastric cancer).

The severe infections which we treated consisted of acute
peritonitis, intra-abdominal abscess, wound infections including
serious burns, sepsis accompanying renal transplantation, and urinary infections associated with cancer (Table 2).

Thirteen cases of a total of twenty-three were successful and
the rate of success was 56.5%. The patients were in serious conditions and the outcome would have been fatal otherwise.

Table 2. Clinical Response

	No. cases	Success (%)
Post-operative peritonitis	9	6 (66.7)
Intra-abdominal abscess	4	1 (25.0)
Wound infections	5	4 (80.0)
Sepsis (with renal transplantation or necrotizing pharyngeal sarcoma)	2	0 (0)
Complicated urinary tract infection (with recurrent rectal cancer)	3	2 (66.7)
Total	23	13 (56.5)

Table 3. Bacteriological Response

Organism	No.strains	MIC to TOB (μg/ml)	Success (%)
Pseudomonas aeruginosa	14	0.4 1.56	9 (64.3)
E. coli	4		2 (50.0)
Ent. cloacae	3	0.8	2 (66.7)
Klebsiella	2	1.56	2 (100)
Citrobacter	2		2 (100)
Rettgerella	1		0 (0)

Fourteen strains of pseudomonas were isolated as a single or mixed pathogen, and nine of them were eliminated after treatment. The rate of elimination was 64.3% (Table 3)

Clinical signs and symptoms such as temperature, leucocytosis, purulent discharge and other clinical chemistry were also checked as criteria of success of the treatment. Of course the background diseases had to be considered as factors influencing the results.

It is quite natural that the patients differ in responses to Tobramycin according to the severity of infections, the background diseases and also the dose and frequency of administration of the drug. However, within our present clinical experience, intramuscular injection of 3 mg/kg of Tobramycin divided into three times a day was a very adequate way to treat a severe infection. All of the cases who received the drug two times a day failed to show successful results, whether two mg/kg or three mg/kg a day. No notable merit in clinical effectiveness was demonstrated for four mg/kg a day or more in our present experience (Table 4).

Table 4. Relationship between Clinical
Response and Daily Dosage

Dose/day (mg/kg)	No. cases	I	II	III	IV times a day
≧1.0	1	1(0)			
≧2.0	12		0(3)	6(3)	
≧3.0	7		0(1)	5(1)	
≧4.0	3		0(1)	1(0)	0(1)
Total	23	1(0)	0(5)	12(4)	0(1) ( ) failure

Table 5

Total Cases	751		
No. of Side Effects	80 (10.7%)		(%)
8th nerve :	15(2.0)	Blood :	5(0.7)
Tinnitus	2	Erythropenia	3
Hearing loss	11	Thrombocytopenia	1
Abnormal audiometry	2	Eosinophilia	1
Renal :	15(2.0)	Others :	27(3.6)
Acute renal failure	1	Pain at	
Increase of BUN	12	injection site	16
Proteinuria	1	Skin rash	6
Cylindruria	1	Nausea	3
Hepatic :	18(2.4)	Anorexia	1
Increase of		Feeling of	
SGOT, SGPT	18	numbness at lip	1

We experienced no remarkable side effect during the administration of Tobramycin in doses of less than five mg/kg a day for
two to fourteen days. However, this does not mean Tobramycin is
totally without side effects, as shown in Table 5, which summarizes
the experiences of investigators in Japan.

SUMMARY

Tobramycin is one of the most effective antibiotics to Gram-
negative bacteria, especially to Pseudomonas aeruginosa in vitro.
However, it must be carefully administered in clinical practice,

because of its potential for side effects such as ototoxicity and nephrotoxicity, especially in high-dose treatment or a long-term treatment.

Our experience indicates that three mg/kg/day in three divided doses was the most adequate regimen.

REFERENCES

1. Chan, R.A., Benner, E.J., and Hoeprich, P.D., Gentamicin therapy in renal failure. Anna Intern. Med. 76: 773-778, 1972.

2. Mehenry, M.D., Ganan, T.L., et al., Gentamicin dosage for renal insufficiency. Ann. Intern. Med. 74: 192-197, 1971.

3. Falco, F.G., Review of bacteriology and preclinical studies and clinical pharmacology of gentamicin sulfate. Therapeutische Umschau Revue Therapeutique Supplementum 1: 8-16, 1969.

EVALUATION OF TOBRAMYCIN

IN SEVERE URINARY TRACT INFECTION

Alan H. Bennett

Harvard Medical School

Boston, Massachusetts   USA

Tobramycin sulfate is a bactericidal aminoglycoside antibiotic which in animal studies has been shown to have lower acute toxicity and lower nephrotoxicity than gentamicin (1,2). Tobramycin has been shown to have more activity in vitro against Pseudomonas sp. than other aminoglycoside antibiotics (3,4). Tobramycin is excreted unchanged in the urine and assayable blood levels are present for at least eight hours. Studies in patients with renal failure showed that the serum half-life was directly related to the degree of renal impairment and that reduced doses were necessary. This antibiotic was found to be effective against infections due to susceptible organisms in the genitourinary system- Pseudomonas sp., Esch. coli, the Klebsiella-Enterobacter-Serratia group, indole-positive and indole-negative Proteus sp., staphylococci and group D streptococci. Early clinical studies showed that Tobramycin was successful in eradicating infections with Pseudomonas sp. which had prior unsuccessful therapy with gentamicin and/or carbenicillin.

This study of twenty-five patients was undertaken to determine the effectiveness of tobramycin sulfate in a dosage schedule of 3mg/kg/day on a bid program in patients with severe urinary tract infection. All patients were treated a minimum of five days if the offending organism was sensitive. No patient with renal impairment was included in the study. Urine cultures were monitored carefully as were CBC, creatinine, BUN and liver function tests during the course of treatment.

Table I indicates the conditions treated. Thirteen patients had uncomplicated infections, three had septicemia with positive blood cultures and nine had urinary tract obstruction caused by prostatism in six and calculi in three.

Table II shows the urinary tract pathogens treated with
Tobramycin. All cultures were collected using strict aseptic
technique, either clean voided or catheterized specimens. Blood
cultures were obtained after a surgical skin prep with Betadine.
E.coli, Proteus sp., and Pseudomonas sp. accounted for the
majority of pathogens (80%). In all of the initial cultures the
organism was sensitive to Tobramycin. One Pseudomonas organism
treated was sensitive to Tobramycin but resistent to gentamicin.
Cultures became negative in most patients (88%) within 48 hours.
In two patients positive cultures persisted for 72 hours and in
one patient 96 hours. Patients were treated an average of 7 days
with a range of 5-9 days.

One patient developed an elevated BUN and creatinine after
three days of treatment. A pretreatment creatinine of 1.1 rose
to 2.3 and had returned to 1.4 within two weeks. This same patient
also exhibited a transient, slight elevation of alkaline phospha-
tase and LDH. Two patients developed a positive urine culture for
monilia while on treatment with Tobramycin. Additional treatment
was not necessary and the monilia disappeared after Tobramycin
was discontinued.

Twelve patients received intravenous injections and no
instances of phlebitis or pain were noted. All twenty-five patients
received intra-muscular injections. Only two complained of minor
discomfort at the injection site. No sterile abscesses occurred
and no systemic side effects or allergic reactions were noted.

A satisfactory clinical response was achieved in 24 of 25
patients (96%). The causative organisms were eliminated in all
twenty-five patients, but one patient with urinary tract infection,
septicemia and a retroperitoneal abscess had an unsatisfactory
clinical response.

Table I

Disease Treated with Tobramycin

Pyelonephritis	6
Cystitis	13
Prostatitis	1
Perinephric abscess	1
Epididymo-orchitis	4

Table II

Pathogens Treated with Tobramycin

E.coli	8
Proteus mirabilis	6
Proteus rettgeri	1
Pseudomonas	5
K. pneumo	2
Enterobacter	1
Enterococcus sp.	1
Streptococcus sp.	1

REFERENCES

1. Meyers, B.R. and Hirschman, S.Z.
    Pharmacologic Studies on Tobramycin and Comparison with
    Gentamicin.
    J. Clin. Pharmacol., 12:321, 1972.

2. DeRosa, F., Buoncristiani, U., etal.
    Tobramycin: Toxicological and Pharmacological Studies in
    Animals and Pharmacokinetic Research in Patients with
    Varying Degrees of Renal Impairment.
    J.Int. Med. Res., 2:100, 1974.

3. Henderson, A. and Byatt, M.E.
    Sensitivity of Pseudomonas to Tobramycin.
    Clin. Med., 81:27, 1974.

4. Klastersky, J., Daneau, D. and deMaertelaer, V.
    Comparative Study of Tobramycin and Gentamicin with Special
    Reference to Anti-Pseudomonas Activity
    Clin. Pharacol. Ther., 14:104, 1973.

BUTIROSIN - PHARMACODYNAMICS AND CLINICAL EXPERIENCE

William E. Kunsman
        Resident, Department of Medicine
William J. Holloway
        Head, Section of Infectious Disease
Wilmington Medical Center
Wilmington, Delaware   USA

Butirosin is a new neomycin-like aminoglycoside antibiotic exhibiting marked activity against many gram-positive and gram-negative bacteria in vitro and in vivo.[1,2,3] The gram-negative spectrum includes the Klebsiella-Enterobacter-Serratia groups as well as Proteus sp. and Pseudomonas sp. Butirosin appears to have less antibacterial potency than gentamicin on a weight basis, but it appears to be less nephrotoxic and considerably less ototoxic in laboratory animals than the older drug.[4] These early reports suggested that this decreased toxicity might compensate for the lower potency resulting in a safe, effective compound for use in man.

This paper reports studies with butirosin carried out at the Wilmington Medical Center. These investigations include a pharmacodynamic study in normal healthy volunteers given a single intramuscular injection of the antibiotic, a laboratory study in which the minimal inhibitory concentration of butirosin was determined against common pathogens, and a clinical study to evaluate the efficacy of butirosin in the treatment of patients with urinary tract infection.

MATERIAL AND METHODS

Butirosin sulfate in a dose of 4 mg/kg was administered via a deep intramuscular injection in twelve healthy male volunteers, all of whom had given informed consent. Samples of plasma for drug assay were obtained prior to

TABLE 1

Patient	Sex	Age	Organism	Concomitant Disorder	Foley Catheter	Blood Culture	Prior Antibiotics
1	M	72	P. aeruginosa	Ca of bladder	No	0**	None***
2	M	71	P. mirabilis	Astrocytoma	Yes	0	None
3	F	71	P. aeruginosa	Hypertensive Cardiovascular Disease, Rheumatoid Arthritis	No	0	Carbenicillin+
4	M	61	E. coli	Cerebral Vascular Accident, Emphysema	Yes	0	None
5	F	60	K. ozoenae	Ca of esophagus	No	0	None
6	F	44	E. coli	Ca of cervix	No	0	None
7	F	52	E. coli	Metastatic Adeno Ca	Yes	0	Gentamicin ++
8*	M	44	E. coli	Pancreatitis	No	0	None
9	F	51	E. coli	Diarrhea and Anemia	Yes	0	None
10	F	40	E. coli	Metastatic Ca	No	0	None
11	M	75	P. rettgeri	Ca of prostate, Diabetes Mellitus, Cerebral Vascular Accident	Yes	0	None

* Drug discontinued because of rising BUN and creatinine after 4 doses.
** 0 = No Growth
*** None = None 3 months prior to butirosin administration
+ Carbenicillin stopped 1 week prior to butirosin administration
++ Gentamicin stopped 6 weeks prior to butirosin administration

and at 1, 2, 4, and 8 hours after administration of butirosin. Aliquots of urine for drug assay were obtained
from hourly specimens during the first, third, and eighth
hours post butirosin administration. Baseline hematologic,
clinical chemistry, and urine profiles were done before
and seventy-two hours after administration of the antibiotic. Drug assays were performed by the agar diffusion
method employing B. subtilis 04555 as the test organism
and butirosin (Rx x42118) as the standard.

In the in vitro study, random isolates were obtained
from the clinical bacteriology laboratories of the Wilmington Medical Center. These isolates included Pseudomonas sp. (100 strains), E. coli (30 strains), Proteus sp.,
indole positive (7 strains), Proteus sp., indole negative
(5 strains), Klebsiella sp. (12 strains), Enterobacter
sp. (12 strains), and Serratia sp. (12 strains). Minimal
inhibitory concentrations were determined by the standard
agar dilution technique with Mueller-Hinton agar, using
a Steers replicator to form reproducible inocula. The
plates were observed for complete growth inhibition after
overnight incubation at 37 degrees. MIC's were determined
for butirosin and gentamicin.

In the clinical study, eleven patients with serious
underlying disease (Table I) in whom urinary tract infection was diagnosed were treated with butirosin at a dose
of 12 mg/kg/day for 7 days. The presence of urinary tract
infection was confirmed by a urine culture with a plate
count greater than 10^5/ml., but no effort was made to determine the extent of upper or lower urinary tract involvement. None of the patients had evidence of obstructive
uropathy or urinary tract calculi. Butirosin sulfate
(provided by Parke Davis and Co.) was administered intramuscularly at a dose of 4 mg/kg every 8 hours (12 mg/kg/
day) for 7 days. Efficacy was determined by clinical improvement and by urine culture repeated on the third and
last day of therapy and two days after completion of therapy. Laboratory studies performed on each patient before,
during and following therapy included blood culture, CBC,
chemistry-12 profile, creatinine, urinalysis and audio-
gram. Butirosin plasma levels were measured in all patients with specimens being obtained prior to administration, and 1, 2, 4 and 8 hours following administration of
the first dose each day.

RESULTS

Nine of the twelve volunteers had peak butirosin

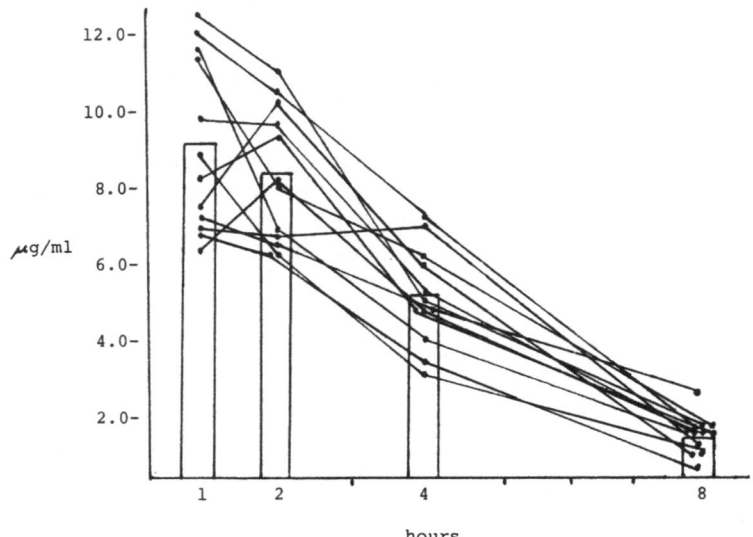

Fig. 1. Butirosin, Volunteer Single Dose IM 4 mg/kg,
Plasma Drug Levels, n = 12

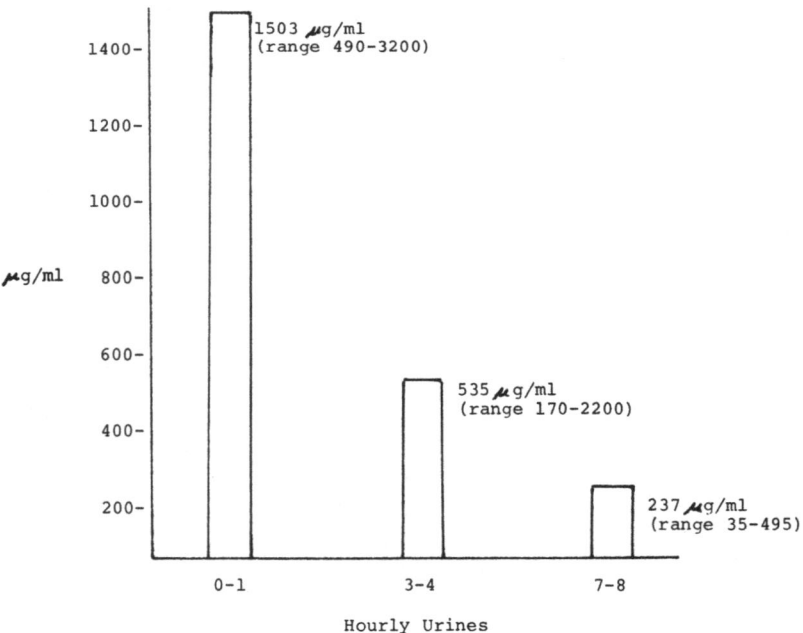

Fig. 2. Butirosin, Volunteer Single Dose IM 4 mg/kg,
Mean Urinary Concentrations in Hourly Urine, n = 9

plasma levels at 1 hour, and three had peak levels at 2
hours (Figure #1). The average concentrations were 9.1
µg/ml (range 6.3-12.3) at 1 hour, 8.2 µg/ml (range 6.3-
10.8) at 2 hours, 4.8 µg/ml (range 2.9-6.9) at 4 hours,
and 1.3 µg/ml (range 0.5-2.3) at 8 hours. The lowest peak
level achieved was 6.8 µg/ml. Nine volunteers submitted
adequately collected hourly urine specimens for analysis.
The average urine concentration during the first hour after butirosin administration was 1503 µg/ml (range 490-
3200), the fourth hour 535 µg/ml (range 170-2200), and
the eighth hour 237 µg/ml (range 35-495) (Figure #2).
Since the urine concentration is related to the urine volume, an analysis of the percentage of the initial intramuscular dose excreted in the urine was done. In the
first hour there was an average of 26 percent excreted
(range 19-41), in the fourth hour 19 percent (range 10-31),
and in the eighth hour 7 percent (range 2-10) (Figure #3).
Analysis of the baseline hematologic, clinical chemistry,
and urine profiles revealed only one change which was a
slight elevation of SGOT from 102 to 139 mU/ml (normal
10-50) in one volunteer. This was felt to be due to ex-
cessive alcohol ingestion during the study period. The
abnormality resolved within one week after the study (and
alcohol ingestion) was completed.

In the in vitro MIC study for 100 strains of Pseudomonas, the geometric mean was 20.75 µg/ml for butirosin
and 2.50 µg/ml for gentamicin (Table #2). Forty-eight
percent of the strains were susceptible to butirosin if
12.5 µg/ml is used as the criteria for susceptibility.
Seventy-three percent were susceptible to gentamicin if
6.25 µg/ml is used as the criteria for susceptibility
(Figure #4). The geometric mean MIC data for the other
organisms tested is summarized in Table #3; of note is the
relative resistance to butirosin of seven strains of indole-positive Proteus.

Ten of the eleven patients in the clinical study were
able to complete therapy while one patient (#8) was dropped
from the study on the second day because of deteriorating
renal function as evidenced by rising BUN and creatinine.
This deterioration was thought to be due to his underlying
disease and not related to butirosin administration.

In eight of the ten patients who received a full
course of butirosin there was eradication of the original
pathogen while in two patients the initial organism persisted despite in vitro susceptibility (Table #4). Among
the eight patients in whom the initial organism was eradicated, only three had sterile urine cultures at the

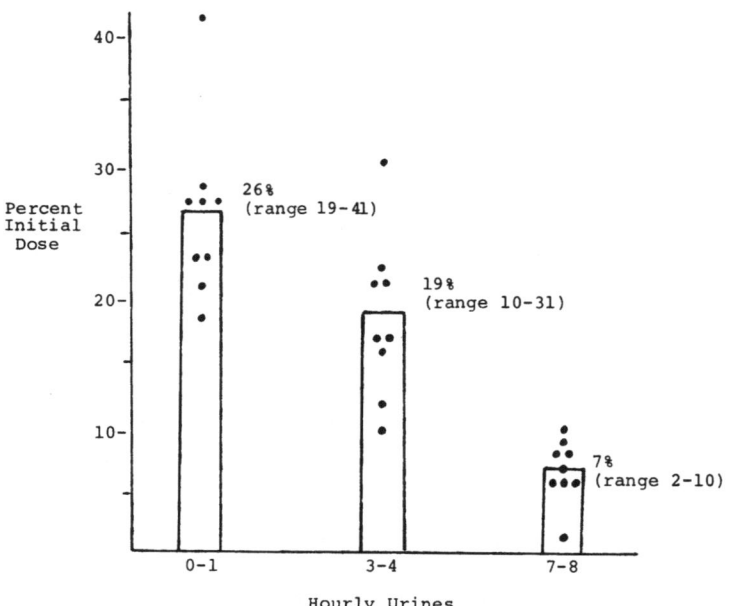

Fig. 3. Butirosin, Volunteer Single Dose IM 4 mg/kg,
Percent Total Dose in Hourly Urine, n = 9

TABLE 2

MIC of 100 Pseudomonas Strains by Agar Dilution

	Geometric Mean mcg/ml	Percent Susceptible
Butirosin	20.75	48 (12.5 mcg/ml)
Gentamicin	2.50	73 (6.25 mcg/ml)

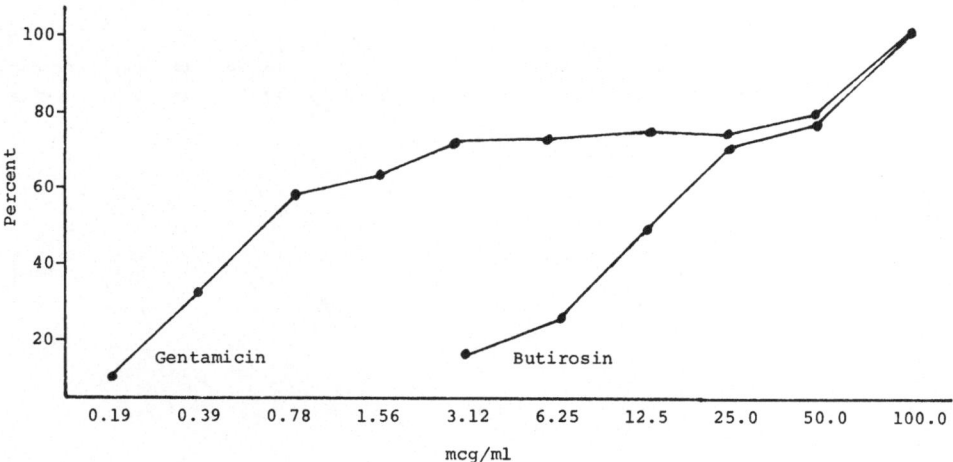

Fig. 4. Cumulative Percent Susceptibility of Pseudomonas to
Two Aminoglycosides

TABLE 3

Geometric Mean MIC by Agar Dilution Comparing
Butirosin with Gentamicin

	# Strains	Butirosin mcg/ml	Gentamicin mcg/ml
E. coli	30	1.09	0.23
Proteus			
Indole positive	7	27.5	2.65
Indole negative	5	7.5	1.56
Klebsiella	12	0.58	<0.19
Enterobacter	12	0.47	<0.19
Serratia	12	3.12	<0.19

TABLE 4. Comparative Activity of Butirosin and Gentamicin vs. Urinary Tract Isolates before and during Butirosin Therapy

Patient Number	Date Isolated	Organism	MIC (µg/ base/ml.)	
			BTN	GTM
1	6-14-74	P. aeruginosa (Type 1)	25	6.3
	6-20-74	" "	25	3.1
	6-24-74	" "	12.5	3.1
	6-26-74	" "	12.5	3.1
2	7-8-74	P. mirabilis	25	3.1
	7-16-74	S. epidermidis	>100	0.1
3	7-9-74	P. aeruginosa (autoagglut.)	12.5	3.1
	7-12-74	" "	12.5	3.1
	7-14-74	" "	6.3	3.1
	7-16-74	" "	1.1	1.6
	7-24-74	" "	12.5	1.6
4	7-18-74	E. coli	12.5	1.6
	7-29-74	S. aureus	50	0.2
5	8-22-74	K. ozoenae	0.8	0.4
6	10-2-74	E. coli	>100	0.4
	10-7-74	Enterococcus	3.1	50
7	1-8-75	E. coli	6.3	1.6
8	1-12-75	E. coli	6.3	0.8
9	1-11-75	E. coli	6.3	0.8
10	2-13-75	E. coli	>100	6.3
	2-26-75	S. epidermidis	>100	0.1
11	3-11-75	P. rettgeri	0.8	0.2
	3-17-75	S. aureus	50	0.4
	3-21-75	S. aureus	50	0.4

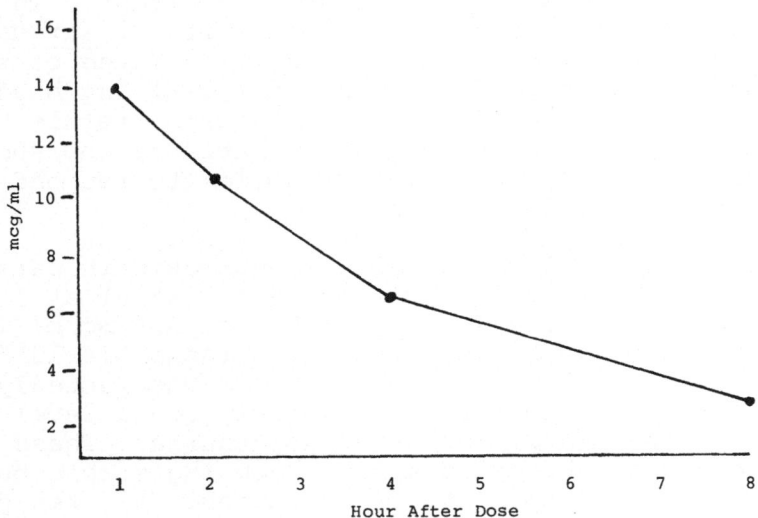

Fig. 5. Plasma Levels of Butirosin, Average from 10 Patients
(Days 1-7)

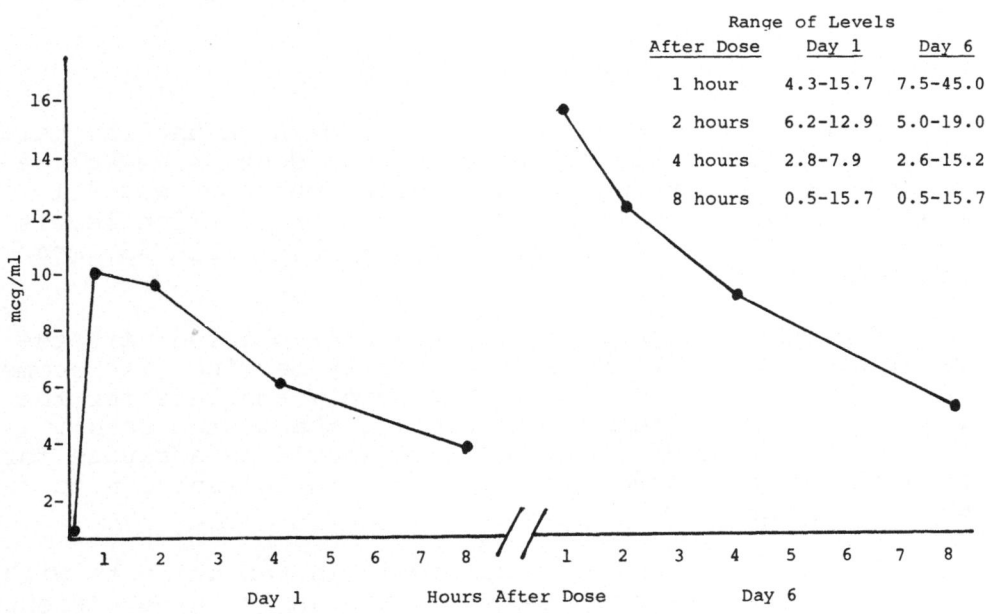

Range of Levels		
After Dose	Day 1	Day 6
1 hour	4.3-15.7	7.5-45.0
2 hours	6.2-12.9	5.0-19.0
4 hours	2.8-7.9	2.6-15.2
8 hours	0.5-15.7	0.5-15.7

Fig. 6. Plasma Levels of Butirosin, Average from 10 Patients

conclusion of the seven day course of therapy. The remaining five patients were colonized with S. aureus (2),
S. epidermidis (2) or enterococcus (1). Three of these
five patients with colonization had indwelling bladder
catheters as did two of the patients with sterile urine at
the completion of the study. Both patients who showed no
response to therapy had likewise failed to respond to
other antibiotics in the past.

The average plasma levels of butirosin in patients
were as follows: 13.9 μg/ml (range 4.3-47.6) at 1 hour,
10.6 μg/ml (range 5.0-41.6) at 2 hours, 6.6 μg/ml (range
2.6-26.5) at 4 hours, and 3.7 μg/ml (range 0.4-13.5) at
8 hours (Figure #5). Two patients had unexpectedly high
plasma levels two to three times their usual level on one
day toward the end of the seven day course. These high
levels could not be explained by sampling errors but may
have been related to state of hydration. All ten patients
showed some elevation of plasma levels at all hours tested
toward the end of the treatment course (Figure #6) suggesting drug accumulation.

None of the patients exhibited evidence of butirosin
toxicity as measured by clinical or laboratory parameters.
Two patients with elevated liver enzymes on admission to
the study showed no significant change during therapy.

COMMENT

A pharmacodynamic study of butirosin in healthy male
volunteers with a single intramuscular dose (4 mg/kg) revealed that the average peak level at one hour was 9.1
mcg/ml, dropping to 1.3 mcg/ml at 8 hours. Urine levels
averaged 1503 mcg/ml during the first hour with 237 mcg/ml
the average at 8 hours.

When the pharmacodynamic data are collated with the
results of the in vitro susceptibility testing, it becomes
apparent that butirosin would be barely adequate for the
treatment of bacteremic patients (in the dosage used).
However, the urine levels achieved should be adequate for
effectiveness in lower urinary tract infections due to susceptible pathogens.

A clinical study with butirosin in ten patients with
urinary tract infections revealed that only three patients
had sterile urine at completion of therapy. In five patients, the original pathogen was replaced with a new organism while in two patients the original pathogen

persisted. The plasma and urine levels of butirosin in patients were similar to those seen in the volunteers. Butirosin was well tolerated with no evidence of toxicity.

In conclusion, this limited study would suggest that butirosin is a well tolerated, safe aminoglycoside at the dosage level employed. However, the marginal therapeutic efficacy seen in this study suggests that higher doses will have to be used for this agent to compete with currently available aminoglycosides.

REFERENCES

1. Dion, H.W., Woo, P.W.K., Willmer, N.E., Kern, D.L., Onaga, J., and Fusari, S.A., "Butirosin, a new aminoglycosidic antibiotic complex: isolation and characterization", Antimicrobial Agents and Chemotherapy, 2:84-88, 1972.

2. Howells, J.D., Anderson, L.E., Coffey, G.L., Senos, G. D., Underhill, M.A., Vagler, D.L., and Ehrlich, J., "Butirosin, a new aminoglycosidic antibiotic complex: bacterial origin and microbiological studies", Antimicrobial Agents and Chemotherapy, 2:78-83, 1972.

3. Heifetz, C.L., Fisher, M.W., Chodubski, J.A. and DeCarlo, M.O., "Butirosin, a new aminoglycosidic antibiotic complex: antibacterial activity in vitro and in mice", Antimicrobial Agents and Chemotherapy, 2:89-94, 1972.

4. Heifetz, C.L., Chodubski, J.A., Pearson, I.A., Silverman, C.A., and Fisher, M.W., "Butirosin compared with gentamicin in vitro and in vivo", Antimicrobial Agents and Chemotherapy, 6:124-135, 1974.

ACTION MECHANISM OF 3,4-DIDEOXYKANAMYCIN B (DKB) ON SOME GRAM-NEGATIVE BACTERIA

SUTEMI OKA (1), KOTARO OIZUMI (2), FUMIO ARIJI (2),
KIYOSHI KONNO (2) and KAZUE FUKUSHI (3)
Inst. of Microbial Chemistry(1), Res. Inst. for Tuberc.,
Leprosy & Cancer,Tohoku Univ.(2),Aomori Central Hosp.(3)
Shinagawa-ku, Tokyo (1), Sendai (2), Aomori, Japan (3)

A new antibiotic, 3',4'-dideoxykanamycin B, abbreviated as DKB, has a broad spectrum of antibacterial activity with a strong selective inhibition on Pseudomonas aeruginosa and kanamycin-resistant Escherichia coli. To study the action modes of DKB, this research was done on the basis of the ultramicroscopic structures and the polypeptide synthesis of the two following bacilli, which had been exposed to DKB.

Klebsiella pneumoniae 602 and Pseudomonas aeruginosa IMA 1007 were used for electron microscopic examination. Cells were subjected to fixation in 1 % osmium tetroxide for 2 hours, then treated with 0.5 % uranylacetate for 1 hour, dehydrated with ethylalchohol, embedded in epoxy resin, and then, sections of the cells were observed with an electron microscope.

In the ultramicroscopic structure of untreated Klebsiella pneumoniae it was shown that the cytoplasm was filled with numerous ribosomes having diameters of about 20 nanometers. There were diffuse fibrillar nuclear components of electron transparent form in the cytoplasm. The cell wall was found to be smooth.

The bacilli exposed to 10 μg/ml of DKB for 1 hour showed a loosing of the cytoplasm, that is, some ribosomes were found to have disappeared, but those remaining did not vary in size. There was a tendency towards the concentration of the nuclear components. The bacilli exposed to 10 μg/ml of DKB for 2 hours, showed a concentration of nuclear components and a decrease in number and an aggregation of the remaining ribosomes. A slight detachment of the cell wall from the cytoplasm was found at some part of the cell. A leakage of the cellular components was also observed.

In the ultramicroscopic structures of Pseudomonas aeruginosa it was shown that the cytoplasm was filled with numerous ribosomes. Diffuse fibrillar nuclear components of electron transparent form were found to exsist dispersedly. Some electron dense granules are seen in the cytoplasm.

The bacilli exposed to 10 μg/ml of DKB for 1 hour showed a concentration of nuclear components and a location of cytoplasm at the peripheral part of the cell, in which a degeneration and an aggregation of ribosomes were seen here and there. The bacilli exposed to 10 μg/ml of DKB for 2 hours showed a degeneration of the cytoplasm and most of ribosome particles were found to be destroyed. A leakage of the cellular substances was also observed on the cell surface. These findings suggested that DKB might inhibit ribosomal activities and consequently affect the adjacent cell wall.

The effects of DKB on the polypeptide synthesis of Klebsiella pneumoniae were studied in the assay system, by measuring the incorporation of ^{14}C-valine into the polypeptide. DKB caused a marked inhibition of ^{14}C-valine incorporation into the polypeptide, when it was added to the reaction mixture in a final concentration of 50 μg/ml.

To asertain the effects of DKB on the ribosomal cycle, the distribution of m·RNA and ribosomal classes of Klebsiella pneumoniae was studied by zonal centrifugation analysis. Stable RNA was labeled with ^{14}C-uracil for 3 hours, then exposed to 50 μg/ml of DKB for 30 minutes, and a pulse labeling with ^3H-uridine was made for 5 minutes. Then, the cells were lysed and the distribution of the ribosomal classes and m·RNA was determined by ultracentrifugation of the lysate and by sucrose density analysis.

The distribution of m·RNA in the untreated bacilli was found to correspond to the polysomes, monosomes and subunits, but when the bacilli were treated with DKB, the polysomes and corresponding m·RNA were found to have disappeared, and similar findings were observed in the bacilli treated with kanamycin.

For these studies, it was supposed that DKB inhibited Klebsiella pneumoniae or Pseudomonas aeruginosa by causing damage to ribosomal activities.

REFERENCES

1) Konno, K., Oizumi, K., Kumano, N. and Oka, S. (1973), Amer. Rev. Resp. Dis., 108, 101.

2) Luzzato, L., Apiron, D. and Schlessinger, D. (1968), Proc. Nat. Acad. Sci., U.S.A., 60, 873.

3) Modolell, J. and Davis, B.D. (1968), Proc. Nat. Acad. Sci.,
    U.S.A., 61, 1279.

4) Umezawa, H., Umezawa, S., Tsuchiya, T. and Okazaki, Y. (1971),
    J. Antibiotics, 24, 485.

USE OF 3,4-DIDEOXYKANAMYCIN B (DKB) IN VARIOUS INFECTIONS

SUTEMI OKA

Institute of Microbial Chemistry

14-23, Kamiosaki 3-chome, Shinagawa-ku, Tokyo, Japan

A new antibiotic, 3',4'-dideoxykanamycin B, discovered by Prof. Umezawa, and abbreviated as DKB, was synthetized on the theory that its mechanism was not apt to succumb to inactivation by bacilli resistant to kanamycin B. Clinical use of DKB, with its commercial preparation named 'Panimycin', was started in January of this year following the acceptance by the Ministry of Welfare of the findings on the animal toxicity, teratogenicity, and human pharmacology of the drug and on double blind clinical trials.

The paper is, however, a result of preliminary studies of DKB in the treatment of various infections, performed in 1972, in co-operation with 22 institutions*, as shown in the slide. The review of the studies seemed to be worthy of presentation in regard to extending the treatment for severe infections, caused by Pseudomonas aeruginosa or Klebsiella pneumoniae, through using the higher dosage of DKB regimens.

DKB was given intramuscularly to 130 patients with various infections in a dosage of 50 mg, twice a day, up to a total dosage of 1,000 - 2,000 mg in most instances. Indications and clinical and bacteriological evaluations were made by doctors in each institution, and the results were classified under different diagnostic groups.

In 21 cases of acute or primary respiratory tract infections, including bronchitis, pneumonia or lung abscess, the overall clinical success rate was 85 % and the bacterial beneficial rate 69 %, but 36 cases of chronic or secondary infection of such underlying lung diseases as bronchiectasis, pulmonary tuberculosis or lung cancer, showed a rate of 41 % and 52 %, respectively.

In 27 cases of simple urinary tract infections, DKB was found to be clinically effective in 100 % and bacteriologically effective in 96 %, but in 23 cases of chronic or complicated urinary tract infections, it was found to be effective in 48 % and 52 %, respectively.

The remaining patients were 7 cases of cholecystitis, 5 cases of infection in leukemia, 6 cases of wound infection of malignant tumors and 5 cases of severe infections, including sepsis, endocarditis and fever of an unknown origin, in which DKB was found to be effective in some instances, but the number of each groupe was too small to evaluate the overall success rate.

Of 130 bacilli strains isolated from the patients, which were assumed to be responsible for the infections, DKB was found to be effective in 64 %, specifically in 46 % of 35 strains of Pseudomonas aeruginosa, in 58 % of 19 strains of Klebsiella pneumoniae and in 86 % of 22 strains of Escherichia coli. It is noteworthy that 6 of 15 strains of Pseudomonas aeruginosa and 2 of 3 strains of Klebsiella so far examined, had revealed resistance to kanamycin before DKB administration.

Relations between the dosage used, the clinical response and the side-effects of DKB are studied. Pain at the site of infection was observed in 21 % of the cases, but not seen in the later studies following improvement of the solvent of DKB. Other side-effects were mild and no case was abandoned for this reason.

On the basis of the above mentioned findings of cooperative studies, we treated 11 of 13 cases of terminal infections due to Pseudomonas aeruginosa or Klebsiella pneumoniae with a higher dosage of DKB, that is, 200 - 300 mg daily for 7 - 28 days. Hereby, although it could be assumed that some isolated strains might be commensals, fever and purulent sputum were found to be have disappeared following the elimination of these strains.

Toxicological assessment thus far undertaken, including liver function tests and full blood and urine tests remained in normal ranges.

In summary, from these findings, DKB is very promising for the treatment of various infections, even of severe infections caused by Pseudomonas aeruginosa or Klebsiella pneumoniae.

* Cooperating Institutions

IInd Dep. of Inter. Med., Nagasaki Univ. School of Med.
Dep. of Inter. Med., Institute of Medical Science, Unit. of Tokyo
Ist Dep. of Inter. Med., Osaka City Univ. Med. School
Senboku National Hospital

IInd Dep. of Inter. Med., Hokkaido Univ. School of Med.
Kawasaki Municipal Hospital
Ist Dep. of Med., Yokohama City Univ. School of Med.
Matsuyama Red Cross Hospital
Dep. of Inter. Med., Dep. of Path and Bacteriol, Shizuoka Central
    Prefectural Hosp.
Aichi Cancer Center
Toyama Prefectural Central Hospital
Dep. of Inter. Med., Juntendo Univ. School of Med., Tokyo
National Medical Center Hospital
Inter. Dep., Tokyo Kyosai Hospital
Dep. of Med., School of Med., Keio Univ.
Dep. of Inter. Med., School of Med., Tokyo Univ.
Res. Inst. For Diseases of the Chest, Faculty of Med., Kyushu Univ.
Ist Dep. of Med., Faculty of Med., Kyushu Univ.
Ist Dep. of Inter. Med., Nihon Univ. School of Med.
Res. Inst. Tuber, Lep. & Cancer, Tohoku Univ.
Dep. of Inter. Med., The Jikei Univ. School of Med.
Hoshigaoka Welfare Pension Hospital

REFERENCES

1) Umezawa, H., Umezawa, S., Tsuchiya, T. and Okazaki, Y. (1971),
    J. Antibiotics, 24, 485.

2) Symposium on New Antibiotics, DKB (3',4'-dideoxykanamycin B)
    (1973), Chemotherapy, 21, 597 (in Japanese).

LIST OF CONTRIBUTORS

Abbate, C.E.
Alagia, I.
Altucci, P.
Ariji, F.
Asscher, A.W.

Bartlett, J.F.
Bell, S.M.
Beltcheva, E.
Bengtsson, E.
Bennett, A.H.
Blowers, R.
Boehni, E.
Broughall, J.M.
Brown, D.F.J.
Brumfitt, W.

Casals, J.B.
Comber, K.R.
Commichau, R.
Cox, C.E.
Craig, W.A.
Csatary, K.N.

Dale, G.A.
Daniels, J.V.
Demierre, G.
Duncan, I.B.R.

Edwards, C.R.W.
Elias, K.S.

Fabius, G.T.J.
Federspil, P.
Finke, K.
Freedman, L.R.
Freerksen, E.
Freiesleben, H.
Fukushi, K.

Geheber, B.S.
Gorbach, S.L.
Greenwood, D.
Gueroguiev, N.

Hall, D.
Hamilton-Miller, J.M.T.
Haranka, K.
Harber, M.J.
Hatala, M.
Heinecke, G.
Henkel, W.
Hince, C.
Holloway, W.J.
Holt, H.A.
Hook, E.W.
Hunter, P.A.

Jarvis, J.D.
Jonsson, M.
Jonsson, S.
Julander, I.

Kerry, D.W.
Kitoshi, K.
Kobata, S.
Kolb, L.B.
Kondo, S.
Kruger, C.
Kunin, C.M.
Kunsman, W.E.
Kutchak, S.N.

Leonessa, V.
Leung, T.
Liska, M.
Louie, T.

461

Malmborg, A-S.
Mangurova, M.
Marinova, R.
Mashimo, K.
Mawer, G.E.
McDonald, P.J.
Mehren, W.
Mergler, G.
Miwa, T.
Mochizuki, I.
Moravek, J.
Moussanwi, M.
Mouton, R.P.
Murata, I.

Nagy, A.E.
Neussel, H.
Ninomiya, K.

O'Grady, F.W.
Ohashi, M.
Oizumi, K.
Oka, S.
Onderdonk, A.B.
Osborne, C.D.

Padeiskaya, E.N.
Perchin, G.N.
Prat, U.
Prounchee, R.B.

Reeves, D.S.
Renner, E.
Rolinson, G.N.
Rosenfeld, M.

Rutgers, A.
Ryan, D.M.

Sack, K.
Scheer, M.
Schoog, M.
Schuck, O.
Shadomy, S.
Shanson, D.C.
Shaw, E.J.
Sherris, J.C.
Spousta, J.
Stone, H.H.
Sugane, K.
Sutherland, R.
Suzuki, S.

Tauberger, G.
Taufer, M.
Temnyalov, N.
Tiesler, E.
Then, R.
Tunevall, G.

Ueno, K.
Utz, C.

Van Klingeren, B.

Watanabe, K.
Watson, R.A.A.
Witting, D.A.

Zanger, J.
Zhelyazkov, D.
Zinner, S.H.